INTERNATIONAL YEARBOOK OF NEPHROLOGY 1990

INTERNATIONAL YEARBOOKS OF NEPHROLOGY

Editor

Vittorio E. Andreucci
University of Naples

Co-editors

Leon G. Fine
University of California, Los Angeles

Carl M. Kjellstrand
Hennepin County Medical Center

Nobuhiro Sugino
Tokyo Women's Medical College

INTERNATIONAL YEARBOOK OF NEPHROLOGY 1990

Editor
Vittorio E. Andreucci
University of Naples
Naples, Italy

Co-editors

Leon G. Fine
Division of Nephrology
University of California, Los Angeles
California, USA

Carl M. Kjellstrand
Department of Medicine
Hennepin County Medical Center, Minneapolis
Minnesota, USA

Nobuhiro Sugino
Department of Medicine
Kidney Center
Tokyo Women's Medical College
Tokyo, Japan

Kluwer Academic Publishers
Boston/Dordrecht/London

Distributors for North America:
Kluwer Academic Publishers
101 Philip Drive
Assinippi Park
Norwell, Massachusetts 02061 USA

Distributors for all other countries:
Kluwer Academic Publishers Group
Distribution Centre
Post Office Box 322
3300 AH Dordrecht, THE NETHERLANDS

Library of Congress Cataloging-in-Publication Data

ISBN-13: 978-1-4612-8802-2 e-ISBN-13: 978-1-4613-1491-2
DOI: 10.1007/978-1-4613-1491-2

ISSN: 0921-9862 (series)

CONTENTS

CONTRIBUTING AUTHORS

Steven A. Atlas,
Cardiovascular Center,
Cornell University Medical College,
New York, New York 10021, USA

Bernard Boudailliez,
Pediatrics Department,
CHU,Hôpital Nord,
80030 Amiens Cedex, France

Jacques J. Bourgoignie,
Division of Nephrology,
Department of Medicine,
University of Miami School of Medicine,
Miami, Florida 33101, USA

Martine Esther Cohen-Solal,
Rheumatology Department,
CHU,Hôpital Nord,
80030 Amiens Cedex, France

Gabriel M. Danovitch,
Division of Nephrology,
Department of Medicine,
UCLA School of Medicine,
10833 La Conte Ave.,
Los Angeles, CA 90024-1689, USA

John B. Eastwood,
Department of Biochemical Medicine,
St George's Hospital Medical School, Tooting
London SW 17, England

Albert Fournier,
Department of Nephrology,
CHU,Hôpital Sud,
80030 Amiens Cedex, France

Malachy J. Gleeson,
Scott Department of Urology,
Baylor College of Medicine,
Houston, Texas 77030, USA

Dollie F. Green,
Division of Nephrology,
Department of Medicine,
University of Miami School of Medicine,
Miami, Florida 33101, USA

Peter Greminger,
Department of Internal Medicine,
University Hospital,
8091 Zurich, Switzerland

Donald P. Griffith,
Scott Department of Urology,
Baylor College of Medicine,
Houston, Texas 77030, USA

Scott M. Grundy,
Center for Human Nutrition,
University of Texas,
Southwestern Medical Center at Dallas,
5323 Harry Hines Boulevard,
Dallas, Texas 75235-9052, USA

Hedvig Hricak,
Uroradiology Section,
Department of Radiology, Box 0628,
University of California,
San Francisco, California 94143-0628, USA

Michel Jadoul,
Cliniques Universitaires St.Luc,
Service de Néphrologie,
1200 Bruxelles, Belgium

David J. Jaffe,
Division of Nephrology,
Department of Medicine,
University of Miami School of Medicine,
Miami, Florida 33101, USA

Priscilla Kincaid-Smith,
Department of Nephrology,
The Royal Melbourne Hospital,
Victoria 3050, Australia

John H. Laragh,
Cardiovascular Center,
Cornell University Medical College,
New York, New York 10021, USA

Raifah Makdassi,
Department of Nephrology,
CHU,Hôpital Sud,
80030 Amiens Cedex, France

Sally M. Marshall,
Medical Department M,
Second University Clinic of Internal Medicine,
Kommunehospitalet,
DK-8000 Aarhus C, Denmark

S. Micheal Mauer,
Department of Pediatrics,
Variety Club Children's Hospital,
University of Minnesota,
Minneapolis, Minnesota 55455, USA

Mathew Mischel,
Division of Nephrology,
Department of Medicine,
UCLA School of Medicine,
10833 La Conte Ave.,
Los Angeles, CA 90024-1689, USA

Carl Erik Mogensen,
Medical Department M,
Second University Clinic of Internal Medicine,
Kommunehospitalet,
DK-8000 Aarhus C, Denmark

Philippe Moriniere,
Department of Nephrology,
CHU,Hôpital Sud,
80030 Amiens Cedex, France

Cynthia C. Nast,
Division of Nephrology,
Department of Medicine,
UCLA School of Medicine,
10833 La Conte Ave.,
Los Angeles, CA 90024-1689, USA

Thomas E. Nevins,
Department of Pediatrics,
Variety Club Children's Hospital,
University of Minnesota,
Minneapolis, Minnesota 55455, USA

Irene de Lourdes Noronha,
Department of Internal Medicine,
University of Heidelberg,
Bergheimer Strasse 56a,
D-6900 Heidelberg, Fed. Rep. Germany

Carmen Ortiz-Interian,
Division of Nephrology,
Department of Medicine,
University of Miami School of Medicine,
Miami, Florida 33101, USA

Victoriano Pardo,
Department of Pathology,
University of Miami School of Medicine,
Miami, Florida 33101, USA

Mark S. Pecker,
Cardiovascular Center,
Cornell University Medical College,
New York, New York 10021, USA

Eberhard Ritz,
Department of Internal Medicine,
University of Heidelberg,
Bergheimer Strasse 56a,
D-6900 Heidelberg, Fed. Rep. Germany

David Roth,
Division of Nephrology,
Department of Medicine,
University of Miami School of Medicine,
Miami, Florida 33101, USA

Jean Luc Sebert,
Rheumatology Department,
CHU,Hôpital Nord,
80030 Amiens Cedex, France

Albert Steiner,
Department of Internal Medicine,
University Hospital,
8091 Zurich, Switzerland

Ernesto Tomei,
University of Rome "La Sapienza",
I-00100 Roma, Italy

Carlos A. Vaamonde, M.D.
Nephrology Section,
Veterans Administration Medical Center
and Department of Medicine,
University of Miami School of Medicine,
Miami, Florida 33125, USA

Charles van Ypersele de Strihou,
Cliniques Universitaires St.Luc,
Service de Néphrologie,
1200 Bruxelles, Belgium

Gloria Lena Vega,
Center for Human Nutrition,
University of Texas,
Southwestern Medical Center at Dallas,
5323 Harry Hines Boulevard,
Dallas, Texas 75235-9052, USA

Wilhelm Vetter,
Department of Internal Medicine,
University Hospital,
8091 Zurich, Switzerland

Rudiger Waldherr,
Department of Pathology,
University of Heidelberg,
Im Neuenheimer Feld 220,
D-6900 Heidelberg, Fed. Rep. Germany

Rowan G. Walker,
Department of Nephrology,
The Royal Melbourne Hospital,
Victoria 3050, Australia

Pierre Francois Westeel,
Department of Nephrology,
CHU,Hôpital Nord,
80030 Amiens Cedex, France

Alan H. Wilkinson,
Division of Nephrology,
Department of Medicine,
UCLA School of Medicine,
10833 La Conte Ave.,
Los Angeles, CA 90024-1689, USA

PREFACE

After the great success of the first issue of the series, the International Yearbook of Nephrology 1989, we were encouraged to proceed in our editorial venture to update nephrologists yearly, on all rapidly-changing areas of nephrology. Thus we have chosen new topics and appointed experts in the field, asking them to give an objective review of the topic, up-dating the readers on the world-wide literature and providing them with a complete, accurate and up-to-date list of important, recent references.

We have decided to maintain the successful format of the International Yearbook of Nephrology 1989. Thus each annual issue will be devided into sections; each section will have a different primary focus every year, depending upon what area is of greatest interest at the time. In other words, the Yearbook will remain different from the numerous books which appear every year covering all aspects of nephrology. In the Yearbooks you will find topics usually anavailable in nephrology textbooks.

In this issue we have improved the printing quality of the book, with a more uniform format throughout the volume, despite the use of camera-ready manuscripts for direct photo-offset reproduction (a procedure mandatory for a rapid publication).

With the aim of having the Yearbook focusing attention on the latest and most important scientific and clinical advances in Nephrology, the Editor and Co-Editors are inviting all readers to suggest topics for next issues of the Yearbook, with potential authors who must be known experts in the field. Your suggestions will be carefully evaluated and eventually included in the list of topics in the series.

The Editor and Co-Editors are deeply grateful to all authors of the present issue for their clear, complete and up-to-date reviews. Special thanks are due to Kluwer Academic Publishers for the rapid publication of this volume.

Vittorio E. Andreucci
Leon G. Fine
Carl M. Kjellstrand
Nobuhiro Sugino

INTERNATIONAL YEARBOOK OF NEPHROLOGY 1990

RENAL PHYSIOLOGY AND PATHOPHYSIOLOGY

1

FLUID AND ELECTROLYTE DISORDERS ASSOCIATED WITH ORTHOTOPIC LIVER TRANSPLANTATION

ALAN H. WILKINSON, GABRIEL M. DANOVITCH, AND MATHEW MISCHEL

Department of Medicine, UCLA School of Medicine, Los Angeles, CA 90024-1689, USA.

INTRODUCTION

Following the NIH Consensus Development Conference on Liver Transplantation (1) in 1984 there has been a rapid increase in the use of transplantation to treat end stage liver disease (2). As a result it has become apparent that a more aggressive approach has to be taken towards the medical management of patients who would previously have been considered terminally ill (3, 4). In addition the operative and postoperative periods are characterised by unique fluid and electrolyte problems (5-11). A number of studies (12-18) have shown that pre-existing renal dysfunction has a significant impact on the post-operative prognosis, and that the need for hemodialysis following transplantation is associated with increased mortality. The various phases of the operation itself and the massive blood transfusions produce calcium and acid-base disorders which necessitate careful intra- and post-operative monitoring.

ELECTROLYTE ABNORMALITIES

Calcium

Most patients with end stage liver disease have a low total serum calcium and normal to low ionised calcium concentration. This is important, as during the operation there is a further profound fall in the ionised calcium level (8, 9). However, although this is usually the case, Gerhardt et al (19) have described hypercalcemia in 16 patients with advanced liver disease. Mild to moderate renal failure was present in 87% of this group. Neither hyperparathyroidism nor hypervitaminosis D was a factor, and none of the patients had granulomatous disease. A small group of patients who have hepatocellular carcinomas (20) is accepted for transplantation. Some of these tumours secrete a parathyroid-type hormone which causes severe hypercalcemia. In our experience the hypercalcemia is strikingly resistant to the usual agents used to treat the hypercalcemia of malignancy, such as mithramycin, etidronate disodium and calcitonin. This hypercalcemia should not be considered a contra-indication to transplantation, but the intra- and postoperative management must include even more careful monitoring of ionised calcium levels.

The liver transplant operation is conventionally divided into three phases: phase I or the preanhepatic phase; phase II or the anhepatic phase; and phase III, the postanhepatic or reperfusion phase. Each phase is characterised by different changes in calcium and other electrolyte levels, the glucose concentration, and acid-base status (8, 9, 21-25). During the preanhepatic phase portal hypertension, abnormal coagulation and thrombocytopenia contribute to massive bleeding and the replacement of large volumes of blood. Packed red cells, whole blood and plasma products all contain citrate which will rapidly chelate and lower the serum ionised calcium. In the presence of normal liver function each mmol of citrate is converted into an equivalent amount of bicarbonate, and there is little effect on ionised calcium levels unless extraordinarily large amounts of citrate overwhelm the capacity of the liver to metabolise citrate. Liver disease, however, reduces this capacity to convert citrate, and by the end of phase I plasma citrate levels reach a maximum. Patients develop a mild hypocalcemia, but it is not usually necessary to give calcium during this period. Theoretically each 1.0 mmol of citrate will bind 0.6 mmol of calcium, but in practice the ionised calcium is maintained within the normal range by the use of ionised calcium-specific electrodes for frequent monitoring, and empiric calcium chloride replacement. Were the entire calculated amount to be given, extremely high levels of hypercalcemia would develop (8). The total dose of calcium given is usually about half of the calculated dose.

During the anhepatic phase, in spite of calcium supplementation, a more profound fall in the ionised calcium level occurs, to as low as 0.6 mmol/l, and at this level there is a high risk of left ventricular dysfunction and myocardial depression (26). Plasma citrate levels may rise dramatically, in the absence of the liver, to as much as 100 times preoperative levels. The use of venovenous bypass adds a hemodilution factor that can further reduce the ionised calcium level. The end of the anhepatic phase and the start of the reperfusion phase are accompanied by the release into the circulation of the donor liver perfusion fluid, which is hypothermic, acidic and which has a high potassium concentration. Unless there has been sufficient calcium and fluid replacement, the patient is now particularly likely to develop systemic hypotension.

During the postanhepatic phase large volumes of plasma are often used, increasing the citrate load, but the donor liver is usually able to convert some of this citrate to bicarbonate, and the ionised calcium level may initially be quite stable. The alkalosis which would result from the metabolism of bicarbonate is neutralised at this stage by the persistent metabolic acidosis, and acid-base changes have little effect on the ionised calcium.

Postoperatively, as the liver metabolises the citrate releasing calcium, marked hypercalcemia can occur. The effect of this is ameliorated by the alkalosis, but levels of ionised calcium are frequently above the reference range. Patients usually become normocalcemic within 36 to 48 hours. The hypercalcemia can be treated by promoting a saline diuresis, taking care not to aggravate the metabolic alkalosis. In the absence of adequate renal function, dialysis against a calcium free dialysate will be necessary to correct the hypercalcemia.

We have observed a similar sequence of events postoperatively when massive bleeding results in the replacement of large volumes of blood and plasma products. Liver function often deteriorates as a consequence of hypotension and the use of vasopressor infusions to maintain the systemic blood pressure. Bleeding may also occur during periods of rejection, or when cyclosporine levels are sufficiently high to cause hepatic dysfunction. The ionised calcium level must be monitored closely as hypocalcemia will impair cardiac function, aggravating any hypotension, with a further risk of hepatic and renal failure. As the factors which impaired liver function are corrected, either by the restoration of systemic blood pressure, treatment of rejection, or reduction in the cyclosporine levels, the citrate is metabolised and a metabolic alkalosis and hypercalcemia may again develop.

One other important complication of these derangements in calcium homeostasis has been described by Munoz et al (27). Soft tissue calcification occurred in seven patients post transplantation. This calcification affected, in order of frequency, the lungs, liver graft, colon, vascular walls, kidneys, adrenal glands and gastric mucosa. In one patient calcification within the lung parenchyma was associated with restricted pulmonary function. All seven patients had elevated parathyroid hormone levels, which peaked during the second week, and which were higher than in patients without calcification. Five of these patients had renal failure, emphasising the importance of correcting hyperphosphatemia, and all patients had received significantly more blood products and elemental calcium. We have not seen this complication in any of our liver transplant patients. This may be because in patients with sufficient renal failure to impair calcium excretion, we have been aggressive in the use of dialysis to correct the hypercalcemia.

Potassium

Mild hypokalemia is common in the pretransplantation period, and in phases I and II of the intraoperative period the potassium level is usually stable (8, 9, 23). Following reperfusion there is frequently a sharp rise as the potassium rich perfusate is flushed into the circulation. This is transient and the serum concentration returns to normal within approximately ten minutes, followed later by a significant decrease in the potassium concentration during the latter half of phase III, presumably as potassium reenters the hepatocytes. In the series reported by the Mayo Clinic, 58% of patients required potassium chloride administration to maintain normal levels. These fluctuations in potassium may in part reflect changes in systemic pH, from an acidosis following reperfusion to an alkalosis as the citrate is converted to bicarbonate.

Atchison et al (21) have reviewed the changes in serum glucose during the three phases of the operation and found that during phase I there is a significant rise in the glucose concentration, the level then remaining steady during phase II, only to rise sharply following reperfusion. There was no correlation between the changes in glucose concentration and the amount of exogenous glucose received. Part of the abrupt rise following reperfusion may have been related to the high glucose concentration in the Euro-Collins solution with which these livers had been flushed. A recent study by El Khoury et al (22), at UCLA, reached similar conclusions. It may be that the glucose concentration varies with the ability of the liver to metabolise it. These changes in glucose and insulin levels may also affect the plasma potassium concentration.

Postoperatively most patients require constant potassium supplementation as a consequence of losses from nasogastric, biliary and ascitic drainage. Renal losses occur in the presence of a saline or diuretic induced diuresis, and are enhanced by the effect of the metabolic alkalosis on tubular potassium excretion. However, even anuric patients on daily dialysis may require potassium supplementation, in addition to being dialysed against dialysates which contain normal potassium concentrations. The hypokalemia may be potentiated by intracellular shifts of potassium in response to insulin infusions, the use of intravenous aminophylline to enhance respiratory muscle function, the metabolic alkalosis, and high doses of steroids.

Hyperkalemia can occur in patients with renal failure when they become septic, are reabsorbing large hematomas, and when they receive large volumes of blood transfusions. Cyclosporine toxicity can cause hyperkalemia and when possible the cyclosporine dose should be reduced. If the elevation in serum potassium concentration is high enough to warrant this, it should be treated in standard fashion with insulin and dextrose, bicarbonate, calcium, potassium exchange resins, and dialysis.

Magnesium

Hypomagnesemia is common in patients with liver disease and during the operation levels have been found to fall further (8, 9). Cyclosporine increases renal magnesium losses and it is important to restore normal serum magnesium concentrations postoperatively, as low magnesium levels have been associated both with convulsions (28-31) and with hypertension (32) in patients receiving cyclosporine. De Groen et al (29, 30) have emphasised not only that hypomagnesemia is an important factor in patients who develop neurologic complications, but also that there is an inverse association between this toxicity and total serum cholesterol levels after transplantation. Other factors involved include hypertension, fluid retention, and high-dose steroids.

However, in patients who develop renal failure, magnesium should be removed from replacement fluids to avoid the development of hypermagnesemia.

Sodium

The total body sodium concentration increases during the operation as a consequence of the infusion of large volumes of blood products, sodium bicarbonate and normal saline (8). Postoperatively this, and the invariable volume overload, can be used in patients with adequate renal function to correct any hypercalcemia by promoting a rapid saline diuresis with furosemide. The majority of patients who continue to require transfusions of large volumes of red blood cells if they continue bleeding, or of fresh frozen plasma to correct coagulation disturbances, develop hypernatremia. Many of these patients have impaired sodium and free water excretion, and dialysis may be required to correct the hypernatremia. Overzealous correction of the hypernatremia can lead to rapid swings between this and hyponatremia. We and others (28) have been concerned that this may have contributed to neurologic changes seen post transplantation in some patients. Autopsy studies have documented the presence of central pontine myelinolysis, a finding which has previously been associated with the too rapid correction of hyponatremia.

Phosphate

Phosphate levels are frequently low prior to the operation. During the operation phosphate levels rise (8), but, except in those patients who develop renal failure, it is more usual to again see hypophosphatemia postoperatively as a consequence of renal phosphate wasting associated with extracellular volume expansion, diuretic use, cyclosporine, and the use of phosphate binding antacids and sucralfate to prevent gastric erosions. The continuous use of the intravenous administration of carbohydrate may also contribute to hypophosphatemia. The bicarbonaturia in the early postoperative phase will promote renal phosphate excretion as the serum ionised calcium falls and parathyroid hormone is released.

ACID-BASE DISTURBANCES

Patients awaiting liver transplantation have the usual acid-base disturbances of chronic liver disease, characterised by a respiratory alkalosis and metabolic acidosis. The use of spironolactone to treat ascites and fluid retention may lead in addition to a renal tubular acidosis with hyperkalemia. However, during the operation the underlying acid-base disorders are rapidly replaced as the patient is artificially ventilated, and by the massive transfusions of stored blood. Hydrogen ion and lactate (9, 23, 24) concentrations increase during the operation, and transfusions of sodium bicarbonate are required to maintain a normal pH. During reperfusion the pH decreases yet further. It is usual to attempt to have the patient in a state of mild metabolic acidosis at the end of the operation in the expectation that a metabolic alkalosis will develop as the donor liver metabolises the citrate load and releases bicarbonate (7, 8). Nasogastric drainage, the metabolism of accumulated lactate, diuretic use, and the hyperaldosteronism associated with the preoperative period, may all contribute to this profound metabolic alkalosis. In those patients who are extubated early, a respiratory alkalosis may persist, adding to the elevation in pH. In others the metabolic alkalosis can impair cellular metabolism and can suppress the respiratory drive, delaying extubation. The ventilator settings should be adjusted to allow as high a pCO_2 as is compatible with adequate oxygenation. The precise pH associated with any elevation in the bicarbonate level will be determined by the pCO_2. The serum bicarbonate concentration should be kept below 30 mmol/l and the arterial pH not allowed to rise above 7.5. The metabolic alkalosis can be treated rapidly by dialysis using a low bicarbonate or sodium chloride dialysate, or by the infusion of hydrochloric acid (HCl) (150 mmol/l) at a rate which maintains the pH below 7.5. Although no complications have been described using HCl infusions at this concentration, Shirer et al (33) have described alterations in breathing and blood pressure, in ponies, following the infusion of 0.3M HCl, even when reductions in systemic arterial pH were prevented. The pulmonary artery pressure and heart rate increased, as a consequence of pulmonary vasoconstriction, and it is postulated that the strong acid causes the local release of a substance which causes these effects. Although this has not been studied in man, it is of theoretic concern, as patients with cirrhosis may already have pulmonary hypertension. In patients in acute renal failure this initial alkalosis still occurs in spite of the absence of acid secretion by the kidneys, and must be corrected by dialysis and sufficient ultrafiltration to allow for the infusion of hydrochloric acid. Continuous arteriovenous hemofiltration may also be used. This procedure results in a net loss of bicarbonate, and the removal of bicarbonate from the replacement solution will provide a slow correction of the systemic alkalosis. As described in the section on calcium disorders, a metabolic alkalosis can develop later in the post operative course as a consequence of the transfusion of large volumes of citrated blood products, diuretic therapy and high concentrations of acetate in parenteral nutrition solutions. This alkalosis should be corrected in exactly the same manner as in the immediate postoperative course, as respiratory depression may otherwise require reintubation.

ACUTE RENAL FAILURE

Although it has been well documented that the hepatorenal syndrome can be reversed by liver transplantation (10), preoperative renal dysfunction correlates significantly with postoperative acute renal failure (ARF) (4, 12, 14-18). In poorly nourished patients with end stage liver disease the serum creatinine may be normal in the presence of a significant reduction in the true glomerular filtration rate (GFR). It is not possible in the face of hepatorenal dysfunction to establish that component of the decline in GFR which is the result of acute tubular necrosis (ATN), or other underlying renal disease. It is our experience that postoperative ARF is seen extremely rarely in pediatric patients (14), but that when it occurs it carries a grave prognosis. In our adult patients the need for postoperative hemodialysis correlates with a preoperative serum creatinine concentration of greater than 130 µmol/l. In our analysis of patients transplanted during the first three years experience at UCLA, 46% of patients required dialysis and a further 20% developed reversible episodes of renal dysfunction.

However, the number of patients requiring dialysis has now fallen to 17%. Of those patients who required dialysis, 55% died, with sepsis and other organ failure as confounding variables. When approached from the opposite perspective, all patients who died required dialysis.

Ellis and Avner (15, 16) have analysed the experience in Pittsburgh in children receiving orthotopic livers. Renal failure occurred in 27 of 146 children referred for transplantation (18.5%). The hepatorenal syndrome was the cause of renal failure in 12 of 15 in whom renal failure preceded the operation, 8 of whom died before transplantation could be performed. In the 19 who had postoperative ARF the survival was significantly lower than in those who had no renal failure (53% vs 81%). The causes of ARF included ATN, cyclosporine nephrotoxicity and other nephrotoxic drugs.

The Pittsburgh group (17) has also reported that noncholestatic cirrhosis was an independent predictor of early postoperative renal impairment in adult patients. In addition to finding that trough cyclosporine levels correlated with renal failure, half the patients had another factor (shock, nephrotoxic drugs and graft failure), and they too noted that preoperative renal impairment was an independent predictor of mortality.

Although the frequency of ARF following liver transplantation is declining, it can be seen from these and other studies that every effort should be made to avoid factors which might contribute to renal failure. In the preoperative period strict attention should be paid to the maintainance of adequate fluid volumes. Dietary sodium restriction should be used to control fluid retention and large doses of diuretics avoided as they may predispose to ARF. Paracentesis should be used when necessary to reduce intraabdominal pressure in an attempt to maintain the GFR (34).

The majority of patients receive a preoperative dose of cyclosporine, and this and hemodynamic factors during the operation contribute to the development of postoperative ATN. Low dose dopamine infusions are used routinely, by us and others (11, 35) in an attempt to prevent ATN. In 34 patients randomised either to receive prophylactic low dose dopamine from before surgery, or to receive dopamine only when clinically indicated (35), the group receiving prophylactic dopamine had a significant reduction in the incidence of ARF, and an increase in postoperative urine output. We have noted that in the immediate postoperative period the measured levels of creatinine and urea nitrogen reflect, in part, the levels of these substances in the large volumes of transfused blood, and that it takes a few hours for the true values to equilibrate. This may mask early renal dysfunction, and the urine output is a better predictor of renal function at this stage.

Cyclosporine nephrotoxicity is a common complication following liver transplantation (36-41). The frequency of renal impairment is highest during the intravenous infusion of cyclosporine (37), and we have switched from infusing the daily cyclosporine dose over 8 hr, to a continuous 24 hr infusion, with a decline in nephrotoxicity. Cyclosporine nephrotoxicity is characterised by a "pre-renal" picture with a low urine output and disproportionately elevated urea nitrogen concentration. The acute effects of cyclosporine on renal function are the consequence of a reduction in renal blood flow. In addition to the use of low dose dopamine to maintain renal function we are studying the effects of calcium channel blocking agents such as verapamil and diltiazem which may prevent the fall in blood flow. This protective effect of calcium antagonists against cyclosporine nephrotoxicity has been well documented in renal transplant recipients (42). These agents also elevate the serum levels of cyclosporine, and equivalent immunosuppression can be achieved at lower doses. The levels of cyclosporine should not be allowed to fall so low as to provide insufficient immunosuppression, and a degree of renal impairment should be tolerated. Although cyclosporine nephrotoxicity is common, it is not often a cause of ARF sufficiently severe to require dialysis, and renal function will usually improve as the serum cyclosporine level declines. All other nephrotoxic agents should be avoided whenever possible, particularly prostaglandin synthetase inhibitors and aminoglycosides. The frequency of bacterial and fungal infections in these patients often necessitates the use of aminoglycoside antibiotics which may be more nephrotoxic in the presence of both cyclosporine and of elevated levels of conjugated bilirubin (43, 44), and of amphotericin, which not only has an inevitable effect on tubule function as the total dose increases, but may cause acute renal failure (45) as the result of a reduction in renal blood flow. This too may be more common in the presence of cyclosporine.

In those patients who already have preoperative renal failure dysfunction, and in those who have a significant decline in renal function in the early postoperative period, cyclosporine can be replaced with the prophylactic use of the anti-T cell monoclonal antibody, OKT3 (Orthoclone OKT3), to protect the recovering kidney from the effects of cyclosporine (46, 47). In one study (47) renal function was significantly better at 14 days in those patients receiving OKT3. Rejection of the graft is susceptible to OKT3 and its use for prophylaxis against renal failure may result in high levels of ant-OKT3 antibodies, diminishing its usefulness in the treatment of subsequent rejection.

A novel approach to the prevention of postoperative renal failure has been reported by Gonwa et al (48), who used combined kidney-liver transplantation in seven patients with combined end organ failure. All seven patients maintained excellent renal function with no apparent episodes of rejection of the donor kidney. We have used a similar approach in a patient with polycystic kidney disease, who now has excellent kidney function nearly one year postoperatively.

Chronic cyclosporine nephrotoxicity has been reported by McDiarmid et al (49, 50), Williams et al (36, 51), and Iwatsuki et al (52). All of these studies showed a significant fall in the GFR of patients on cyclosporine. Cyclosporine has been discontinued or reduced to preserve renal function, without loss of the graft to acute rejection. In studies of our renal transplant patients we have found that on low dose cyclosporine the GFR of these patients has remained steady for up to 3 yr post transplant (53, 54), and with a reduction in the doses being used for liver transplantation, and the early use of OKT3, the GFR of liver transplant patients may be better preserved.

Other complications have been described in liver patients receiving cyclosporine (36, 41, 51). Hypertension has occurred in 60% to 70% of patients, and neurotoxicity, which was described in as many as 17% of patients in earlier studies, still occurs. Cyclosporine associated hypertension (32) is dose related but correlates poorly with serum cyclosporine levels. Hypomagnesemia is frequently seen in hypertensive patients and urinary magnesium wasting may make it difficult to restore magnesium levels to normal. Sodium restriction and diuretics may be used in the treatment of this hypertension, but excessive diuresis may contribute to the pre-renal azotemia induced by cyclosporine. Calcium antagonists may prove to be the therapy of choice.

DISORDERS OF VOLUME REGULATION

Renal free water excretion is usually impaired in end-stage liver disease, predisposing patients to the accumulation of edema, ascites and extravascular lung water. During the operation it is extremely difficult to maintain patients in normal fluid balance and, in spite of the large volumes of blood lost, patients are usually hypervolemic at the end of the procedure. Rettke et al (8) have described the changes in hemodynamics during transplantation. Cirrhotic patients have a hyperdynamic circulation, with a high cardiac output and low systemic vascular resistance. During the first two phases of the operation the systemic blood pressure is stable, but then falls significantly following reperfusion. The cardiac output declines during the anhepatic phase, increases significantly following reperfusion, and then returns to baseline values within an hour. The systemic vascular resistance is stable initially, falls significantly following reperfusion, and then increases during phase III. Although patients have an excess of total body water at the end of the procedure, the pulmonary capillary wedge pressure falls during phases I and II, rises significantly immediately following reperfusion, and then falls steadily during the rest of phase III. From these data it can be seen that the most unstable period follows reperfusion. The cause of the reperfusion syndrome is unknown but thought to be related to the release into the circulation of acid metabolites, potassium, and the cold perfusate. Although vasoactive substances may be released from the donor liver, Khoury et al (55) have shown that neither neurotensin nor vasoactive intestinal peptide levels are increased. We routinely use intraoperative hemodialysis and ultrafiltration for those patients in whom renal function is so impaired as to make it impossible to maintain adequate fluid balance. Tuman et al (56) used intraoperative continuous arteriovenous hemofiltration (CAVH), and assessed the effects of this on cardiopulmonary function and on oxygen transport during and in the first 24 hr after transplantation. CAVH prevented increases in pulmonary shunting and permitted lower positive end expiratory pressures and inspired oxygen concentrations. Postoperative cardiac filling pressures were lower, and systemic peripheral resistances were more normal than in patients not being treated by CAVH.

The correction of volume overload should be gradual unless there is evidence of pulmonary edema, as intravascular dehydration is more prone to cause ARF in patients on cyclosporine. We feel that it is safer to use either CAVH or intermittent ultrafiltration than to induce a massive diuresis with diuretics. Any volume overload should be corrected in patients about to receive OKT3 as they are at particular risk of developing pulmonary edema.

REFERENCES

1. National Institutes of Health Consensus Development Conference on Liver Transplantation. Hepatology, 4(S1): 1S-110S, 1984.
2. Busuttil RW, Colonna JO, Hiatt JR, Brems JJ, el Khoury G, Goldstein LI, Quinones WJ, Abdul-Rasool IJ, Ramming KP: The first 100 liver transplants at UCLA. Ann Surg, 206: 387-402, 2987.
3. O'Grady JG, Williams R: Management of acute liver failure. Schweiz Med Wochenschr, 116: 541-544, 1986.
4. Dindzans VJ, Schade RR, Van Thiel DH: Medical problems before and after transplantation. Gastroenterol Clin North Am, 17: 19-31, 1988.
5. Grenvik A, Gordon R: Postoperative care and problems in liver transplantation. Trans Proc, 19(S4): 17-20, 1987.
6. Moulin D, Paris E, Kalenga M, Francois G, Reynaert M, Tremouroux J, Carlier MA, Veyckemans F, Scholtes JL, Gouverneur JM: Intensive care course after orthotopic liver transplantation in children. Acta Anaesthesiol Belg, 36: 214-221, 1985.
7. Rettke SR, Chantigian RC, Janossy TA, Burritt MF, Van Dyke RA, Harper JV, Ilstrup DM, Taswell HF, Wiesner RH, Krom RAF: Anesthesia approach to hepatic transplantation. Mayo Clin Proc, 64: 224-231, 1989.

8. Rettke SR, Janossy TA, Chantigian RC, Burritt MF, Van Dyke RA, Harper JV, Ilstrup DM, Taswell HF, Wiesner RH, Krom RAF: Hemodynamic and metabolic changes in hepatic transplantation. Mayo Clin Proc, 64: 232-240, 1989.
9. Wu AH, Bracey A, Bryan-Brown CW, Harper JV, Burritt MF: Ionized calcium monitoring during liver transplantation. Arch Pathol Lab Med, 111: 935-938, 1987.
10. Wood RP, Ellis D, Starzl TE: The reversal of the hepatorenal syndrome in four pediatric patients following successful orthotopic liver transplantation. Ann Surg, 205: 415-419, 1987.
11. Veyckemans F, Carlier M, Scholtes JL, Gouverneur JM, Decocq L, Gribomont BF, Otte JB, Kestens PJ, de Hemptinne B, Reynaert M: Anesthetic experience in adult and pediatric liver transplantation. Acta Anaesthesiol Belg, 37: 77-87, 1986.
12. Brems JJ, Hiatt JR, Colonna JO, el Khoury G, Quinones WJ, Ramming KP, Ziomek S, Busuttil RW: Variables influencing the outcome following orthotopic liver transplantation. Arch Surg, 122: 1109-1111, 1987.
13. Ceurvas-Mons V, Starzl TE, Van Thiel DH: Prognostic value of preoperatively obtained clinical and laboratory data in predicting survival following orthotopic liver transplantation. Hepatology, 6: 922-927, 1986.
14. Danovitch GM, Wilkinson AH, Colonna JO, Busuttil RW: Determinants of renal failure in patients receiving orthotopic liver transplants. Kidney Int, 31: 195, 1987.
15. Ellis D, Avner ED: Renal failure and dialysis therapy in children with hepatic failure in the perioperative period of orthotopic liver transplantation. Clin Nephrol, 25: 295-303, 1986.
16. Ellis D, Avner ED, Starzl TE: Renal failure in children with hepatic failure undergoing transplantation. J Pediatr, 108: 393-398, 1986.
17. Rimola A, Gavaler JS, Schade RR, el Lankany S, Starzl TE, Van Thiel DH: Effects of renal impairment on liver transplantation. Gastroenterology, 93: 148-156, 1987.
18. Stock PG, Belani K, Estrin J: Prognostic perioperative factors in outcome following liver transplantation. Transplant Proc, 19: 2427-2428, 1987.
19. Gerhardt A, Greenberg A, Reilly JJ, Van Thiel DH: Hypercalcemia. A complication of advanced chronic liver disease. Arch Intern Med, 147: 274-277, 1987.
20. Sealey MM: Severe hypercalcemia due to a parathyroid-type hormone-secreting tumour of the liver treated by hepatic transplantation. Anaesthesia, 40: 170-177, 1985.
21. Atchison SR, Rettke SR, Fromme GA, Janossy TA, Kunkel SE, Williamson KR, Perkins JD, Rakela J: Plasma glucose concentrations during liver transplantation. Mayo Clin Proc, 64: 241-245, 1989.
22. El Khoury GF, Klandorf H, Brems J, Busuttil RW: Pancreatic hormonal responses to hyperglycemia during orthotopic liver transplantation in man. Transplantation, 47: 891, 1989.
23. Fortunato FL, Kang Y, Aggarwal S, Freeman JA, Pinsky MR: Acid-base status during and after orthotopic liver transplantation. Transplant Proc, 19(4S3): 59-60, 1987.
24. Gray TA, Buckley BM, Sealey MM, Smith SC, Tomlin P, McMaster P: Plasma ionized calcium monitoring during liver transplantation. Transplantation, 41: 335-339, 1986.
25. Ickx B, Walter S, Farman JV: Ionised calcium levels during liver transplantation. Eur J Anaesthesiol, 4: 421-427, 1987.
26. Marquez J, Martin D, Virji MA, Kang YG, Warty VS, Shaw B, Sassano JJ, Waterman P, Winetr PM, Pinsky MR: Cardiovascular depression secondary to ionic hypocalcemia during hepatic transplantation in humans. Anesthesiol, 65: 457-461, 1986.
27. Munoz SJ, Nagelberg SB, Green PJ, Angstadt JD, Yang SL, Jarrell BE, Maddrey WC: Ectopic soft tissue calcium deposition following liver transplantation. Hepatology, 8: 476-483, 1988.
28. Vogt DP, Lederman RJ, Carey WD, Broughan TA: Neurologic complications of liver transplantation. Transplantation, 45: 1057-1061, 1988.
29. de Groen PC, Aksamit AJ, Rakela J, Forbes GS, Krom RAF: Central nervous system toxicity after liver transplantation. New Eng J Med, 317: 861-866, 1987.
30. de Groen PC: Cyclosporine, low-density lipoprotein, and cholesterol. Mayo Clin Proc, 63: 1012-1021, 1988.
31. Deierhoi MH, Kalayoglu M, Sollinger HW, Belzer FO: Cyclosporine neurotoxicity in liver transplant recipients. Transplant Proc, 20: 116-118, 1988.
32. Bennet WM, Porter GA: Cyclosporine-associated hypertension. Am J Med, 85: 131-133, 1988.
33. Shirer HW, Erichsen DF, Orr JA: Cardiorespiratory responses to HCl vs lactic acid infusion. J Appl Physiol, 65: 534-540, 1988.
34. Savino JA, Cerabona T, Agarwal N, Byrne D: Manipulation of ascitic fluid pressure in cirrhotics to optimize hemodynamic and renal function. Ann Surg, 208: 504-511, 1988.

35. Polson RJ, Park GR, Lindrop MJ, Farman JV, Calne RY, Williams R: The prevention of renal impairment in patients undergoing orthotopic liver grafting by infusion of low dose dopamine. Anaesthesia, 42: 15-19, 1987.
36. O'Grady JG, Forbes A, Rolles K, Calne RY, Williams R: An analysis of cyclosporine efficacy and toxicity after liver transplantation. Transplantation, 45: 575-579, 1988.
37. Powell-Jackson PR, Young B, Calne RY, Williams R: Nephrotoxicity of parenterally administered cyclosporine after orthotopic liver transplantation. Transplantation, 36: 505-508, 1983.
38. Gonwa TA, Poplawski SC, Husberg BS, Nery JR, Klintmalm GB: Cyclosporine nephrotoxicity in orthotopic liver transplantation. Trans Proc, 20(S3): 401-404, 1988.
39. Iwatsuki S, Esquival CO, Klintmalm GB, Gordon RD, Shaw BW, Starzl TE: Nephrotoxicity of cyclosporine in liver transplantation. Trans Proc, 17(S1): 191-195, 1985.
40. Klintmalm GB, Klingensmith WC, Iwatsuki S, Schroter GP, Starzl TE: 99mTc-DTPA and I131-Hippuran findings in liver transplant recipients treated with cyclosporine A. Radiology, 142: 199-202, 1982.
41. Grant D, Wall W, Duff J, Stiller C, Ghent C, Keown P: Adverse effects of cyclosporine therapy following liver transplantation. Transplant Proc, 19: 3463-3465, 1987.
42. Neumayer HH, Wagner K: Prevention of delayed graft function in cadaver kidney transplants by diltiazem: outcome of two prospective randomised clinical trials. J Cardiovasc Pharm, 10: S170-S177, 1987.
43. Desai TK, Tsang TK: Aminoglycoside nephrotoxicity in obstructive jaundice. Am J Med, 85: 47-50, 1988.
44. Lietman PS: Liver disease, aminoglycoside antibiotics and renal dysfunction. Editorial. Hepatology, 8: 966-968, 1988.
45. Sacks PS, Fellner SK: Recurrent reversible acute renal failure from Amphotericin. Arch Intern Med, 147:593-595, 1987.
46. Gordon RD, Tzakis AG, Iwatsuki S, Todo S, Esquivel CO, Marsh JW, Stieber A, Molowka L, Starzl TE: Experience with OKT3 monoclonal antibody in liver transplantation. Am J Kidney Dis, 11: 141-144, 1988.
47. Millis JM, McDiarmid SV, Hiatt JR, Brems JJ, Colonna JO, Klein AS, Ashizawa T, Hart J, Lewin K, Goldstein LI, Busuttil RW: Randomised prospective trial of OKT3 for early prophylaxis of rejection after liver transplantation. Transplantation, 47: 82-88, 1989.
48. Gonwa TA, Nery JR, Husberg BS, Klintmalm GB: Simultaneous liver and renal transplantation in man. Transplantation, 46: 690-693, 1988.
49. McDiarmid SV, Ettenger RB, Senguttvan P, Hawkins R, Busuttil RW, Ament ME: The impairment of the true GFR in pediatric liver transplant recipients. Transplantation, 1989 (in press).
50. McDiarmid SV, Ettenger RB, Fine RN, Busuttil RW, Ament ME: Serial decrease in glomerular filtration rate in long-term pediatric liver transplant survivors treated with cyclosporine. Transplantation, 47: 314-318, 1989.
51. Williams R, Blackburn A, Neuberger J, Calne RY: Long-term use of cyclosporine in liver grafting. Q J Med, 224: 897-905, 1985.
52. Iwatsuki S, Starzl TE, Shaw BW, Yank SL, Zitelli BJ, Gartner JC, Malatack JJ: Long term use of cyclosporine in liver recipients. Reduction of dosages in the first year to avoid nephrotoxicity. Transplantation, 36: 641-643, 1983.
53. Wilkinson AH, Ross EA, Hawkins RA, Danovitch GM: Measurement of the true GFR in renal transplant patients receiving cyclosporine. Transplant Proc, 19: 1739-1741, 1987.
54. Slomowitz LA, Wilkinson AH, Hawkins RA, Danovitch GM: Evaluation of kidney function in renal transplant patients receiving long-term cyclosporine. Am J Kidney Dis, 1989 (in press).
55. Khoury GF, Kaufman RD, Musich JA, Mogard M: Neurotensin and vasoactive intestinal peptide levels during orthotopic liver transplantation.Anesth Analg, 65: S79-S79, 1986.(Abstract)
56. Tuman KJ, Spiess BD, McCarthy RJ, Logas WG, Williams JW, Sankary HN: Effects of continuous arteriovenous hemofiltration on cardiopulmonary abnormalities during anesthesia for orthotopic liver transplantation. Anesth Analg, 67: 363-369, 1988.

2

ATRIAL NATRIURETIC FACTOR AND ITS CLINICAL IMPLICATIONS

MARK S. PECKER, STEVEN A. ATLAS AND JOHN H. LARAGH

Cardiovascular Center, Cornell University Medical College, New York, New York 10021, U.S.A.

In 1961, de Wardener and his colleagues triggered the search for a natriuretic hormone by demonstrating that changes in glomerular filtration rate and mineralocorticoid activity did not account for the natriuresis which occurs after a saline load (1). Twenty years later, de Bold et al. showed the existence of a natriuretic factor derived from the atria of the heart (2), leading to the discovery of the only natriuretic hormonal substance clearly identified to date. The groundwork for de Bold's discovery lay in two series of observations. First, a large body of evidence had accumulated indicating that the atria were involved in extracellular volume regulation, since atrial distention was shown to provoke diuresis, natriuresis and suppression of renin, vasopressin and aldosterone release (3, 4). The second series of observations were anatomic: electron micrographs of atrial tissue revealed the presence of granules identical to secretory granules found in endocrine cells (5, 6). Further, the density of these granules varied with changes in fluid balance (7, 8). De Bold and his co-workers synthesized these findings by demonstrating that injection of atrial extracts produced a marked natriuresis and diuresis in the rat (2).

Since de Bold's seminal work, the "atrial natriuretic factor" has been purified, its gene cloned and the peptide synthesized (9-13). The major circulating form of ANF is now known to comprise the C-terminal 28 amino acids of a 126 residue precursor. In addition to the heart, low levels of ANF have been found in a variety of tissues including the brain, where it may function as a neurotransmitter. Recently, an additional series of peptides, homologous to but clearly distinct from ANF and having similar biologic activities, has been isolated from porcine brain and termed "brain natriuretic peptides" (14).

The diverse actions of ANF, somewhat different from the original concept of a natriuretic hormone, may serve to protect the organism against intravascular volume expansion. Major gaps in our present knowledge concern the relative importance of the various actions of ANF and of their contribution to volume homeostasis in health and disease.

ACTIONS OF ANF

Renal Effects

The striking natriuresis and diuresis which occur after ANF administration make ANF unique among endogenous natriuretic substances. The basis of this response is complex and appears to involve both hemodynamic and direct tubular actions.

Hemodynamic effects

Studies in isolated perfused kidneys (15) and intact animals and humans (16-21) indicate that ANF increases glomerular filtration rate (GFR) by 15 to 50% found during sustained, high-dose infusions. The increase in GFR is all the more remarkable since it can occur in the face of falls in both arterial blood pressure and renal blood flow. In the isolated kidney perfused without vasoconstrictors, the increase in GFR caused by ANF is associated with an increase in renal vascular resistance and filtration fraction (15). This renal vasoconstrictor effect develops slowly and is dependent on extracellular calcium. Low extracellular calcium levels also abolish the increases in GFR and sodium excretion (15). In the vasoconstricted kidney, however, ANF lowers resistance, while the increases in GFR and in filtration fraction are maintained (15). In intact animals, ANF transiently increases renal blood flow, and decreases renal vascular resistance, after which resistance returns to or above control levels, despite maintained increases in GFR, filtration fraction, and water and sodium excretion (16, 18). The increase in GFR appears to be secondary to an increase in glomerular capillary hydrostatic pressure related to an increase in efferent arteriolar tone (16, 18, 22, 23). Afferent arteriolar tone may also decrease, since, in general, renal resistance does not rise. The effect on afferent arteriolar tone may be direct or secondary to an autoregulatory response to a fall in renal perfusion pressure. ANF may affect capillary permeability (see below), and increases in the filtration coefficient, K_f, have been observed in some studies, although not achieving statistical significance (22, 23). ANF also inhibits angiotensin II-induced contractions of mesangial cells (24), and this inhibition would decrease K_f.

A second hemodynamic effect of ANF is a medullary washout (15, 18, 25, 26). This enhances natriuresis by decreasing sodium reabsorption in the thin ascending limb of Henle's loop and volume flow through the thick ascending limb (27). This effect would also disrupt load-reabsorption balance in the distal nephron and thereby enhance the natriuretic effect of an increase in GFR.

Effects on tubular transport

Micropuncture studies and studies with isolated perfused tubules indicate that ANF does not directly inhibit sodium reabsorption in the proximal tubule, loop of Henle, distal convoluted tubule or cortical collecting duct (28-31). An effect of ANF on sodium transport in the medullary collecting duct has been proposed based on several lines of evidence. First, sodium reabsorption in the papillary collecting duct does not increase in proportion to load after ANF administration (32, 33). Second, in outer medullary collecting duct, ANF inhibits oxygen consumption sensitive to both ouabain and amiloride (34), compatible with an effect on sodium transport. Studies showing that ANF depolarizes the cell membrane in transporting outer medullary collecting duct support this view (35). The mechanisms of the load-reabsorption imbalance in this segment is unclear. One possibility is an effect on the amiloride-sensitive sodium channel, but an indirect effect mediated by an increase of medullary interstitial fluid pressure has not been ruled out (32, 36).

Mechanism of the natriuresis

The importance of hemodynamic mechanisms to the ANF-induced natriuresis is suggested by the demonstration that the natriuretic response can be obliterated by preventing the increase in GFR by clamping the aorta or renal artery (37, 38). Although natriuresis has been observed to occur without apparent changes in GFR (2, 29, 37-39), such findings must be interpreted cautiously for several reasons. Among these is the difficulty of measuring small changes in GFR (40). Thus, changes which could provide an absolute increase in the filtered load of sodium sufficient to more than account for the natriuresis are within the error of most methods. Further difficulties involve the problem of measuring GFR under non-steady state conditions such as after boluses of ANF (which has a short half-life), or during abrupt changes in renal blood or urine flow rate (40). Nevertheless, it is clear that similar degrees of natriuresis can occur under conditions where the induced changes in GFR vary widely (38, 39). Thus, an increase in GFR is not the sole basis for the natriuresis induced by ANF. It should be emphasized that the medullary washout will amplify the effect of any increase in filtered load.

Studies in water-loaded subjects have shown that free water clearance increases during ANF administration (19, 20), indicating that sodium reabsorption by the thick ascending limb of Henle's loop is increased. This finding could be due to several different effects, including an increase in GFR (with an accompanying disruption of glomerular tubular balance), medullary washout, or an effect on proximal tubular sodium reabsorption. While confirming the importance of events in the proximal nephron, clearance studies do not rule out a distal effect.

The relative contributions of hemodynamic effects and direct effects on the collecting duct are uncertain, and may vary under different conditions. However, it is noteworthy that in all studies, ANF increases load to the base of the papillary collecting duct, and that absolute levels of sodium reabsorption in this segment are maintained (29, 30). In addition, the effects of ANF and amiloride on sodium reabsorption *in vivo* or in the isolated kidney are at least additive (39), supporting the hypothesis that the principal site of action of ANF is not identical to that of amiloride. Further, unlike inhibitors of sodium transport in the collecting duct, ANF does not provoke hyperkalemia or acidosis. The natriuresis therefore seems to depend on an increase in distal delivery of sodium, related largely to hemodynamic factors, augmented by diminished sodium reabsorption in the collecting duct.

Effects on the Renin-Angiotensin-Aldosterone System

ANF antagonizes the renin-angiotensin system at multiple points, and this antagonism may prove to be an important mode of its action.

Inhibition of renin secretion

In both animals and humans, low dose infusions of ANF suppress plasma levels of renin (16, 18, 20, 41). This may be a direct effect or may be mediated by increased distal delivery of sodium chloride with consequent suppression of the macula densa signal to renin release. Several lines of evidence support the latter hypothesis. Unilateral renal artery constriction, which stimulates ipsilateral renin secretion, abolishes the acute renin suppression and natriuresis due to ANF in that kidney (42). Similarly, in pathologic states such as congestive heart failure or cirrhosis, ANF fails to produce a natriuresis or to lower plasma renin activity (PRA) (20, 43). Although ANF infusion can lower PRA in normal subjects without significantly increasing sodium excretion, a rise in distal sodium supply can be inferred from the concurrent rise in free water clearance (20). In addition, ANF does not decrease renin secretion in the non-filtering kidney (44). Finally, high dose infusions of ANF, which significantly lower blood pressure and cardiac output, may be associated with an increase in PRA (20).

Results of *in vitro* studies on renin release by dispersed or cultured juxta-glomerular cells (45, 46), isolated afferent arterioles (47), isolated glomeruli (48), or kidney slices (49, 50) have yielded conflicting results. Studies have shown either no effect (46-48), suppression (45, 50) or even stimulation at high doses (46, 49). Although the impressive inhibitory effect noted in one study suggests the existence of a direct mechanism at physiologic concentrations (45), the results in intact animals noted above suggest that any direct effect of ANF on renin release can be readily overcome by other stimuli for renin release, such as activation of the macula densa or baroreceptor signals.

Inhibition of aldosterone production

As expected based on its ability to lower plasma renin levels, ANF also lowers circulating aldosterone concentrations (18, 20, 41, 51). However, the effect is not solely due to suppression of plasma renin, since direct inhibition of basal and agonist-induced aldosterone release by isolated adrenal cell has been demonstrated *in vitro* (52-57). In intact humans, stimulation of aldosterone secretion by angiotensin II is blocked by low-dose infusion of ANF (58). Interestingly, in the same study, stimulation of aldosterone secretion by ACTH was not altered by ANF (58), and this may explain the occasional failure of ANF to lower aldosterone levels. ANF also has been reported to blunt the aldosterone response to potassium infusion in rats (59).

The *in vitro* studies cited above showed that ANF decreases aldosterone release secretion stimulated by angiotensin II, potassium, ACTH and cAMP analogues, but suggest a more profound inhibition of angiotensin-stimulated release (56), consistent with *in vivo* findings (51, 58). The cellular basis of ANF's effects on the zona glomerulosa is not well defined, but may involve inhibition of cAMP and perhaps other unidentified mechanisms (57).

In addition to its effects on mineralocorticoid production, ANF infusion may decrease cortisol levels in man (20), an effect not found in dogs (18). The effect is small and not consistently found, although the rise in cortisol after cessation of the infusion may be dramatic. Inhibition of ACTH secretion might contribute to this effect, since ANF has been reported to inhibit cAMP formation and ACTH release in cultured anterior pituitary cells (60, 61). In addition, direct inhibition of glucocorticoid production by ANF has been reported in bovine and human, but not rat, adrenal cells (52, 54, 62), in accord with the distribution of ANF receptors in these species (54, 63).

Antagonism of angiotensin II

In addition to its effects on renin and aldosterone release, ANF is a functional antagonist of angiotensin II in other target organs. As noted above, although ANF lowers aldosterone release in response to a variety of stimuli, the inhibition of the response to angiotensin II is particularly powerful. A similar situation exists in vascular smooth muscle where, while ANF relaxes preparations contracted by a variety of stimuli including high potassium and norepinephrine, the antagonism of contractions induced by angiotensin II involves not only a shift in the dose response curve of tension to the right but also a decrease in the maximum tension elicited by angiotensin II (64). Similarly, ANF has a marked antihypertensive effect during the renin dependent phase of two-kidney, one-clip Goldblatt hypertension in rats while having lesser effects, and only at higher infusion rates, in rats with DOCA-salt hypertension, a model in which angiotensin II levels are extremely low (65).

In addition, angiotensin II has a direct action on the proximal tubule to promote sodium reabsorption (66). ANF is reported to antagonize this effect by some workers (67), but not by others (68). Thus, antagonism of angiotensin II could make a contribution to the acute natriuresis induced by ANF. Finally, intracerebroventricular administration of ANF has been shown to antagonize the effects of central angiotensin II on thirst, blood pressure, and vasopressin and ACTH release (67, 69-71).

Effects on Vascular Smooth Muscle

ANF relaxes precontracted smooth muscle preparations without affecting resting tension. The vasorelaxant effect is non-specific, but as noted above the antagonism of angiotensin-induced contraction is particularly marked (64). This effect is pronounced in arteries or in artery-like vessels such as the rabbit facial vein, but is minimal in veins (72, 73). The vasorelaxation is not dependent on an intact endothelium (74), but similar to the action of endothelium derived relaxing factor, it is probably mediated by cGMP (see below).

In intact animals, peripheral vasodilatation is not the major mechanism underlying ANF's blood pressure-lowering effect under basal conditions (see below). In certain circumstances, however, such as in renin-dependent hypertensive models (65), or heart failure (20, 43) ANF can decrease systemic vascular resistance.

Effects on Fluid Shifts Between Compartments

In the first report of the effects of atrial extract infusion, a rise in hematocrit was noted (2), a finding that has been repeatedly confirmed. This hemoconcentration is not solely due to renal fluid losses, since it also occurs in nephrectomized rats (75-77). ANF leads to redistribution of fluid from the intravascular to the interstitial space, without changing intracellular water (77). The mechanism of this effect is unclear; it may due to increased capillary bed hydraulic permeability, owing to an increase in effective surface area or to a direct effect on hydraulic conductivity of capillary endothelium, where ANF receptors have been localized (63). Alternatively, it may be due to alterations in Starling forces. Whatever the mechanism, this effect of ANF can cause significant intravascular volume contraction, an effect which probably contributes to the decreases in central venous pressures and in cardiac output which is often observed (20, 65, 78, 79).

Effects on Vasopressin

Systemic ANF infusion inhibits vasopressin release induced by hemorrhage or dehydration in rats (80). This effect has also been demonstrated with intraventricular administration of ANF (81), and the antagonism of vasopressin release mediated by centrally administered angiotensin II is particularly pronounced (71). Recent work suggests that ANF exerts its effect at the level of the hypothalamus and not directly on the posterior pituitary (82).

TRANSDUCTION OF THE ANF SIGNAL

Like other peptide hormones, ANF binds to specific receptors on cell surfaces. Two classes of ANF receptors have been identified with molecular weights of 130 kD and 66 kD (83). The former represent about 1% of the total receptors and have a K_d of 10^{-10} to 10^{-9} M (compared to normal circulating levels of

ANF in the range of 10^{-11} M)(84). These receptors co-purify with the membrane-bound ("particulate") form of guanylate cyclase, suggesting that, unlike adenylate cyclase-coupled receptors, this ANF receptor is a single protein containing both hormone-binding and catalytic domains (85). Binding to this class of receptors is thought to mediate many of the biological actions of ANF.

The 66 kD receptor is of similar affinity, but is of unknown biological function (83). It has been proposed that these receptors serve a storage or clearance function, since biologically inert analogues of ANF which retain affinity for this class of receptor raise circulating levels of ANF (84).

The stimulation of particulate guanylate cyclase by ANF (74), is an action which is unique among known mammalian hormones. Other substances including nitrates and EDRF also increase cellular cGMP levels, but by activating the soluble (cytosolic) form of guanylate cyclase (83). Although ANF increases cGMP production in all known target tissues, it has not been established that cGMP production can account for all of its effects (e.g. on adrenal (57)). The extent to which other actions, such as inhibition of adenylate cyclase (60), mediate effects of ANF is not certain.

Changes in plasma or urine levels of cGMP have been used as an index of ANF action. Acute elevations of plasma ANF levels during saline infusion, water immersion, atrial tachycardia or exercise are also associated with elevations of plasma cGMP levels (86). The relationship between plasma ANF and plasma cGMP is maintained during chronic elevation of plasma ANF levels such as in congestive heart failure (87, 88), suggesting that if tolerance to the effects of ANF occurs, it does so at a site distal to cGMP production. Urinary cGMP also increases with increasing levels of plasma ANF. Following marked stimulation of ANF secretion, the fractional excretion of cGMP can exceed 1.0 (86), suggesting a renal source of urinary cGMP. However, given the ability of endogenous substances other than ANF to stimulate cGMP production, and the possibility of non-specific effects (such as increases in urine flow) on urinary cGMP, changes in nucleotide levels cannot be used as an unequivocal index of ANF activity.

SECRETION OF ANF

Although immunoreactive ANF and ANF messenger RNA are detectable in other tissues, ANF secretion has only been demonstrated from the heart. ANF messenger RNA is most abundant in atrial myocytes, but is also detectable in ventricular muscle (89). Under normal conditions in mammals, secretory granules are found only in atrium; however, ventricular mRNA and immunoreactive ANF levels increase in states of pressure or volume overload of the ventricle (89, 90), in which situations granules have occasionally been observed. Secretion of ANF by ventricular muscle has not as yet been demonstrated, however.

The major stimulus for ANF release is atrial stretch (91). Plasma ANF levels rise in response to acute volume expansion (92, 93), water immersion (94) and mechanical distension of the atria (95). Stimulation of ANF by vasoconstrictor agents most often is related to induced increases in atrial pressure (96, 97). It is probable, however, that release can be modulated independently of atrial distension. For example, increased sympathetic nervous system outflow after baroreceptor denervation in rats (98) or deactivation in humans (99) is associated with reduced ANF release. ANF levels also increase during intravenous infusion of subpressor doses of angiotensin II (100) or after central nervous system administration of angiotensin II (101) are less clear. A direct osmotic stimulus for ANF release *in vivo* seems unlikely (102).

CLINICAL IMPLICATIONS OF ANF

Actions of ANF to cause natriuresis, increase GFR, suppress renin and aldosterone secretion, and antagonize angiotensin II are similar to the effects of intravascular volume expansion. The effects of infusing ANF to attain levels approximating those found after interventions or in disease states have been studied. Such studies probably underestimate the contributions of ANF since the resulting hemodynamic milieu is markedly different from that in which endogenous secretion occurs, i.e. infusions decrease central blood volume thereby activating counter-regulatory mechanisms which would oppose its effects, whereas ANF is usually secreted during central blood volume expansion. Endocrine ablation models have been approximated by studying the effects of atrial appendectomy (103, 104) and immunization against ANF (105). Both these models have serious limitations. In the former, the atrium, which has volume regulatory functions in addition to ANF secretion, is disrupted and ANF secretion only blunted. In the latter, immunization against ANF may produce additional effects. For example, if the antibody-ANF complex binds to 66 kD receptors, which are numerous in the glomerulus (84), disruption of glomerular function might result independently inactivation of plasma ANF.

Circulating levels of immunoreactive ANF in normal humans are usually less than 30 pM (90 ngm/l) (20, 106). The plasma half-life of ANF is about 3 minutes (107). Plasma ANF levels increase with recumbency (108, 109), exercise (110), saline infusions (93), or water immersion (94). In the latter intervention, levels of ANF correlate well with the degree of natriuresis, but not of renin or aldosterone suppression (94). Infusions of ANF which yield levels comparable to those found during these interventions also suppress renin and aldosterone and, often, increase sodium excretion (20, 41, 111, 112). Percentage changes in these parameters are similar on either high or low salt intake, but absolute changes in natriuresis are greater, and in renin and aldosterone smaller, on a high salt intake (113). In animals, either removal of the atrial appendages (103, 104) or immunization against ANF (105) diminishes the natriuretic response to acute volume expansion. These results therefore suggest a role for ANF in modulating the response to acute changes in intravascular volume.

The results in longer term studies are less clear. In normal humans, ANF levels increase about two-fold after three to five days of increasing sodium intake from low to high levels (109, 114, 115), and the increases are maintained after 14 days of high sodium intake (116). Longer term studies in mildly hypertensive subjects suggest that smaller increases are maintained after 4 weeks of high sodium intake (117). The significance of these results is unclear. ANF infusions which yield such modest increases do not cause the same degree of natriuresis or renin suppression as does high salt intake. In animals, neither atrial appendectomy nor immunization against ANF grossly disturb the ability to achieve sodium balance (104, 105). In studies of escape from the sodium retention due to mineralocorticoid excess, ANF levels rise (118, 119), but auto-immunization against ANF does not alter the changes in sodium excretion during mineralocorticoid escape (105).

Levels of ANF are elevated in some patients with hypertension (120), often in association with left ventricular hypertrophy (121). ANF levels increase to a similar extent after saline infusion in hypertensive subjects as in normal subjects, and levels correlate poorly with the degree of natriuresis (122). ANF may still play a role in the phenomenon of exaggerated natriuresis of hypertension, however, since hypertensive subjects may be more sensitive to ANF than are normals. High dose ANF infusions lower blood pressure in hypertensive subjects, and the effects are sustained for hours after the end of the infusion despite the short half-life of ANF (123). Thus, ANF-like substances may have therapeutic potential in this disorder.

ANF levels are also elevated in chronic renal failure (124), and fluctuate with intravascular volume status, falling after dialysis (125). A close correlation exists between ANF levels and increases in single nephron GFR in rats with renal ablation (126), indicating that ANF may play a role in the hyperfiltration of surviving nephrons in progressive renal failure. ANF infusions also ameliorates post-ischemic damage in acute renal failure (127, 128).

Plasma ANF levels are also increased in patients with edematous disorders, especially congestive heart failure (20, 43, 106). In contrast to hypertension or chronic renal failure (129), patients with edematous disorders have, in general, been found to be refractory to the natriuretic and renin lowering effects of endogenous or exogenous ANF (20, 43), consistent with results in animal models of underperfused kidneys caused by renal artery constriction (37, 38). Thus, ANF cannot overcome the powerful salt retaining stimuli present in these disorders. Small absolute effects such as observed during ANF administration to sodium-restricted normal subjects would of course be of little benefit in removing large amounts of sodium in edematous subjects. A possible role for ANF in promoting edema formation owing to its effect to shift fluid out of the intravascular space in combination with refractoriness to its natriuretic actions is intriguing but speculative to date. Such an effect would be more likely in heart failure where levels are extremely high, than in cirrhosis (106) or nephrosis (130) where elevations are modest. Despite the failure to accelerate sodium loss, ANF infusions can lower systemic resistance and pulmonary capillary wedge pressure in patients with heart failure (20, 43), suggesting that the hormone may play a protective role in this disorder.

In summary, ANF occupies a strategic position in the network of systems which maintain intravascular volume homeostasis. While elevated levels of ANF in clinical situations reflect central blood volume expansion, the precise physiologic role of ANF remains to be delineated. It is likely that an inhibitor will be necessary to definitively ascertain the place of ANF in regulation of the circulation. Potential therapeutic uses of ANF in hypertension, acute renal failure and heart failure are currently being defined.

REFERENCES

1. de Wardener HE, Mills IH, Clapham WF, Hayter CJ: Studies on the efferent mechanism of the sodium diuresis which follows the administration of intravenous saline in the dog. Clin Sci Mol Med, 21: 249-258, 1961.

2. de Bold AJ, Borenstein HB, Veress AT, Sonnenberg H: A rapid and potent natriuretic response to intravenous injection of atrial myocardial extract in rats. Life Sci, 28: 89-94, 1981.
3. Gauer OH, Henry JP: Circulatory basis of fluid volume control. Physiol Rev, 43: 423-481, 1963.
4. Goetz KL, Bond GC, Bloxham DD: Atrial receptors and renal function. Physiol Rev, 55: 157-205, 1975.
5. Kisch, B. Electron microscopy of the atrium of the heart. I. Guinea pig. Exp Med Surg, 114: 99-112, 1956.
6. Jamieson JD, Palade GE, Specific granules in atrial muscle cells. J Cell Biol, 23: 151-172, 1964.
7. de Bold AJ: Heart atria granularity: effects of change in water-electrolyte balance. Proc Soc Exp Biol Med, 161: 508-511, 1979.
8. Marie JP, Guillemot H, Hatt PY: Le degree de granulation des cardiocytes auriculaires. Etude planimetrique au cours de differents apports d'eau et du sodium chez le rat. Pathol Biol, 24: 549-554, 1976.
9. de Bold AJ: Atrial natriuretic factor: A hormone produced by the heart. Science, 230: 767-770, 1985.
10. Cantin M, Genest, J: The heart and the atrial natriuretic factor. Endocr Rev, 6: 107-127, 1985.
11. Maack T, Camargo MJF, Kleinert HD, Laragh JH, Atlas SA: Atrial natriuretic factor: Structure and functional properties. Kidney Int, 27: 607-615, 1985.
12. Needleman P, Adams SP, Cole BR, Currie MG, Geller DM, Michener ML, Saper CB, Schwartz D, Standaert DG: Atriopeptins as cardiac hormones. Hypertension, 7: 469-482, 1985.
13. Matsuo, H, Nakazato H: Molecular biology of atrial natriuretic peptides. Endocrinol Metab Clin N Amer, 16: 43-61, 1987.
14. Sudoh T, Kangawa K, Minamino N, Matsuo H: A new natriuretic peptide in porcine brain. Nature, 332: 78-81, 1988.
15. Camargo MJF, Kleinert HD, Atlas SA, Sealey JE, Laragh JH, Maack T: Ca-dependent hemodynamic and natriuretic effects of atrial extract in isolated rat kidney. Am J Physiol, 246: F447-F456, 1984.
16. Burnett JC, Jr, Granger JP, Opgenorth TJ: Effects of synthetic atrial natriuretic factor on renal function and renin release. Am J Physiol, 247: F863-F866, 1984.
17. Huang CL, Lewicki J, Johnson LK, Cogan MG: Renal mechanism of action of rat atrial natriuretic factor. J Clin Invest, 75: 769-773, 1985.
18. Maack T, Marion DN, Camargo MJF, Kleinert HD, Laragh JH, Vaughan ED, Jr, Atlas SA: Effects of auriculin (atrial natriuretic factor) on blood pressure, renal function, and the renin-aldosterone system in dogs. Am J Med, 77: 1069-1075, 1984.
19. Weidmann P, Hasler L, Gnadinger MP, Lang RE, Uehlinger DE, Shaw S, Rascher W, Reubi FC: Blood levels and renal effects of atrial natriuretic peptide in normal man. J Clin Invest, 77: 734-742, 1986.
20. Cody RJ, Atlas SA, Laragh JH, Kubo SH, Covit AB, Ryman KS, Shaknovich A, Pondolfino K, Clark M, Camargo JF, Scarborough RM, Lewicki JA: Atrial natriuretic factor in normal subjects and heart failure patients: plasma levels and renal, hormonal and hemodynamic responses to peptide infusion. J Clin Invest, 78: 1362-1372, 1986.
21. Hirata Y, Ishii M, Sugimoto T, Matsuoka H, Sugimoto T, Kangawa K, Matsuo H: The effects of human atrial 28-amino acid peptide on systemic and renal hemodynamics in anesthetized rats. Circ Res, 57: 634-9, 1985.
22. Dunn BR, Ichikawa I, Pfeffer JM, Troy JL, Brenner BM: Renal and systemic hemodynamic effects of synthetic atrial natriuretic peptide in the anesthetized rat. Circ Res, 59: 237-246, 1986.
23. Fried TA, McCoy RN, Osgood RW, Stein JH: Effect of atriopeptin II on determinants of glomerular filtration in the *in vitro* perfused dog glomerulus. Am J Physiol, 250: F1119-F1122, 1986.
24. Appel RG, Wang J, Simonson MS, Dunn MJ: A mechanism by which atrial natriuretic factor mediates its glomerular actions. Am J Physiol, 251: F1036-F1042, 1986.
25. Borenstein HB, Cupples WA, Sonnenberg H, Veress AT: The effect of a natriuretic atrial extract on renal hemodynamics and urinary excretion in anaesthetized rats. J Physiol, 334: 133-140, 1983.
26. Hirata Y, Ganguli M, Tobian L: Dahl S rats have increased natriuretic factor in atria but are markedly hyporesponsive to it. Hypertension, 6: I148-I155, 1984.

27. Reineck HJ, Parma B: Effect of medullary hypertonicity on urine sodium in the rat. J Clin Invest, 69: 971-978, 1982.
28. Sonnenberg H, Cupples WA, de Bold AJ, Veress AT: Intrarenal localization of the natriuretic effect of cardiac atrial extract. Can J Physiol Pharmacol, 60: 1149-1152, 1982.
29. Briggs JP, Steipe B, Schubert G, Schnermann J: Micropuncture studies on the renal effects of atrial natriuretic substance. Pflugers Arch, 395: 271-276, 1982.
30. Baum M, Toto R: Lack of a direct effect of atrial natriuretic factor in the rabbit proximal tubule. Am J Physiol, 250: F66-F69, 1986.
31. Kondo Y, Imai M, Kangawa K, Matsuo H: Lack of a direct action of beta-human atrial natriuretic polypeptide on the *in vitro* perfused segments of Henle's loop isolated from rabbit kidney. Pflugers Arch, 406: 273-278, 1986.
32. Sonnenberg H, Honrath U, Chong CK, Wilson DR: Atrial natriuretic factor inhibits sodium transport in medullary collecting duct. Am J Physiol, 250: F963-F966, 1986.
33. van de Stolpe A, Jamison RL: Micropuncture study of the effect of ANP on the papillary collecting duct in the rat. Am J Physiol, 254: F477-F483, 1988.
34. Zeidel ML, Seifter JL, Lear S, Brenner BM, Silva P: Atrial peptides inhibit oxygen consumption in kidney medullary collecting duct cells. Am J Physiol, 251: F379-F383, 1986.
35. Zeidel ML, Kikeri D, Burrowes M, Silva P, Brenner BM: Atrial natriuretic peptide inhibits conductive sodium uptake in rabbit inner medullary collecting duct cells. J Clin Invest, 82: 1067-1074, 1988.
36. Mendez RA, Dunn BR, Troy JL, Brenner BM: Atrial natriuretic peptide and furosemide effects on hydraulic pressure in the renal papilla. Kidney Int, 34: 36-42, 1988.
37. Sosa RE, Volpe M, Marion DN, Atlas SA, Laragh JH, Vaughan ED, Jr, Maack T: Relationship between renal hemodynamics and natriuretic effects of atrial natriuretic factor. Am J Physiol, 250: F520-F524, 1986.
38. Salazar FJ, Fiksen-Olsen MJ, Opgenorth TJ, Granger JP, Burnett JC, Jr, Romero JC: Renal effects of ANP without changes in glomerular filtration rate and blood pressure. Am J Physiol, 251: F532-F536, 1986.
38a. Camargo MJF, Atlas SA, Maack, T: Role of increased glomerular filtration rate in atrial natriuretic factor-induced natriuresis in the rat. Life Sci, 38: 2397-2404, 1986.
39. Seino M, Abe K, Nushiro N, Omata K, Yoshinaga K: The effects of atrial natriuretic peptide and amiloride on renal haemodynamics and the renal kallikrein-kinin system. J Hypertension, 6: 321-327, 1988.
40. Maack T: Renal clearance and isolated kidney perfusion techniques. Kidney Int, 30: 142-151, 1986.
41. Cuneo RC, Espiner EA, Nicholls MG: Renal, hemodynamic, and hormonal responses to atrial natriuretic factor in normal man, and effect of sodium intake. J Clin Endocrinol Metab, 63: 946-953, 1986.
42. Sosa RE, Volpe M, Marion DM: Effect of atrial natriuretic factor on renin secretion, plasma renin and aldosterone in dogs with acute unilateral renal artery constriction. J Hypertension, 3 (suppl. 3): S299-S302, 1985.
43. Crozier IG, Ikram H, Gomez HJ, Nicholls MG, Espiner EA, Warner NJ: Haemodynamics of atrial peptide infusion in heart failure. Lancet, ii: 1242-1245, 1986.
44. Opgenorth TJ, Burnett JC, Granger JP, Scriven TA: Effects of atrial natriuretic peptide on renin secretion in nonfiltering kidney. Am J Physiol, 250: F798-F801, 1986.
45. Kurtz A, Della-Bruna R, Pfeilschifter J, Taugner R, Bauer C: Atrial natriuretic peptide inhibits renin release from juxtaglomerular cells by a cGMP-mediated process. Proc Natl Acad Sci (USA), 83: 4769-4773, 1986.
46. Takagi M, Takagi M, Franco-Saenz R, Mulrow PJ: Effect of atrial natriuretic peptide on renin release in a superfusion system of kidney slices and dispersed juxtaglomerular cells. Endocrinology, 122: 1437-1442, 1988.
47. Itoh S, Abe K, Nushiro N, Omata K, Yasujima M, Yoshinaga K: Effect of atrial natriuretic factor on renin release in isolated afferent arterioles. Kidney Int, 32: 493-497, 1987.
48. Rodriguez PD, Arriba G, Blanchart A, Santos JC, Caramelo C, Fernandez-Cruz A, Hernando L, Lopez-Novoa JM: Lack of a direct regulatory effect of atrial natriuretic factor on prostaglandins and renin release by isolated rat glomeruli. Biochem Biophys Res Commun, 138: 496-501, 1986.
49. Hiruma M, Ikemoto F, Yamamoto K: Rat atrial natriuretic factor stimulates renin release from renal cortical slices. Eur J Pharmacol, 125: 151-153, 1986.

50. Obana K, Naruse M, Naruse K, Sakurai H, Demura H, Inagami T, Shizume K: Synthetic rat atrial natriuretic factor inhibits *in vitro* and *in vivo* renin secretion in rats. Endocrinology, 117: 1282-1284, 1985.
51. Vari RC, Freeman RH, Davis JO, Villarreal D, Verburg KM: Effect of synthetic atrial natriuretic factor on aldosterone secretion in the rat. Am J Physiol, 251: R48-R52, 1986.
52. Atarashi K, Mulrow PJ, Franco-Saenz R, Snajdar R, Rapp J: Inhibition of aldosterone production by an atrial extract. Science, 224: 992-994, 1984.
53. Goodfriend TL, Elliott M, Atlas SA: Actions of synthetic atrial natriuretic factor on bovine adrenal glomerulosa. Life Sci, 35: 1675-1682, 1984.
54. De Lean A, Racz K, Gutkowska J, Nguyen TT, Cantin M, Genest J: Specific receptor-mediated inhibition by synthetic atrial natriuretic factor of hormone-stimulated steroidogenesis in cultured bovine adrenal cells. Endocrinology, 115: 1636-1638, 1984.
55. Kudo T, Baird A: Inhibition of aldosterone production in the adrenal glomerulosa by atrial natriuretic factor. Nature, 312: 756-757, 1984.
56. Aguilera G: Differential effects of atrial natriuretic factor on angiotensin II- and adrenocorticotrophin-stimulated aldosterone secretion. Endocrinology, 120: 299-304, 1987.
57. Barrett PQ, Isales CM: The role of cyclic nucleotides in atrial natriuretic peptide-mediated inhibition of aldosterone secretion. Endocrinology, 122: 799-808, 1988.
58. Cuneo RC, Espiner EA, Nicholls MG, Yandle TG, Livesey JH: Effect of physiological levels of atrial natriuretic peptide on hormone secretion: inhibition of angiotensin-induced aldosterone secretion and renin release in normal man. J Clin Endocrinol Metab, 65: 765-772, 1987.
59. Takagi M, Franco-Saenz R, Mulrow PJ: Effect of atrial natriuretic factor on the plasma aldosterone response to potassium infusion in rats: *in vivo* study. Life Sci, 39: 359-364, 1986.
60. Anand-Srivastava MB, Franks DJ, Cantin M, Genest J: Atrial natriuretic factor inhibits adenylate cyclase activity. Biochem Biophys Res Commun, 121: 855-862, 1984.
61. Shibasaki T, Naruse M, Yamauchi N, Masuda A, Imaki T, Naruse K, Demura H, Ling N, Inagami T, Shizume K: Rat atrial natriuretic factor suppresses proopiomelanocortin-derived peptides secretion from both anterior and intermediate lobe cells and growth hormone release from anterior lobe cells of rat pituitary *in vitro*. Biochem Biophys Res Commun, 135: 1035-1041, 1986.
62. Naruse M, Obana K, Naruse K, Yamaguchi H, Demura H, Inagami T, Shizume K: Atrial natriuretic polypeptide inhibits cortisol secretion as well as aldosterone secretion *in vitro* from human adrenal tissue. J Clin Endocrinol Metab, 64: 10-16, 1987.
63. Bianchi C, Gutkowska J, Thibault G, Garcia R, Genest J, Cantin M: Radioautographic localization of 125-I-atrial natriuretic factor (ANF) in rat tissues. Histochemistry, 82: 441-452, 1985.
64. Kleinert HD, Maack T, Atlas SA, Januzewicz A, Sealey JE, Laragh JH: Atrial natriuretic factor inhibits angiotensin-, norepinephrine-, and potassium-induced vascular contractility. Hypertension, 6: 1143-1147, 1984.
65. Volpe M, Sosa RE, Muller FB, Camargo MJ, Glorioso N, Laragh JH, Maack T, Atlas SA: Differing hemodynamic responses to atrial natriuretic factor in two models of hypertension. Am. J. Physiol, 250: H871-H878, 1986.
66. Schuster VL, Kokko JP, Jacobson HR: Angiotensin II directly stimulates sodium transport in rabbit proximal convoluted tubules. J Clin Invest, 73: 507-515, 1984.
67. Harris PJ, Thomas D, Morgan TO: Atrial natriuretic peptide inhibits angiotensin-stimulated proximal tubular sodium and water reabsorption. Nature 326: 697-698, 1987.
68. Liu FY, Cogan MG: Atrial natriuretic factor does not inhibit basal or angiotensin II-stimulated proximal transport. Am J Physiol, 255: F434-F437, 1988.
69. Antunes-Rodrigues J, McCann SM, Rogers LC, Samson WK: Atrial natriuretic factor inhibits dehydration- and angiotensin II-induced water intake in the conscious, unrestrained rat. Proc Nat'l Acad Sci, USA, 82: 8720-8723, 1985.
70. Katsuura G, Nakamura M, Inouye K, Kono M, Nakao K: Regulatory role of atrial natriuretic poly-peptide in water drinking in rats. Eur J Pharmacol, 121: 285-287, 1986.
71. Yamada T, Nakao K, Morri N, Itoh H, Shiono S, Sakamoto M, Sugawara A, Saito Y, Ohno H, Kanai A: Central effect of atrial natriuretic polypeptide on angiotensin II-stimulated vasopressin secretion in conscious rats. Eur J Pharmacol, 125: 453-456, 1986.
72. Winquist RJ, Faison EP, Nutt RF: Vasodilator profile of synthetic atrial natriuretic factor. Eur J Pharmacol, 102: 169-173, 1984.

73. Kleinert HD, Volpe M, Atlas SA, Camargo MJF, Laragh JH, Maack T: Blood vessels vary in sensitivity to atrial natriuretic factors (ANF): Circulation (Abstract) 70: II-333, 1984.
74. Winquist RJ, Faison EP, Waldman SA, Scwartz K, Murad F, Rapoport RM: Atrial natriuretic factor elicits an endothelium-independent relaxation and activates particulate guanylate cyclase in vascular smooth muscle. Proc Nat Acad Sci USA, 81: 7661-7664, 1984.
75. Almeida FA, Suzuki M, Maack T: Atrial natriuretic factor increases hematocrit and decreases plasma volume in nephrectomized rats. Life Sci, 39: 1183-1189, 1986.
76. Fluckiger JP, Waeber B, Matsueda G, Delaloye B, Nussberger J, Brunner HR: Effect of atriopeptin III on hematocrit and volemia of nephrectomized rats. Am J Physiol, 251: H880-H883, 1986.
77. Vidal NA, Arranz CT, Mones-Sias MC, Herrmann AP, Martinez-Seebur A: Atrial natriuretic factor and body water distribution. Arch Int Physiol Biochem, 95: 329-332, 1987
78. Ackermann U, Irizawa TG, Milojevic S, Sonnenberg H: Cardiovascular effects of atrial extracts in anesthetized rats. Can J Physiol Pharmacol: 62: 819-826, 1984.
79. Kleinert HD, Volpe M, Odell G, Marion D, Atlas SA, Camargo MJF, Laragh JH, Maack T: Cardiovascular effects of synthetic atrial natriuretic factor in anesthetized and conscious dogs. Hypertension, 8: 312-316, 1986.
80. Samson WK: Atrial natriuretic factor inhibits dehydration and hemorrhage-induced vasopressin release. Neuroendocrinology, 40: 277-279, 1985.
81. Lee J, Malvin RL, Claybaugh JR, Huang BS: Atrial natriuretic factor inhibits vasopressin secretion in conscious sheep. Proc Soc Exp Biol Med, 185: 272-276, 1987.
82. Standaert DG, Cechetto DF, Needleman P, Saper CB: Inhibition of the firing of vasopressin neurons by atriopeptin. Nature, 329: 151-153, 1987.
83. Murad F, Waldman S, Molina C, Bennett B, Leitman D: Regulation and role of guanylate cyclase-cyclic GMP in vascular relaxation. Prog Clin Biol Res, 249: 65-76, 1987.
84. Maack T, Suzuki M, Almeida FA, Nussenzveig D, Scarborough RM, McEnroe GA, Lewicki JA: Physiological role of silent receptors of atrial natriuretic factor. Science, 238: 675-678, 1987.
85. Kuno T, Andersen JW, Kamisaki Y, Waldman SA, Chang LY, Saheki S, Leitman DC, Nakane M, Murad F: Co-purification of an atrial natriuretic factor receptor and guanylate cyclase from rat lung. J Biol Chem, 261: 5817-5823, 1986.
86. Sala C, Pecker M, Laragh J, Muller F, Epstein M, Cody R, Atlas S: Relationship of endogenous or exogenous ANF to plasma cGMP in humans. (Abstract) 2nd World Congress on Biologically Active Atrial Peptides, NY, NY, 1987, p.181.
87. Hirata Y, Ishii M, Matsuoka H, Sugimoto T, Iizuka M, Uchida Y, Serizawa T, Sato H, Kohmoto O, Mochizuki T, Sugimoto T, Miyata A, Kangawa K, Matsuo H: Plasma concentrations of alpha-human atrial natriuretic polypeptide and cyclic GMP in patients with heart disease. Am Heart J, 113: 1463-1469, 1987.
88. Riegger GAJ, Elsner D, Kromer EP, Daffner C, Forssmann WG, Muders F, Pascher EW, Kochsiek K: Atrial natriuretic peptide in congestive heart failure in the dog: plasma levels, cyclic guanosine monophosphate, ultrastructure of atrial myoendocrine cells, and hemodynamic, hormonal, and renal effects. Circulation, 77: 398-406, 1988.
89. Lattion AL, Michel JB, Arnauld E, Corvol P, Soubrier F: Myocardial recruitment during ANF mRNA increase with volume overload in the rat. Am J Physiol, 251: H890-H896, 1986.
90. Day ML, Schwartz D, Wiegand RC, Stockman PT, Brunnert SR, Tolunay HE, Currie MG, Standaert DG, Needleman P: Ventricular atriopeptin. Unmasking of messenger RNA and peptide synthesis by hypertrophy or dexamethasone. Hypertension, 9: 485-491, 1987.
91. Brooks SE, Zimmerman RS, Schwab TR, Heublein DM, Burnett JC, Jr: Atrial stretch, not pressure, is the principal determinant controlling the acute release of atrial natriuretic factor. Circ Res, 62: 191-195, 1988.
92. Lang RE, Tholken H, Ganten D, Luft FC, Ruskoaho H, Unger TH: Atrial natriuretic factor-a circulating hormone, stimulated by volume loading. Nature, 314:264-266, 1985.
93. Sagnella GA, Shore AC, Markandu ND, MacGregor GA: Effects of changes in dietary sodium and saline infusion on immunoreactive atrial natriuretic peptide in human plasma. Lancet, ii: 1208-1211, 1985.
94. Epstein M, Loutzenhiser R, Friedland E, Aceto RM, Camargo MJF, Atlas SA: Relationship of increased plasma ANF and renal sodium handling during imersion-induced central hypervolemia in normal humans. J Clin Invest, 79: 738-745, 1985.

95. Ledsome JR, Wilson N, Courneya CA, Rankin AJ: Release of atrial natriuretic peptide by atrial distension. Can J Physiol Pharmacol, 63: 739-742, 1985.
96. Manning PT, Schwartz D, Katsube NC, Holmberg SW, Needleman P: Vasopressin-stimulated release of atriopeptin: endocrine antagonists in fluid homeostasis. Science Wash. DC, 229: 395-397,1985.
97. Uehlinger DE, Zaman T, Weidmann P, Shaw S, Gnadinger MP: Pressure dependence of atrial natriuretic peptide during norepinephrine infusion in humans. Hypertension, 10: 249-253, 1987.
98. Morris M, Alexander N: Baroreceptor influences on plasma atrial natriuretic peptide (ANP): sinoaortic denervation reduces basal levels and the response to an osmotic challenge. Endocrinology, 122: 373-375, 1988.
99. Volpe M, De Luca N, Atlas SA, Camargo MJ, Indolfi C, Lembo G, Trimarco B, Condorelli M, Laragh JH: Reduction of atrial natriuretic factor circulating levels by endogenous sympathetic activation in hypertensive patients. Circulation, 77: 997-1002, 1988.
100. Volpe M, Sosa RE, Atlas S, Sealey J, Laragh JH: Angiotensin II stimulates atrial peptide secretion which modulates aldosterone and renal responses to angiotensin II. (Abstract) Hypertension, 12: 346, 1988.
101. Itoh H, Nakao K, Yamada T, Morii N, Shiono S, Sugawara A, Saito Y, Mukoyama M, Arai H, Imura H: Brain renin-angiotensin. Central control of secretion of atrial natriuretic factor from the heart. Hypertension, 11: 157-161, 1988.
102. Salazar FJ, Granger JP, Joyce ML, Burnett JC, Jr, Bove AA, Romero JC: Effects of hypertonic saline infusion and water drinking on atrial peptide. Am J Physiol, 251: R1091-R1094, 1986.
103. Veress AT, Sonnenberg H: Right atrial appendectomy reduces the renal response to acute hypervolemia in the rat. Am J Physiol, 247: R610-R613, 1984.
104. Garcia R, Cantin M, Thibault G: Role of right and left atria in natriuresis and atrial natriuretic factor release during blood volume changes in the conscious rat. Circ Res, 61: 99-106, 1987.
105. Greenwald JE, Sakata M, Michener ML, Sides, SD, Needleman P: Is atriopeptin a physiological or pathophysiological substance? J Clin Invest, 81: 1036-1041, 1988.
106. Shenker Y, Sider RS, Ostafin EA, Grekin RJ: Plasma levels of immunoreactive atrial natriuretic factor in healthy subjects and in patients with edema. J Clin Invest, 76: 1684-1687, 1985.
107. Yandle TG, Richards AM, Nicholls MG, Cuneo R, Espiner EA, Livesey JH: Metabolic clearance rate and plasma half life of alpha-human atrial natriuretic peptide in man. Life Sci, 38: 1827-1833, 1986.
108. Hollister AS, Tanaka I, Imada T, Onrot J, Biaggioni I, Robertson D, Inagami T: Sodium loading and posture modulate human atrial natriuretic plasma levels. Hypertension, 8: II106-II111, 1986.
109. Solomon LR, Atherton JC, Bobinski H, Green R: Effect of dietary sodium chloride and posture on plasma immunoreactive atrial natriuretic peptide concentrations in man. Clin Sci, 72: 201-208, 1987.
110. Freund BJ, Claybaugh JR, Dice MS, Hashiro GM: Hormonal and vascular fluid responses to maximal exercise in trained and untrained males. J Appl Physiol, 63: 669-75, 1987.
111. Richards AM, Tonolo G, Montorsi P, Finlayson J, Fraser R, Inglis G, Towrie A, Morton JJ: Low dose infusions of 26- and 28-amino acid human atrial natriuretic peptides in normal man. J Clin Endocrinol Metab, 66: 465-72, 1988.
112. Anderson JV, Donckier J, Payne NN, Beacham J, Slater JDH, Bloom SR: Atrial natriuretic peptide: evidence of action as a natriuretic hormone at physiologic plasma concentrations in man. Clin Sci, 72: 305-312, 1987.
113. Weidmann P, Hellmueller B, Uehlinger DE, Lang RE, Gnaedinger MP, Hasler L, Shaw S, Bachmann C: Plasma levels and cardiovascular, endocrine, and excretory effects of atrial natriuretic peptide during different sodium intakes in man. J Clin Endocrinol Metab, 62: 1027-36, 1986.
114. Sagnella GA, Markandu ND, Shore AC, Forsling ML, MacGregor GA: Plasma atrial natriuretic peptide: its relationship to changes in sodium intake, plasma renin activity and aldosterone in man. Clin Sci, 72: 25-30, 1987.
115. Wambach G, Gotz S, Bonner G, Degenhardt S., Kaufmann W: Modulation of atrial natriuretic peptide, renin, and aldosterone by dietary sodium intake in normotension and essential hypertension. J Hypertension, 4 (suppl. 6): S564-S566, 1986.

116. Sagnella GA, Markandu ND, Shore AC, MacGregor GA: Plasma immunoreactive atrial natriuretic peptide and changes in dietary sodium intake in man. Life Sci, 40: 139-143, 1987.
117. Pecker MS, James GD, Laragh JH, Di Fabio B, Sealey JE, Atlas SA: Effect of changes in sodium intake on plasma atrial natriuretic factor levels in mild hypertension. (Abstract) Am J Hypertension, 1: 142A, 1988.
118. Ballerman, BJ, Bloch KD, Brenner BM: Atrial natriuretic peptide transcription, secretion, and glomerular receptor activity during mineralocorticoid escape in the rat. J Clin Invest, 78: 840-843, 1986.
119. Zimmerman RS, Edwards BS, Schwab TR, Heublein DM, Burnett JC, Jr: Atrial natriuretic peptide during mineralocorticoid escape in the human. J Clin Endocrinol Metab, 64: 624-627, 1987.
120. Sagnella GA, Markandu ND, Buckley MG, Shore AC, Sugden AL, Singer DRJ, MacGregor GA: Plasma atrial natriuretic peptide in essential hypertension: Comparisons with normotensive subjects and effects of changes in dietary sodium intake. Am J Hypertension, 1: 112-118, 1988.
121. Montorsi P, Tonolo G, Polonia J, Hepburn D, Richards AM: Correlates of plasma atrial nariuretic factor in health and hypertension. Hypertension, 10: 570-576, 1987.
122. Pecker MS, Cody RJ, Laragh JH, Sala C, Atlas SA: Atrial natriuretic factor response to saline infusion in hypertensive and normotensive subjects. Proceedings of the 19th Annual Meeting of the American Society of Nephrology: 125A, 1986.
123. Weder AB, Sekkarie M, Takiyyuddin M, Schork NJ, Julius S: Antihypertensive and hypotensive effects of atrial natriuretic factor in men. Hypertension, 10: 582-589, 1987.
124. Suda S, Weidmann P, Saxenhofer H, Cottier C, Shaw CG, Ferrier C: Atrial natriuretic factor in mild to moderate chronic renal failure. Hypertension, 11: 483-490, 1988.
125. Rascher W, Tulassay T, Lang RE: Atrial natriuretic peptide in plasma of volume-overloaded children with chronic renal failure. Lancet, ii: 303-305, 1985.
126. Smith S, Anderson S, Ballerman BJ, Brenner BM: Role of atrial natriuretic peptide in adaptation of sodium excretion with reduced renal mass. J Clin Invest, 77: 1395-1398, 1986.
127. Nakamoto M, Shapiro JI, Shanley PF, Chan L, Schrier RW: *In vitro* and *in vivo* protective effect of atriopeptin III on ischemic acute renal failure. J Clin Invest, 80: 698-705, 1987.
128. Shaw SG, Weidmann P, Hodler J, Zimmermann A, Paternostro A: Atrial natriuretic peptide protects against acute ischemic renal failure in the rat. J Clin Invest, 80: 1232-1237, 1987.
129. Cole BR, Kuhnline MA, Needleman P: Atriopeptin III: A potent natriuretic, diuretic, and hypotensive agent in rats with chronic renal failure. J Clin Invest, 76: 2413-2415, 1985.
130. Tulassay T, Rascher W, Lang RE, Seyberth HW, Scharer K: Atrial natriuretic peptides and other vasoactive hormones in nephrotic syndrome. Kidney Int, 31: 1391-1395, 1987.

GLOMERULONEPHRITIS

3

RECURRENCE OF GLOMERULONEPHRITIS AFTER RENAL TRANSPLANTATION

ROWAN G. WALKER AND PRISCILLA KINCAID-SMITH

Department of Nephrology, The Royal Melbourne Hospital, Victoria 3050, Australia.

INTRODUCTION

In 1989, the expectation of good results in renal transplantation is taken for granted. This improvement in renal allograft survival since the early 1960's when renal transplantation as a way of managing patients with end-stage renal failure (ESRF) became widely accepted, can largely be attributed to the improved quality of immunosuppression and particularly the introduction of cyclosporine (CyA). One feature of patients on ESRF programmes around the world which has remained constant over the three decades of renal transplantation is the importance of glomerulonephritis as the major cause of renal failure. Glomerulonephritis still accounts for nearly 40% of all underlying renal diagnoses in patients on most dialysis programmes (1).

Recurrence of glomerulonephritis in a renal allograft recipient was reported quite early in the renal transplant literature (2) and has been the subject of several reviews since (3-6). As immunosuppression improves, and transplant rejection diminishes, recurrent glomerulonephritis in renal allografts will perhaps assume greater importance as it becomes a relatively more prevalent cause of subsequent graft loss. Certainly, the less favorable graft survival in those patients whose primary disease is glomerulonephritis compared to those in whom reflux nephropathy is the cause, has been attributed, at least in part, to a recurrence of glomerulonephritis in the allografts of the glomerulonephritic group (Table 1), although recurrent glomerulonephritis probably accounts for less than 2% of all graft failures (7, 8).

Glomerular lesions are seen not infrequently in renal biopsies of allografts. Rejection and drugs (particularly CyA) which may cause chronic vascular changes and glomerular ischemia, sometimes make the clear differentiation of glomerular lesions more difficult but essentially four main types of lesions may be observed:

- recurrent glomerulonephritis
- *de novo* glomerulonephritis
- transplant glomerulopathy
- glomerulonephritis in the donor kidney

The purpose of this chapter is primarily to review the prevalence and nature of recurrent glomerulonephritic disease in the renal allograft recipient.

Table 1 Primary cadaveric graft percent survival. Australia (1971-1986)

	6 months	1 year	5 years	10 years	
Reflux nephropathy	78%	73%	56%	44%	n=369
Glomerulonephritis	69%	64%	43%	34%	n=1263

[Table derived from data in Reference 1]

RECURRENT GLOMERULONEPHRITIS

A number of authors have stressed the importance of renal biopsy if an accurate diagnosis of the primary disease causing ESRF and the true nature of subsequent recurrent disease are to be assessed (3-6, 9). Individual unit policy in relation to performing a renal biopsy will affect the accuracy of diagnosis and will have an important influence of the reported incidence of recurrent glomerulonephritis which by definition involves identifying the same disease process in the allograft as was present in the native kidney (3, 6).

Although nearly all histologically classified forms of glomerulonephritis have been reported to recur following renal transplantation, the likelihood and severity of recurrence varies enormously even within one histological classification.

Focal and segmental hyalinosis and sclerosis (focal glomerulosclerosis, FSGS)

FSGS is the most important form of glomerulonephritis causing renal failure in childhood and in adult patients, is the most important cause of ESRF associated with the nephrotic syndrome (1). It is also the glomerular disease which is most frequently reported as recurring in renal allografts.

Recurrence of FSGS in a renal allograft was first reported in 1972 (10) and numerous other reports appeared subsequently (reviewed in 3). Difficulties have been encountered in accurate histological and clinical definition but from larger series of both adult and pediatric patients, the recurrence rate of FSGS varies between less than 10% and greater than 60%. However, most authors agree that the recurrence rate is approximately 30% - 40% and actual graft losses due to recurrent FSGS occur in about half of these cases (6, 11-16).

Recurrent FSGS is invariably associated with the re-development of the nephrotic syndrome (11-16). Proteinuria may occur immediately post-transplantation but may occur weeks or months later. Histological and clinical differentiation between early FSGS and minimal lesion nephrotic syndrome can be extremely difficult and as with primary FSGS in native kidneys, early renal biopsies from transplanted kidneys may show only foot process fusion on ultrastructural studies. Subsequent biopsies however, reveal focal and segmental hyalinotic and sclerotic lesions of the glomeruli on light microscopy and with advancing renal failure progressive interstitial fibrosis.

Attempts have been made to define those characteristics of the FSGS affecting the native kidneys which might predict recurrence in the allograft. Mesangial expansion or proliferation certainly seems to be an unfavorable predictive feature (12, 15-17) and if the interval between the onset of nephrotic syndrome and the subsequent development of ESRF is less than 3 years, the recurrence rate in the allograft is at least 2x higher than if the interval is greater than 3 years (11-13, 15-18). The age of the patient at presentation also tends to predict outcome (6, 13). In addition, recurrence in the first allograft predicts a very high chance of recurrence in second and subsequent grafts, so much so that it is suggested that living related kidney donation in this setting should be avoided (16).

As with primary FSGS, a number of therapeutic strategies have been employed for recurrent FSGS in allografts with very variable (Figure 1) but generally with only modest success. Corticosteroids, cyclophosphamide, antiplatelet agents, plasma exchange, meclofenamate and cyclosporine have all been employed with the latter two reported as reducing proteinuria and perhaps prolonging remission in some patients (3, 6, 13, 19-22). CyA which seems to be beneficial in prolonging graft survival in patients whose primary disease is glomerulonephritis (23, 24) has generally been disappointing in the treatment of recurrent FSGS in renal allografts (22, 25). It should be remembered, however, that recurrence of FSGS is not inevitably associated with deterioration of renal function and occasional spontaneous remissions occur.

Cases of *de novo* FSGS have also been documented (12, 26)

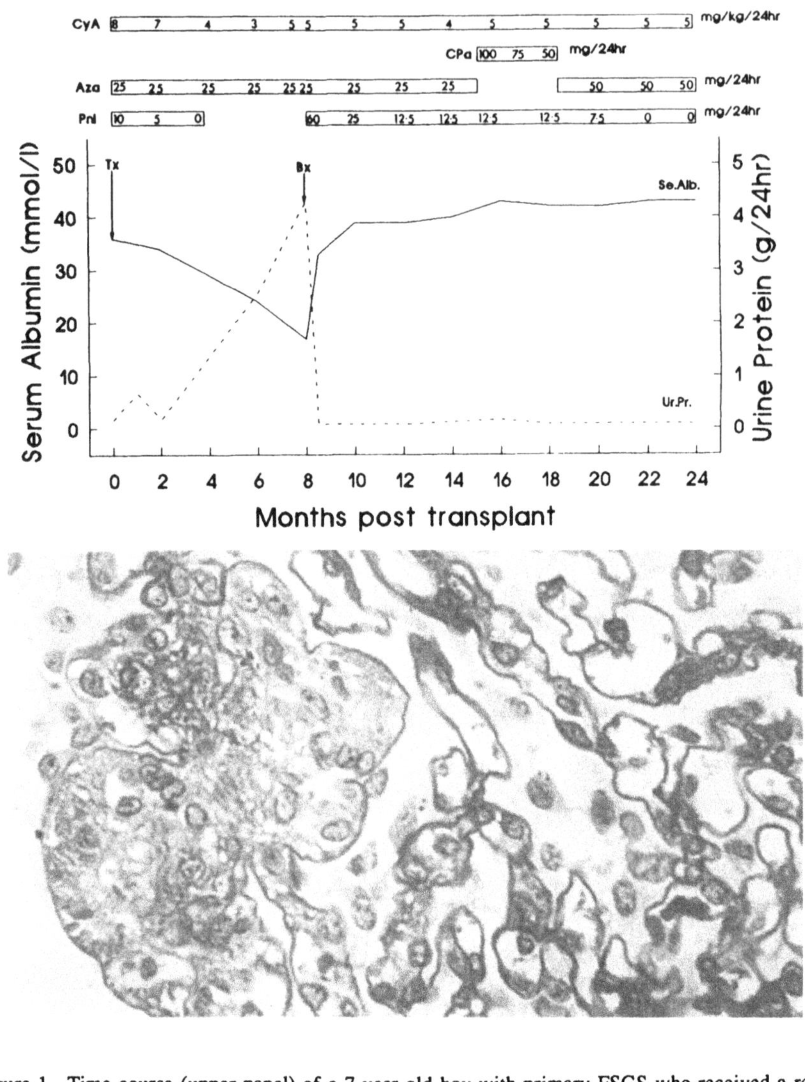

Figure 1. Time course (upper panel) of a 7 year old boy with primary FSGS who received a renal allograft (Tx). He was initially treated with prednisolone (Pnl), azathioprine (Aza) and cyclosporine (CyA). Coincident with dosage reduction of CyA and weaning from Pnl, he developed nephrotic syndrome. An increase in CyA from 3 mg/kg/24hr to 5 mg/kg/24hr for 4 weeks had no effect. Renal allograft biopsy (Bx) confirmed the presence of early sclerotic lesions of recurrent FSGS (lower panel). Pnl was re-introduced in high doses with rapid resolution of the nephrotic syndrome. Cyclophosphamide (CPa) was given 6 months later and Pnl was gradually reduced then ceased. No relapse has occurred. The case illustrates the problem of strict clinical and morphological definition of recurrent FSGS and the variable and unpredictable response to therapy.

Membranous glomerulonephritis

This form of glomerulonephritis is a relatively rare cause of ESRF (1). Its recurrence in the renal allograft is also rare and has been controversial because cases have been confused with a relatively high incidence of *de novo* membranous glomerulonephritis (27-34) in renal allografts. The reasons for the difficulties in separating true recurrent disease from *de novo* cases of glomerulonephritis have been carefully reviewed by both Cameron (3) and Mathew (7). Perhaps the most persuasive evidence in favour of genuine cases of recurrent membranous nephritis is the evaluation showing the incidence of membranous glomerulonephritis in allografts being 3x greater in patients whose primary lesion was membranous glomerulonephritis than in the group comprising all other causes of renal failure (7). Furthermore, the two groups may be distinguished by a more rapid appearance of nephrotic range proteinuria in the recurrent group compared to the *de novo* group (3, 7).

Proteinuria is invariable and the eventual development of nephrotic syndrome is usual in recurrent membranous glomerulonehritis in renal allografts. Bearing in mind the very small number of patients with truly recurrent membranous glomerulonephritis (27-34) reported in the literature (less than 15 cases), from which conclusions may be drawn, one possible risk factor for recurrence is a history of a rapid course in the primary disease. The overall outcome of the graft with recurrent membranous glomerulonephritis shows that 60% reached ESRF within 10 years (7). This contrasts with the overall prognosis in membranous glomerulonephritis which suggests that over 80% of patients survive for 10 years or more without renal failure (35).

IgA glomerulonephritis

IgA glomerulonephritis (IgA GN) is the most common form of glomerulonephritis and the most frequent cause of ESRF (1), but it is noteworthy that only 20% of patients with IgA GN progress to ESRF and the progression usually occurs over a median period of 17 years (36).

Of ESRF patients with IgA GN as the cause, recurrence of IgA deposits in the glomerular mesangium is very common in renal allografts (37) and recurrent IgA GN with associated proteinuria and/or microscopic hematuria probably occurs in up to 50% of patients (37, 38). However, actual progression of recurrent disease to ESRF is relatively rare (39), and in this respect, the time course of progressive IgA GN may be as important in the renal allograft as it is in native kidneys. The high incidence of recurrent disease in living related donor kidneys has been linked to a genetic susceptibility of certain HLA types (specifically HLA B35 and DR4) (37, 39-41).

One particular problem with the assessment of the incidence of IgA GN in the renal allograft is the unsuspected presence of mesangial IgA deposits in the donor kidney. In some units including our own, a renal biopsy is carried out on all cadaveric donor kidneys at the time of transplantation to the recipient. At least 3% of all these donor kidney biopsies contain mesangial IgA deposits, although these deposits disappear in most cases on subsequent biopsies. This is similar to the reported incidence of mesangial IgA deposits detected on renal biopsy in the populations of South East Asia (42).

Henoch Schonlein purpura nephritis (HSP)

As with IgA GN, recurrence of IgA deposits in the glomerular mesangium occurs variably but quite commonly in the renal allograft of HSP patient recipients. Not surprisingly, much of the reported incidence of recurrence of disease comes from pediatric populations, where despite the presence of glomerular deposits, urinary abnormalties (proteinuria and/or hematuria) are relatively uncommon as are systemic manifestations (purpura) (6, 39, 43, 44). However, clinical recurrences of HSP can be severe and crescentic nephritis and graft failure have been reported usually with concurrent purpura. A consensus view seems to be to avoid transplantation until 12 months after purpura has subsided (3, 7).

Mesangiocapillary glomerulonephritis (Type I) [MCGN]

MCGN is a disease with a declining incidence and therefore importance and it accounts for only very small numbers of patients on ESRF programmes in western countries (1) Careful histological evaluation should distinguish recurrence of MCGN from the mesangiocapilllary-type glomerulopathy seen in association with allograft rejection. The key feature is the presence of electron dense sub-endothelial deposits in recurrent glomerulonephritis (7, 9).

The actual incidence of MCGN recurrence is not clear but Mathew (7) estimates it to be approximately 30%, and progressive disease to loss of the graft probably occurs in up to 10% of recurrent cases of MCGN (3, 4). Clinical recurrence is usually characterized by nephrotic range proteinuria but florid crescentic disease may occur (3, 4, 7). Recurrent disease may also occur in successive grafts (45, 46).

Mesangiocapillary glomerulonephritis (Type II)

Recurrence of the electron dense ribbon like material in the glomerular basement membrane which characterizes mesangiocapillary glomerulonephritis (Type II) or Dense Deposit Disease (DDD) occurs in virtually 100% (47) of renal allograft recipients although this is some times detectable only on electron microscopy. However, progression of the lesion to renal failure and loss of the graft occurs much less frequently (approximately 10% of cases) (3) except in one series (50% of cases) (48).

Hypocomplementemia (low C_3 complement), neither accurately predicts the likelihood of recurrence (49), as was previously suggested (50), nor does it predict progression of recurrent disease to renal failure. Despite a relatively equal sex distribution for DDD as a primary lesion, a predominance of males with recurrence has been reported although male sex did not predict progression of the disease (48).

From a clinical point of view, recurrence of the nephrotic syndrome and/or the presence of crescents superimposed on the DDD lesion would be causes for concern (3).

Anti-glomerular basement membrane (GBM) nephritis

As a primary lesion, anti-GBM nephritis is the most fulminating form of crescentic glomerular disease. The natural history of anti-GBM disease is considered to be resolution and eventual disappearance of the circulating anti-GBM antibody over weeks or months (51). Plasma exchange has dramatically improved patient and renal survival for cases involving kidneys alone and kidneys and lungs, but anuric patients and those with a high proportion of glomeruli involved with crescents will progress rapidly to ESRF if plasma exchange and concomitant immunosuppression is not instituted early (52).

Anti-GBM nephritis accounts for relatively small numbers of patients on ESRF programmes (1). The resolution of circulating anti-GBM antibody for a period of 6 to 12 months has been used as a criterion for safely undertaking renal transplantation (3, 4). However, in practice, the relationship between circulating anti-GBM antibody and clinical activity is not clearly established and recurrence of anti-GBM disease has occurred both in patients in whom antibody is detected and in others in whom it is not detected (53, 54).

The overall experience suggests that the risk of recurrence of anti-GBM disease in renal allografts is very low (probably less than 5%) (3) although the presence of linear IgG on glomerular basement membranes on immunofluorescence studies is considerably higher (50%) (55, 56). Bilateral nephrectomy (57) and plasma exchange (58) have been used for recurrent disease but the former treatment has virtually no credibility in 1989 (3). *De novo* crescentic anti-GBM nephritis has also been reported in renal allografts especially in patients with Alport's syndrome (59-62).

Idiopathic rapidly progressive (crescentic) glomerulonephritis (RPGN)

Only very few cases of true recurrence of RPGN have been reported (3, 18). Crescentic nephritis is more often seen with anti-GBM disease or MCGN. *De novo* RPGN occurs rarely (63) (Figure 2).

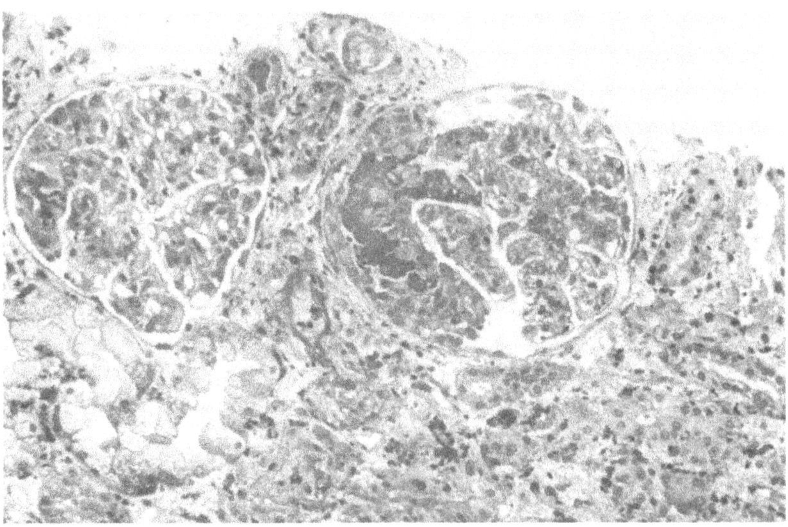

Figure 2. Renal allograft biopsy of a 52 year old woman who developed idiopathic *de novo* crescentic glomerulonephritis 3 months post-transplantation. Many glomeruli showed fibrin in glomerular capillaries and fibrin and crescents in Bowman's space.

Systemic lupus erythematosus (SLE)

Recurrence of SLE in a renal allograft had not been reported until relatively recently (64, 65). It remains an unusual occurrence (66) and it is probable that the concurrent immunosuppression modifies the renal histology to such a degree that the clinical implications of recurrent SLE are trivial.

Wegener's granulomatosis and microscopic polyarteritis

These two vasculitides are very infrequent causes of ESRF (1). Recurrence of Wegener's granulomatosis has only rarely been described (67). Immunosuppression with cyclophosphamide (and steroids) may be preferable to CyA for allograft recipients with Wegener's granulomatosis (68).

NON-GLOMERULONEPHRITIC RECURRING GLOMERULAR LESIONS

Although not glomerulonephritic diseases, there are a number of metabolic/systemic disorders which may recur in the renal allografts. The recurrent lesions in these diseases are most often not confined to the glomeruli. Several of these disease processes are worthy of at least brief mention in a review of recurrent glomerulonephritis in renal allografts.

Diabetic nephropathy

The increasing population of patients with ESRF due to diabetes (69), suggests that any tendency for this lesion to recur warrants comment. Vascular lesions (arteriolar hyalinization) may be relatively early and quite prominent in the renal allograft (70, 71) and the recurrence of classical nodular glomerulosclerosis has been reported (72). HLA B8/DR3 is associated with an increased predilection for diabetic microangiopathy and vascular disease and predisposes to the development of accelerated diabetic lesions in the donor kidney with similar HLA typing (72). Linear staining for IgG on immunofluorescence, similar to that seen in anti-GBM nephritis may also be a feature (72) not only of the glomerular basement membranes but also along tubular basement membranes. However, for the most part the development of recurrent diabetic glomerulosclerosis leading to ESRF probably runs a time course similar to that in primary diabetic nephropathy. Interest awaits confirmation as to whether simultaneous pancreatic transplantation will protect against the development of recurrent diabetic nephropathy in an allograft (73).

Amyloidosis

This metabolic disorder (primary or secondary) is a rare cause of ESRF and recurrent disease which occurs in approximately 1/3 of cases is not usually associated with significant clinical manifestations. However, nephrotic syndrome and progressive renal failure may sometimes occur (74, 75).

Fabry's disease

Transplantation for this rare x-linked inherited metabolic disease, characterized by a lack of the enzyme α-galactosidase A, has been disappointing (76). Long-term graft survival is very poor and recurrence of Fabry's disease deposits in glomerular but mostly tubulo-interstitial areas may be especially likely in living-related donor kidneys (i.e. heterozygous for Fabry's) (77).

Hemolytic-uremic syndrome (HUS)

HUS is a rare cause of ESRF (1) affecting mainly children. It is a disease characterized by microangiopathic hemolytic anemia, thrombocytopenia and renal failure. Renal histology shows micro-thrombi of small vessels and glomerular capillaries. Recurrence of HUS in renal allograft recipients has been recognized for many years (78) but the introduction of CyA, a drug which alters coagulation and renal prostaglandin production and may also cause long-term renal vascular damage, has raised the suggestion about this agent may increase the chance of recurrence in some patients. One group has stated that its use should be avoided in renal transplant recipients with HUS (79). Prior to the widespread use of CyA, the recurrent rate of HUS was approximately 10% (7) (Figure 3).

CONCLUDING REMARKS

The renal biopsy has provided us with much information about the incidence of recurrence of glomerular disease in the renal allograft recipient. Although histopathological features of glomerulonephritis in the renal allograft recipient are common, the number of cases with progressive renal failure appear to be much less common. In certain forms of recurrent glomerulonephritis such as FSGS, MCGN Type I and DDD, the histological features on renal biopsy may provide additional information about the likelihood of progression of the glomerulopathy.

For diseases, such as anti-GBM nephritis, HSP and HUS additional clinical and serological guidelines are evolving as to the relative safety under which transplantation may be performed specifically in relation to the likelihood of recurrence. However, it is perhaps ironical that for patients with certain glomerular diseases, the recognised HLA associations of these diseases may be predisposing these same patients to develop recurrent or *de novo* disease in an allograft. In most units, HLA tissue typing forms the very basis for allocation of cadaveric/living-related donor kidneys for transplantation and it is possible that individuals with a genetic susceptibility for a particular glomerular disease are being transplanted with organs genetically susceptible to the development of those same diseases.

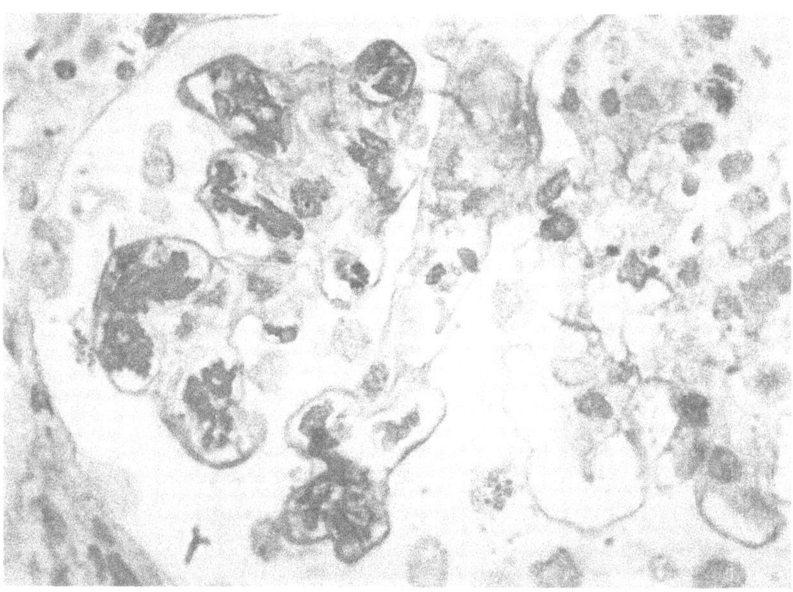

Figure 3. Renal allograft biopsy, 2 weeks post-transplantation of a 9 year old boy with recurrent HUS. Glomerular capillaries show numerous micro-thrombi. Other glomeruli showed congestion and early infarction. Widespread micro-thrombi were also seen in arterioles. The patient had not been treated with CyA.

ACKNOWLEDGEMENTS

The authors wish to acknowledge the contributions of Mrs V. Kuek and Mr D. Mathews in the preparation of this manuscript.

REFERENCES

1. Tenth Report of the Australia and New Zealand Combined Dialysis and Transplant Registry (ANZDATA)(Ed. APS Disney), Queen Elizabeth Hospital, South Australia. 1987, pp 24-29.
2. Glassock RJ, Feldman R, Reynolds ES, Dammin GJ, Merrill JP: Human renal isografts: a clinical and pathologic analysis. Medicine, 47: 411, 1968.
3. Cameron JS: Glomerulonephritis in renal transplants. Transplantation, 34: 237-245, 1982.
4. Morzycka M, Croker BP, Seigler HF, Tisher CG: Evaluation of recurrent glomerulonephritis in kidney allografts. Am J Med,72: 588, 1982.
5. Leumann EP, Briner J: Rezidive der Grundkrankheit im Nieren transplantat. Klin Wochenschr, 62: 289-298, 1984.
6. Habib R, Antignac C, Hinglais N: Glomerular lesions in the transplanted kidney in children, Am J Kidney Dis, 10: 198-207, 1987.
7. Mathew TH: Recurrence of disease following renal transplantation. Am J Kidney Dis, 12: 89-96, 1988.
8. Seventh Report of the Australia and New Zealand Combined Dialysis and Transplant Registry (ANZDATA)(Ed. APS Disney), Adelaide, Queen Elizabeth Hospital, South Australia, 1984, pp 35-36.
9. Mathew TH, Mathews DC, Hobbs JB, Kincaid-Smith P: Glomerular lesions after renal transplantation. Am J Med, 59: 177-190, 1975.
10 Hoyer JR, Raij L, Vernier RL, Simmons RL, Najarian JS, Michael AF: Recurrence of idiopathic nephrotic syndrome after renal transplantation. Lancet, ii: 343-348, 1972.
11. Leumann EP, Briner J, Donckerwolcke RAM, Kuijten R, Largiader F: Recurrence of focal segmental glomerulosclerosis in the transplanted kidney. Nephron, 25: 65-71, 1980.
12. Maizel SE, Sibley RK, Horstman JP, Kjellstrand CM, Simmons RL: Incidence and significance of recurrent focal segmental glomerulosclerosis in renal allograft recipients. Transplantation, 32: 512-516, 1981.
13. Pinto J, Lacerda G, Cameron JS, Turner DR, Bewick M, Ogg CS and the Physicians, Paediatricians and Pathologists of the South East Thames Renal Units: Recurrence of focal segmental glomerulosclerosis in renal allografts. Transplantation, 32: 83-89, 1981.
14. Cheigh JS, Muoradian J, Soliman M, Tapia L, Riggio RR, Stenzel KH, Rubin AL: Focal segmental glomerulosclerosis in renal transplants. Am J Kidney Dis, 2: 449-455, 1983.
15. Axelsen RA, Seymour AE, Mathew TH, Fisher G, Canny A, Pascoe V: Recurrent focal glomerulosclerosis in renal transplants. Clin Nephrol, 21: 110-114, 1984.
16. Striegel JE, Sibley RK, Fryd DS, Mauer SM: Recurrence of focal segmental sclerosis in children following renal transplantation. Kidney Int, 30: 544-550, 1986.
17. Habib R, Hebert D, Gagnadoux MF, Broyer M: Transplantation in idiopathic nephrosis. Transpl Proc, 14: 489-495, 1982.
18. Hamburger J, Crosnier J, Noel LH: Recurrent glomerulonephritis after renal transplantation. Ann Rev Med, 19: 67-72, 1978.
19. Munoz J, Sanchez R, Perez-Garcia R, Anaya F, Valderrabano F: Recurrent focal glomerulosclerosis in renal transplants. Proteinuria relapsing following plasma exchange. Clin Nephrol, 24: 213-214, 1985.
20. Zimmerman SW: Plasmapheresis and dipyridamole for recurrent focal glomerulosclerosis. Nephron, 40: 241-245, 1985.
21. Torres VE, Velosa JA, Holley KE, et al: Meclofenamate treatment of recurrent idiopathic nephrotic syndrome with focal segmental glomerulosclerosis after renal transplantation. Mayo Clin Proc, 59: 146-152, 1984.
22. Voets AJ, Hoitsma AJ, Koene RAP: Recurrence of nephrotic syndrome during cyclosporin treatment after renal transplantation. Lancet, i: 266-267, 1986.
23. Cats S, Perdue S, Terasaki PI, Mickey MR: Preferential effectiveness of cyclosporin in patients receiving kidney tranpslants after glomerulonephritis. Lancet,i: 490-491, 1985.

24. Tomlanovich S, Vincenti F, Amend W, Biava C, Melzer J, Feduska N, Salvatierra O: Is cyclosporine effective in preventing recurrence of immune-mediated glomerular disease after renal transplantation. Transpl Proc, 20(Suppl 4): 285-288, 1988.
25. Pirson Y, Squifflet JP, Marbaix E, et al: Recurrence of focal glomerulosclerosis despite cyclosporin treatment after renal trans-plantation. Br Med J, 292: 1336, 1986.
26. Woolley AC, Rosenberg ME, Burke BA, Nath KA: *De novo* focal glomerulosclerosis after kidney transplantation. Am J Med, 84: 310-314, 1988.
27. Briner J, Binswanger U, Largiader F: Recurrent and *de novo* membranous glomerulonephritis in renal cadaver allotransplants. Clin Nephrol, 13: 189-196, 1980.
28. Dische FE, Herbertson BM, Melcher DH, Morley AR: Membranous glomerulonephritis in transplant kidneys: recurrent or *de novo* disease in four patients. Clin Nephrol, 15: 154-163, 1981.
29. Iskandar SS, Jennette JC: Recurrence of membranous glomerulopathy in an allograft. Case Report and Review of the Literature. Nephron, 29: 270-273, 1981.
30. Verani R, Dan M: Membranous glomerulonephritis in renal transplant. Am J Nephrol, 2: 316-320, 1982.
31. Cosyns JP, Pirson Y, Squifflet JP, Alexandre GPJ, van Ypersele de Strihou, Pinn VW, Sweet SJ, Shapiro KS, Cho S, Harrington JT: *De novo* membranous nephropathy in human renal allografts: Report of nine patients. Kidney Int, 22: 177-183, 1982.
32. Berger BE, Vincenti F, Biava C, Amend WJ Jr, Feduska N, Salvatierra O: *De novo* and recurrent membranous glomerulopathy following kidney transplantation. Transplantation, 35: 315-319, 1983.
33. Obermiller LE, Hoy WE, Eversole M, Sterling WA: Recurrent membranous glomerulonephritis in two renal transplants. Trans-plantation, 40: 100-102, 1985.
34. Ward HJ, Koyle MA: Immunopathologic features of *de novo* membranous nephropathy in renal allografts. Transplantation, 45: 524-529, 1988.
35. Murphy BF, Fairley KF, Kincaid-Smith P: Idiopathic membranous glomerulonephritis: long-term follow-up in 139 cases. Clin Nephrol, 30: 175-181, 1988.
36. Nicholls KM, Fairley KF, Dowling JP, Kincaid-Smith P: The clinical course of mesangial IgA nephropathy. Quart J Med, 53: 227-250, 1984.
37. Berger J: Recurrence of IgA nephropathy in renal allografts. Am J Kidney Dis, 12: 371-372, 1988.
38. Petterson E, Honkanen E, Tornroth T: Recurrence of IgA nephropathy with nephrotic syndrome in renal allograft. Nephron, 41: 114-117, 1985.
39. Bachman U, Biava C, Amend W, Feduska N, Mezzer J, Salvatierra O, Vincenti F: The clinical course of IgA nephropathy and Henoch Schonlein purpura following renal transplantation. Transplantation, 42: 511-515, 1986.
40. Berger J, Noel LH, Nabarra B: Recurrence of mesangial IgA nephropathy after renal transplantation. Contrib Nephrol, 40: 195-197, 1984.
41. Brensilver JM, Mallat S, Scholes J, McCabe R: Recurent IgA nephropathy in living-related donor transplantation: recurrence on transmission of familial disease. Am J Kidney Dis, 12: 147-151, 1988.
42. Sinniah R, Pwee HS, Lim CH: Glomerular lesions in asymptomatic microscopic haematuria on routine medical examination. Clin Nephrol,5: 216-228, 1976.
43. Baliah T, Kim KH, Anthone S, et al: Recurrence of Henoch Schonlein purpura glomerulonephritis in transplanted kidneys. Transplantation, 18: 343-346, 1974.
44. Nast CC, Ward HJ, Koyle MA, Cohen AH: Recurrent Henoch Schonlein purpura following renal transplantation. Am J Kidney Dis, 9: 39-43, 1987.
45. Zimmerman SW, Hyman LR, Vehling DT, Burkholder PM: Recurrent membranoproliferative glomerulonephritis with glomerular properdin deposition in allografts. Ann Intern Med, 80: 169-175, 1974.
46. Glicklich D, Matas AJ, Sablay LB, Senitzer D, Tellis VA, Soberman R, Veith FJ: Recurrent membranoproliferative glomerulonephritis type I in successive renal transplants. Am J Nephrol, 7: 143-149, 1987.
47. Turner DR, Cameron JS, Bewick M, Sharpstone P, Melcher D, Ogg CS, Evans DJ, Trafford AJP, Leibowitz S: Transplantation in mesangiocapillary glomerulonephritis with intramenbranous dense "deposits": recurrence of disease. Kidney Int, 9: 439-448, 1976.
48. Eddy A, Sibley R, Mauer SM, Kim Y: Renal allograft failure due to recurrent dense intramembranous deposit disease. Clin Nephrol, 21: 305-313, 1984.
49. Leibowitch J, Halbwachs L, Wattel S, Gaillard MH, Droz D: Recurrence of dense deposits in transplanted kidney. II. serum complement and nephritic factor profiles. Kidney Int, 15: 396-403, 1979.

50. Berthoux FC, Ducrot F, Colon S, Blanc-Brunat N, Zech PY, Traeger J: Renal transplantation in mesangioproliferative glomerulonephritis (MPGN): relationship between the high frequency of recurrent glomerulonephritis and hypocomplementemia. Kidney Int, 7: S323-S327, 1975.
51. Lockwood CM, Peters DK: Plasma exchange in glomerulonephritis and related vasculitides. Ann Rev Med, 31: 167, 1980.
52. Walker RG, Scheinkestel C, Becker GJ, Owen JE, Dowling JP, Kincaid-Smith P: Clinical and morphological aspects of the management of crescentic anti-glomerular basement membrane antibody (anti-GBM) nephritis/Goodpasture's syndrome. Q J Med, 54: 75-89, 1985.
53. Almkuist RD, Buckalew VM, Hirszel P, Maher JF, James PM, Wilson CB: Recurrence of antiglomerular basement membrane antibody mediated glomerulonephritis in an isograft. Clin Immunol Immunopathol, 18: 54, 1981.
54. Couser WG, Wallace A, Monaco A, Lewis EJ: Successful renal transplantation in patients with anti-GBM antibody to glomerular basement membrane. Clin Nephrol, 1: 381-388, 1973.
55. Cameron JS, Turner DR: Recurrent glomerulonephritis in allografted kidneys. Clin Nephrol, 7: 47, 1977.
56. Wilson CB, Dixon FJ: Anti-glomerular basement membrane antibody induced glomerulonephritis. Kidney Int, 3: 74-89, 1973.
57. Bergrem H, Jervell J, Brodwall EK, Flatmark A, Mellbye O: Goodpasture's syndrome: a report of seven patients including long-term follow-up of three who received a kidney transplant. Am J Med, 68: 54-58, 1980.
58. Cove-Smith JR, McLeod AA, Blamey RW, Knapp MS, Reeves WG, Wilson CB: Transplantation, immunosuppression and plasmapheresis in Goodpasture's syndrome. Clin Nephrol, 9: 126, 1978.
59. Milliner DS, Pierides AM, Holley KE: Renal transplantation in Alport's syndrome. Anti-glomerular basement membrane glomerulonehritis in the allograft. Mayo Clin Proc, 57: 35-43, 1982.
60. McCoy RC, Johnson HK, Stone WJ, Wilson CB: Absence of nephritogenic GBM antigen(s) in some patients with hereditary nephritis. Kidney Int, 21: 642-652, 1982.
61. Teruel JL, Liano F, Mampaso F, Moreno J, Serrano A, Quereda C, Ortuno J: Allograft antiglomerular basement membrane glomerulonephritis in a patient with Alport's syndrome. Nephron, 46: 43-44, 1987.
62. Boyce N, Holdsworth S, Atkins R, Dowling J: *De novo* anti-GBM-antibody-induced glomerulonephritis in a renal transplant. Clin Nephrol, 23: 148-151, 1985.
63. Ihle BU, d'Apice AJF, Dowling J, Kincaid-Smith P: *De novo* crescentic glomerulonephritis in a renal transplant. Transplantation Proc, 15: 2147-2151, 1983.
64. Amend WJC, Vincenti F, Feduska NJ, Salvatierra O, Johnston WH, Jackson J, Tilney N, Garovoy M, Burwell EL: Recurrent systemic lupus erythematosus involving renal allografts. Ann Intern Med, 94: 444, 1981.
65. Yakub YN, Freeman RB, Pabico RC: Renal transplantation in systemic lupus erythematosus. Nephron, 27: 197-201, 1981.
66. Kumano K, Sakai T, Mashimo S, Endo T, Koshiba K, Elises JS, Iitaka K: A case of recurrent lupus nephritis after renal transplantation. Clin Nephrol, 27,: 94-98, 1987.
67. Steinman TI, Jaffe BF, Monaco AP, Wolff SM, Fauci A: Recurrence of Wegener's granulomatosis after kidney transplantation. Successful re-induction of remission with cyclophosphamide. Am J Med, 68: 458-460, 1980.
68. Lazarouits AI: Recurrence of Wegener's granulomatosis in a renal transplant recipient treated with cyclosporin. Clin Invest Med, 8: A224, 1985.
69. Eighth Report of the Australia and New Zealand Combined Dialysis and Transplant Registry (ANZDATA) (Ed. APS Disney), Queen Elizabeth Hospital, South Australia, pp 109-129, 1985.
70. Najarian JS, Sutherland DE, Simmons RL et al: Ten year's experience with renal transplantation in juvenile onset diabetes. Ann Surg, 1900: 487-501, 1979.
71. Mauer SM, Barbosa J, Vernier RC et al: Development of diabetic vascular lesions in a normal kidney transplanted into a patient with diabetes mellitus. N Eng J Med, 2395: 916-919, 1976.
72. Maryniak RK, Mendoza N, Clyne D, Balakrishnan K, Weiss MA: Recurrence of diabetic nodular glomerulosclerosis in a renal transplant. Transplantation, 39: 35-38, 1985.
73. Bohman SO, Wilczek H, Tyden G et al: Recurrent diabetic nephropathy in renal allografts placed in diabetic patients and protective effect of simultaneous pancreatic transplantation. Transpl Proc, 19: 2290-2293, 1987.
74. Helin H, Pasternack A, Falck H, Huhlback B: Recurrence of renal amyloid and *de novo* membranous glomerulonephritis after transplantation. Transplantation, 32: 6-9, 1981.

75. Dorman SA, Gammelli RL, Benzinger JR et al: Systemic amyloidosis involving two renal transplants. Hum Pathol, 12: 735-748, 1981.
76. Maizel SE, Simmons RL, Kjellstrand C, Fryd DS: Ten-year experience in renal transplantation for Fabry's disease. Transpl Proc, 13: 57-59, 1981.
77. Popli S, Molna ZV, Leehey DJ, Daugirdas JT, Roth DA, Adams MB, Cheng JC, Ing TS: Involvement of renal allograft by Fabry's disease. Am J Nephrol, 7: 316-318, 1987.
78. Cerilli GJ, Welsen C, Dorfman L: Renal monotransplantation in infants and children with the hemolytic uremic syndrome. Surgery 71:66-71, 1972.
79. Hebert D, Sibley RK, Mauer SM: Recurrence of hemolytic uremic syndrome in renal transplant recipients. Kidney Int, 30: S51-S58,1986.

4

MANAGEMENT OF THE HYPERLIPIDEMIA OF THE NEPHROTIC SYNDROME

SCOTT M. GRUNDY AND GLORIA LENA VEGA

Center for Human Nutrition, University of Texas, Southwestern Medical Center at Dallas, Dallas, Texas 75235, USA

The nephrotic syndrome is a renal disorder characterized by proteinuria, hypoalbuminemia, sometimes edema, and hyperlipidemia. A variety of diseases of the glomerulus can produce the nephrotic syndrome. The major primary causes of this syndrome are membranous nephropathy, focal sclerosis, and minimal change disease (1). In addition, a common cause of the nephrotic disease in adults is diabetes mellitus. The hyperlipidemia of the nephrotic syndrome can consist of hypercholesterolemia, hypertriglyceridemia or both (mixed hyperlipidemia). An elevation of serum total cholesterol (and low density lipoprotein LDL-cholesterol) usually is the first form of hyperlipidemia to develop (2, 3). Later in the course of the disease, hypertriglyceridemia will appear (4).

There is growing evidence that the hyperlipidemia of the nephrotic syndrome can accelerate the development of atherosclerosis and thereby increase the risk for coronary heart disease (5, 6). It must be noted that atherogenesis is a life-long process, and the development of the nephrotic syndrome later in life, with its accompanying hyperlipidemia, may not cause a sufficient increase in atherosclerosis to produce the clinical manifestations of atherosclerotic disease. However, if nephrotic hyperlipidemia is of prolonged duration, this abnormality may be sufficient to induce coronary heart disease. Moreover, if nephrotic hyperlipidemia is superimposed on other conditions that accelerate atherosclerosis (e.g. aging, diabetes mellitus, hypertension, smoking) then it could be an important contributing factor in the causation of coronary heart disease. Because of difficulty in carrying out a prospective study in a large number of nephrotic patients, it has not been possible to define with precision the incidence of nephrotic hyperlipidemia on coronary risk. However, there is abundant evidence that the same pattern of dyslipidemia due to primary causes will increase the risk for coronary heart disease, and thus, the same should occur with the nephrotic syndrome. This reasoning taken with currently available clinical data strongly suggest that nephrotic hyperlipidemia can predispose to coronary heart disease; and if so, there is a justification for treatment of the hyperlipidemia for the purpose of reducing coronary risk.

MECHANISMS OF NEPHROTIC HYPERLIPIDEMIA

Hypercolesterolemia

The hypercholesterolemia of the nephrotic syndrome basically represents an increase in serum LDL-cholesterol. This increase theoretically could be the result of either: (a) an overproduction of lipoproteins containing apolipoprotein B-100 (apo B) by the liver, and (b) a defective clearance of LDL via LDL receptors. The precise mechanism for elevated LDL levels in human nephrosis has not been determined with certainty. However, it can be said that hypercholesterolemia is related to hypoalbuminemia. Indeed, correction of reduced levels of serum albumin will cause the hypercholesterolemia to resolve (3, 7, 8). Studies in laboratory animals have shown that induction of hypoalbuminemia will stimulate the synthesis of both lipids and proteins in the liver (9-13). A similar response has been shown in cultured hepatocytes, i.e. reducing the oncotic pressure of the media will increase the secretion of lipoproteins into the media (14, 15). This finding is consistent with reports of increased secretion of apo B-containing lipoproteins as demonstrated by several techniques (9-11). Thus, overproduction of lipoproteins by the liver appears to be a major cause of nephrotic hypercholesterolemia.

Another factor that may contribute to an increase in LDL levels is a reduction in activity of LDL receptors. A decrease in LDL receptor activity can have two causes: (a) a genetic deficiency of LDL receptors and (b) downregulation of LDL receptor synthesis.

A genetic deficiency of receptors occurs in the hereditary disorder called heterozygous familial hypercholesterolemia (16). Normally, one gene encoding for synthesis of LDL receptors is inherited from each parent, and the function of both genes is required to maintain a normal level of LDL-cholesterol. In the disorder heterozygous familial hypercholesterolemia, one gene is defective, and the affected patient thus has half the normal number of LDL receptors, LDL-cholesterol levels are twice normal. Heterozygous familial hypercholesterolemia occurs in one in 500 people in the population.

A more common cause of hypercholesterolemia appears to be a down regulation of the synthesis of LDL receptors. It has been shown that the activity of the gene encoding for LDL receptors is regulated by the cholesterol content of the cells, particularly liver cells (17). When the cholesterol content of the cells is increased, the synthesis of LDL receptors decreases; and conversely, a reduction of cellular cholesterol leads to a stimulation of synthesis of receptors. Through this mechanism, the cell regulates the uptake of the LDL-cholesterol and thereby maintains cellular content of cholesterol at a constant level. If the nephrotic syndrome results in an increased synthesis of cholesterol this could overload the liver with cholesterol, and thereby downregulate the synthesis of LDL receptors. This effect in turn will raise the serum level of LDL-cholesterol.

Hypertriglyceridemia

As the nephrotic syndrome worsens, patients often develop hypertriglyceridemia or mixed hyperlipidemia. One cause of elevated triglycerides could be an overproduction of VLDL particles by the liver. However, it is of interest that early in the course of the nephrotic syndrome hypercholesterolemia frequently exists without hypertriglyceridemia (2-4). Thus, if high LDL levels in nephrosis are due in part to overproduction of lipoproteins, this response will not necessarily produce hypertriglyceridemia. If an excessive input of triglyceride-rich lipoproteins occurs early in the course of the disease, lipolytic mechanisms may be adequate to prevent the development of elevated serum triglycerides.

If the above reasoning holds, the increase in triglyceride levels with advancing nephrosis may be due to the breakdown of normal lipolytic mechanisms. In fact, several lines of evidence support this concept. For example, isotope kinetic studies from our laboratory indicate that clearance of triglyceride-rich lipoproteins in nephrotic patients is markedly delayed (18). This abnormality could have several causes. First, there could be a deficiency of apo C-II, the activator of lipoprotein lipase (19); second, the activity of lipoprotein lipase could be reduced; or third, there could be a deficiency of LDL receptors leading to a decrease in direct removal of VLDL remnants. In the nephrotic syndrome, some apo C-II is lost in urine, but studies in nephrotic animals show that apo C-II levels are sufficient to activate lipoprotein lipase (19-21). A more likely cause of nephrotic hypertriglyceridemia is decreased activity of lipoprotein lipase, and/or possibly hepatic triglyceride lipase (22-24). Depressed lipase activities have been reported in laboratory animals (23), and circulating inhibitors of lipoprotein lipase have been reported for patients with renal disease (24). Since hypertriglyceridemic patients with uremia have a defect in lipolysis of VLDL triglycerides, a similar defect may exist in patients with advanced nephrotic syndrome. Finally, we have reported that enhancement of LDL receptor activity by drug therapy will increase clearance of VLDL and mitigate hypertriglyceridemia in nephrotic patients (18); this finding raises the possibility that a reduced activity of LDL receptors may be one cause of elevated VLDL triglycerides in nephrotic patients.

DRUG TREATMENT OF NEPHROTIC HYPERLIPIDEMIA

Although circumstantial evidence implicates nephrotic hyperlipidemia in the genesis of coronary atherosclerosis and coronary heart disease, the link has not been proven with the certainty that exists for various primary hyperlipidemias. Even so, available evidence does appear strong enough to justify efforts to modify lipoprotein levels in nephrotic patients by active medical therapy. In general, the first mode of treatment of hyperlipidemia is dietary therapy. The diet approach includes reduction in dietary intakes of saturated fatty acids and cholesterol and weight reduction to achieve a desirable body weight (25). To date no dietary trials have been carried out to determine effectiveness of dietary modification in nephrotic patients with hypercholesterolemia. In all probability, however, dietary change will not cause a major reduction in cholesterol levels; nonetheless, changes in diet are justified to induce a modest decrease in LDL levels and to potentiate the action of cholesterol-lowering drugs. In most cases, however, to obtain a meaningful reduction in LDL levels, drug therapy will be required.

Five categories of lipid-lowering drugs are available for treatment of hyperlipidemia. These are bile acid-binding resins, nicotinic acid, competitive inhibitors of 3-hydroxy-3-methylglutaryl coenzime A (HMG CoA) reductase, fibric acids, and probucol. Only a limited number of studies have been carried out to determine actions of these drugs in therapy of nephrotic hyperlipidemia, but the results are consistent enough to give a fairly good picture of their therapeutic efficacy in this condition. Each category will be discussed in terms of their mode of action, and then their specific effects in nephrotic patients will be summarized.

Bile acid resins

The resins are nonabsorbable drugs having quaternary amine groups that bind to negatively charged bile acids (26). Currently available resins are cholestyramine and colestipol. By binding bile acids in the intestine, the resins reduce the absorption of cholesterol and decrease their return to the liver. This effect releases the feedback inhibition of bile acids on hepatic conversion of cholesterol to bile acids, and thus hepatic cholesterol concentrations are reduced by increased degradation of cholesterol into bile acids. The result of less hepatic cholesterol content is a stimulation of LDL receptor synthesis which promotes the removal of LDL from the circulation. The LDL level is further reduced by enhanced clearance of VLDL remnants, which are precursor of LDL (27). In patients with primary hypercholesterolemia, LDL-cholesterol levels generally is reduced by 15 to 25% by bile acid resins. The degree of reduction is limited to some extent by a compensatory increase in synthesis of cholesterol which partially restores cholesterol content.

The bile acid resins can have two additional effects on lipoprotein levels. They often cause modest elevations of high density lipoproteins (HDL), which may be an added benefit (28). But in addition, the resins can raise VLDL-triglyceride concentrations. The effect is due to stimulation of hepatic synthesis of VLDL triglycerides (29); and in patients who have an inherent defect in lipolysis of serum triglycerides, the result can be a marked increase in triglyceride concentrations (30).

A major advantage to use of bile acid resins is that they have proven to be safe and effective for reducing risk for coronary heart disease in a large clinical trial - the Lipid Research Clinics Coronary Primary Prevention Trial (28, 31). In this trial approximately 4000 hypercholesterolemic men were divided into two groups - cholestyramine and placebo - and they were treated for seven years. At the end of the trial, the cholestyramine treatment group had a significantly lower rate of coronary events than the placebo group. This benefit was not associated with significant side effects in the cholestyramine group. Thus, cholestyramine, and most likely colestipol, can safely reduce coronary risk in patients with primary hypercholesterolemia, although the degree of reduction is limited because bile acids do not produce major reductions in LDL levels.

Bile acids have been tested in two studies for cholesterol lowering in patients with nephrotic syndrome (32, 33). In one investigation, Valeri et al (32) examined the action of colestipol on plasma cholesterol levels in seven patients with the nephrotic syndrome. Patients were given colestipol in doses of 15 to 25 grams per day in divided doses. Results are shown in Table 1.

In this study, colestipol therapy caused a 20.2% decrease in total cholesterol and a 31.9% decrease in LDL-cholesterol, both statistically significant reductions. No other changes were significant, although colestipol had a tendency to increase VLDL-cholesterol. Moreover, in spite of the significant decrease in LDL-cholesterol, the levels remained elevated during drug therapy. Thus, bile acid resins do not normalize LDL levels in many nephrotic patients.

Table 1. Colestipol therapy in the nephrotic syndrome*

Lipid Parameter	Pre-Drug Control	Colestipol Therapy	Post-Drug Control
		mmol/liter±SEM	
Total cholesterol	10.3±0.7	8.2±0.9	10.0±1.2
Triglyceride	2.9±0.5	3.2±0.7	3.5±0.8
VLDL cholesterol	1.4±0.4	1.8±0.8	1.9±0.5
LDL cholesterol	7.7±0.5	5.2±0.5	6.9±2.4
HDL cholesterol	1.2±O.1	1.2±0.2	1.1±0.2

* Data of Valeri et al (32)

More recently, Rabelink et al (33) reported on effects of cholestyramine in patients with nephrotic syndrome. Eight patients were studied, and cholestyramine, 8 grams twice daily, was used. Treatment periods were six weeks. Results of this study are given in Table 2.

In this trial, the only statistically significant change was a 19% reduction in LDL-cholesterol levels ($p < 0.005$). Again, this report indicates that bile acids will lower LDL-cholesterol levels in patients with the nephrotic syndrome, but levels usually are not normalized. Therefore, in spite of the proven safety and effectiveness of bile acid resins, it will be necessary to consider use of other drugs if the aim of therapy is to reduce LDL-cholesterol levels to the desirable range.

Nicotinic acid

Another cholesterol-lowering drug is nicotinic acid (niacin). The major action of nicotinic acid appears to reduce the secretion of apo B-containing lipoproteins by the liver. The drug partially inhibits release of free fatty acids from adipose tissue, which may limit their availability for synthesis of VLDL triglycerides (34). However, this action alone probably cannot account fully for the reduced hepatic secretion of lipoproteins. The mechanisms whereby nicotinic acid directly inhibits the synthesis of apo B-containing lipoproteins in the liver have not been determined.

Table 2. Cholestyramine therapy in nephrotic syndrome.

Parameter	Placebo	Cholestyramine
	mmol/liter±SEM	
Total cholesterol	10.13±0.90	9.35±0.67
Triglyceride	4.28±0.55	5.19±1.42
LDL cholesterol	7.30±0.91	5.90±0.77
HDL cholesterol	0.90±0.07	1.11±0.14
Total apo B (g/l)	1.67±0.13	1.56±0.12

* Data of Rabelink et al (33)

Because of this action to interfere with lipoprotein synthesis, nicotinic acid has a favorable effect on all lipoprotein levels. The drug lowers both VLDL and LDL levels. Moreover, the fall in VLDL triglycerides is accompanied by an increased level of HDL cholesterol. These changes appear to be more favorable than noted with any other form of drug therapy. The beneficial effect of nicotinic acid on lipoprotein levels is reflected in coronary heart disease rates by the results of the Coronary Drug Project (35); this study demonstrated that in patients with previous myocardial infarction nicotinic acid reduced recurrence rates for myocardial infarction. In addition, in a 15-yr follow up of participants of the Coronary Drug Project, total death rates were lower in patients who had received nicotinic acid than in the placebo group (36). Thus, nicotinic acid seemingly has a favorable effect on lipoprotein levels that is reflected in a reduced coronary risk.

Even though nicotinic acid appears to directly counteract the lipoprotein defects occurring in the nephrotic syndrome, i.e. hepatic overproduction of lipoproteins, the drug has not been used systematically in therapy in nephrotic patients. Certainly nicotinic acid should favorably affect nephrotic hyperlipidemia, but this possibility remains to be proven. Furthermore, another crucial question regarding use of nicotinic acid in nephrotic patients is whether it will be well tolerated. Nicotinic acid is known to have several side effects. The two most bothersome are skin reactions (flushing, itching, and rash) and gastrointestinal upsets. But of greater concern for nephrotic patients may be metabolic side effects; these include hepatotoxicity manifested by abnormal function tests, deterioration in glucose tolerance, and increase in uric acid levels. These metabolic side effects may be more common and more serious in patients with renal disease, and clearly clinical investigation is needed to resolve this question.

HMG CoA reductase inhibitors

The recent introduction of a new class of cholesterol-lowering drugs - the HMG CoA reductase inhibitors - may offer a new opportunity for effective treatment of severe hypercholesterolemia (37). These drugs have been shown to be effective for several different forms of hypercholesterolemia. Their primary site of action appears to be in the liver where they reduce synthesis of cholesterol by competitively inhibiting the rate-limiting enzyme in cholesterol formation, namely, HMG CoA reductase. The major response to a reduction in cholesterol synthesis is an increase in the formation of LDL receptors (17). Studies in laboratory animals have shown that reductase inhibitors increase messenger RNA for LDL receptors in liver cells (38) and increase the number of receptors expressed on the surface of liver cells (39). Investigations of lipoprotein kinetics in humans are consistent with the concept that these agents increase the activity of LDL receptors (40). For example, patients who are completely devoid of LDL receptors, namely, those with receptor-negative, homozygous familial hypercholesterolemia, fail to respond to reductase-inhibitor therapy with a decrease in LDL-cholesterol levels (41). Therefore, the bulk of the evidence indicates that the major action of HMG CoA reductase inhibitors on lipoprotein levels is to increase the activity of LDL receptors.

Several studies now have demonstrated that reductase inhibitors also will lower triglyceride levels in some patients (42, 43). One mechanism whereby this could occur would be through enhanced direct removal of VLDL and VLDL remnants by increased LDL-receptor activity in liver cells. This effect should decrease the conversion of VLDL to LDL; and in fact, a decreased formation of LDL has been reported in patients treated with reductase inhibitors (44). Although enhanced clearance of VLDL could be one explanation for a reduced input of LDL, a decreased production of apo B-containing lipoproteins by the liver could be another. Indeed, Ginsberg et al (45) have postulated that reductase inhibitors reduce the synthesis of apo B-containing lipoproteins, perhaps secondarily to a decrease in hepatic cholesterol content. This possibility certainly has not been ruled out, and it could be a second mechanism whereby HMG CoA reductase inhibitors lower plasma levels of VLDL and LDL.

A recent study from our laboratory (18) indicates that one reductase inhibitor, lovastatin, will reduce cholesterol levels in hypercholesterolemic patients with the nephrotic syndrome. We carried out an investigation in three nephrotic patients in which lovastatin therapy was compared to a control period. The results for plasma lipids and lipoproteins are presented in Table 3.

Table 3. Lovastatin therapy in nephrotic syndrome.

	Total	Total	Lipoprotein-cholesterol		
Patient	Cholesterol	Triglyceride	VLDL	LDL	HDL
		mmol/liter±SD*			
No.1					
Control	9.8±0.3	3.5±0.1	2.6±0.3	6.4±0.40	0.8±0.05
Lovastatin	6.7±0.5°	2.1±0.1°	1.6±0.2°	4.3±0.20°	0.9±0.08°
No.2					
Control	7.4±0.2	3.4±0.4	2.1±0.2	4.3±0.05	0.9±0.09
Lovastatin	5.0±0.1°	2.5±0.4°	1.5±0.1°	2.3±0.20°	1.2±0.10°
No.3					
Control	14.1±0.7	7.1±2.5	6.3±0.3	7.6±0.70	0.3±0.05
Lovastatin	9.8±0.7°	3.9±0.4°	2.9±0.4°	6.2±0.10°	0.6±0.05°

* Mean±SD for four 3-day pools of fasting plasma over a 14-day period.
° Significantly different from control by Student's t-test ($p<0.05$).

In all these patients, lovastatin produced a marked reduction in total-cholesterol and LDL-cholesterol levels. Of interest, the drug also lowered levels of triglycerides and VLDL-cholesterol, and significantly raised HDL-cholesterol concentrations. In this same study, we carried out determinations of LDL-apo B kinetics, and the findings are presented in Table 4.

Table 4. Effects of lovastatin on LDL-apo B kinetics.

Patient	LDL-apo B		
	Concentration	FCR*	Input Rate°
	mg/dl	pools/day	mg/kg/day
No1			
Control	171	0.28	21.1
Lovastatin	117	0.26	14.3
No.2			
Control	125	0.20	11.5
Lovastatin	72	0.24	5.2
No.3			
Control	228	0.29	25.6
Lovastatin	158	0.28	18.2
Normal man (n = 14)	101	0.30	13.5
(mean±SEM)	±5	±0.01	±0.7
(Ref. 46)			

* FCR = fractional catabolic rate
° Input rate = transport rate or production rate

The data show that lovastatin markedly reduced LDL-apo B levels in all patients. One patient (No. 2) did not have a striking elevation of LDL-apo B levels, and in this patient, production (input) rates of LDL were relatively normal in the control period. In contrast, the other two patients (Nos. 1 and 3) did have very high LDL-apo B levels, and the major cause of their high concentrations was an increased production (input) rate of LDL-apo B. This overproduction of LDL may have been secondary to excessive hepatic secretion of apo B-containing lipoproteins, because fractional catabolic rates for LDL were not strikingly reduced. The major effect of lovastatin therapy was to decrease the input rate for LDL. Although this change might have been due to a decreased synthesis of apo B-containing lipoproteins, it also could have been secondary to enhanced direct removal of VLDL, the precursor of LDL, resulting from an increased activity of LDL receptors.

In this same study, kinetics of VLDL-apo B also were determined. The data from these measurements are given in Table 5.

In all three patients, lovastatin therapy lowered concentrations of VLDL-apo B. It also increased the fractional catabolic rate for VLDL-apo B in all patients, but did not decrease input rates for VLDL-apo B. These results suggest that the major action of lovastatin is to promote the clearance of VLDL, via enhanced LDL-receptor activity, and not to decrease the synthesis of apo B-containing lipoproteins. It should be noted, however, that input of LDL-apo B often exceeded the total input of VLDL-apo B, and thus some LDL was derived from pathways other than through measured circulating VLDL (48). Presumably, some nascent lipoproteins can be converted to LDL without entering the circulating pool of VLDL. Therefore, it is not possible to be certain that lovastatin does not decrease the formation of apo B-containing lipoproteins in nephrotic patients.

Table 5. Effects of lovastatin therapy on VLDL-apo B kinetics.

Patient	VLDL-apo B		
	Concentration	FCR*	Input Rate°
	mg/dl	pools/day	mg/kg/day
No.1			
Control	33	0.92	9.7
Lovastatin	23	1.82	18.5
No.2			
Control	26	0.53	8.8
Lovastatin	14	0.88	7.8
No.3			
Control	60	0.77	18.4
Lovastatin	21	2.12	16.9
Normal men (n=5) (mean±SEM) (Ref. 47)	14.5 ±1.0	3.33 ±0.46	12.5 ±2.2

* FRC = fractional catabolic rate
° Input rate = transport rate or production rate

More recently, Rabelink et al (33) have reported the effects of another HMG CoA reductase inhibitor, simvastatin, on lipid levels in eight patients with the nephrotic syndrome. Compared to a placebo period, results of simvastatin therapy are shown in Table 6.

The results of this study are similar to those reported from our laboratory with lovastatin treatment (18). Simvastatin therapy produced a 36% lowering in total cholesterol levels, 39% in triglycerides, 39% for LDL cholesterol, and 30% for total apo B. Simvastatin treatment clearly was more effective for lowering cholesterol and triglycerides levels than cholestyramine therapy in the same patients (Table 2). Reductase inhibitors thus appear to be highly-promising drugs for the treatment of hyperlipidemia of the nephrotic syndrome.

Table 6. Effects of simvastatin in the nephrotic syndrome*

	Placebo	Simvastatin
	mmol/liter±SEM	
Total cholesterol	10.01±0.70	6.44±0.59°
Triglycerides	4.45±0.60	2.73±0.43°
LDL-cholesterol	7.02±0.60	4.28±0.56°
HDL-cholesterol	0.99±0.11	1.20±0.11
Total apo B (g/l)	1.60±0.15	1.12±0.18

* From Rabelink et al (33)
° Difference significant at $p<0.05$, compared to placebo period.

An important question about HMG CoA reductase inhibitors is whether they will be well tolerated in chronic therapy in nephrotic patients. Some patients treated with these drugs develop mild abnormalities in liver-function tests, but overt hepatotoxicity has not been reported. Perhaps of more concern is development of proximal myopathy. This side effect occurs in 2% to 10% of patients, depending on how the syndrome is defined. Most patients have modest increases of creatine kinase or mild muscle pain or weakness. These findings disappear when the drug is discontinued. More rarely, severe myopathy may develop, and is manifest by muscle weakness, marked increases of creatine kinase concentration, and myoglobinuria

(49). A few patients have even developed acute tubular necrosis. This side effect would be particularly unfortunate in patients with underlying renal disease.

The development of myopathy appears to be a result of increased blood levels of lovastatin. The reductase inhibitors are excreted through the liver, and factors that interfere with drug excretion can substantially increase risk for severe myopathy. Such factors are underlying liver disease, concomitant nicotinic acid therapy, cyclosporin, and possibly aging and female sex hormones. Another cause of severe myopathy is concomitant use of fibric acids (49), which themselves can have muscle toxicity.

Fibric acids

Several drugs in this category are available in various countries. These include clofibrate, gemfibrozil, fenofibrate, bezafibrate, and ciprofibrate. They have been used widely for treatment of hyperlipidemia for well over two decades. Although their precise mechanisms of action have not been determined, they affect the metabolism of both triglycerides and cholesterol (50). Two actions on triglyceride metabolism have been reported: (a) an increase in the activity of lipoprotein lipase, enhancing clearance of VLDL-triglycerides, and (b) a decrease in secretion of VLDL-triglycerides; both changes can reduce concentrations of VLDL-triglycerides, and secondarily raise HDL-cholesterol levels. The fibric acids also have been reported to inhibit the synthesis of cholesterol, which may increase LDL receptor activity (51). They also enhance the secretion of cholesterol in bile, which can increase risk for gallstone formation. A recent report (52) indicates that one fibric acid, gemfibrozil, significantly decreases risk for coronary heart disease in patients with primary hypercholesterolemia.

There is limited experience with fibric acids for treatment of hypercholesterolemia in patients with the nephrotic syndrome. In one study, Bridgeman et al (53) reported that clofibrate produced myopathy in several patients with the nephrotic syndrome. Indeed, muscular pain, stiffness, and general malaise occurred in five of six patients treated with clofibrate. The authors suggested that because of reduced albumin levels, excessive amounts of clofibrate were free in serum, unbound to albumin. There are no reports yet on use of gemfibrozil, but the same side effect might occur. Therefore, the fibric acids should be used cautiously in patients with the nephrotic syndrome. In particular, they probably should not be used in combination with HMG CoA reductase inhibitors because of the already high risk of severe myopathy with the latter.

Probucol

This drug has a moderate cholesterol-lowering action. Its major action is to reduce LDL-cholesterol concentrations, and it appears to enhance removal of LDL from the circulation (54). Probucol also reduces HDL-cholesterol levels. The latter effect at first was considered to negate the usefulness of probucol. However, a recent study (55) indicates that probucol will retard the development of atherosclerosis in hypercholesterolemic rabbits, possibly by inhibiting the oxidation of LDL in the arterial wall. If this effect occurs in man, probucol might have a greater utility in prevention of atherosclerosis than previously realized.

Valeri et al (32) have examined actions of probucol in five hypercholesterolemic patients with the nephrotic syndrome. They reported that probucol therapy caused a 22.6% decrease in total cholesterol, a 23.8% decrease in LDL cholesterol, and a 12.2% reduction in HDL cholesterol. Overall, probucol was well tolerated by the patients. More recently, Iida et al (56) carried out a similar study in 12 hypercholesterolemic, nephrotic patients. In this study, probucol therapy reduced total cholesterol levels by 30%, triglycerides by 28%, LDL cholesterol by 25%, and HDL cholesterol by 25%. Again, no side effects were noted. Thus, in two studies, probucol proved to be moderately effective for treatment of hypercholesterolemia in nephrotic patients.

COMBINED DRUG THERAPY

Because of the severe hypercholesterolemia and often mixed hyperlipidemia in patients with the nephrotic syndrome, use of lipid-lowering drugs in combination were worthy of consideration. To date, however, no such studies have been carried out. Even so, from studies in primary hyperlipidemia, the HMG CoA reductase inhibitors combined with either fibric acids or nicotinic acid would appear to be contraindicated in routine practice bacause of the danger of severe myopathy. Use of nicotinic acid or fibric acids with bile acid binding resins do not pose the same risk, and either combination can be tried. The combination of resin with nicotinic acid is particularly attractive. Another excellent combination is an HMG CoA reductase inhibitor plus resin, which together are highly effective in patients with primary hypercholesterolemia. Probucol appears to be safe to use in combination with other drugs, and if future studies reveal that it directly prevents atherosclerosis in humans, it could be a valuable addition to cholesterol-lowering therapy. Therefore, we suggest that investigation of combined drug therapy for hyperlipidemia of the nephrotic syndrome may be particularly rewarding.

REFERENCES

1. Collaborative study of the adult idiopathic nephrotic syndrome. A controlled study of short-term prednisone treatment in adults with membranous nephropathy. N Eng J Med, 301: 1301-1306, 1979.
2. Baxter JH: Hyperlipoproteinemia in nephrosis. Arch Intern Med, 109: 742-757, 1962.
3. Zilleruelo G, Hsia SL, Freundlich M, Gorman HM, Strauss J: Persistence of serum lipid abnormalities in children with idiopathic nephrotic syndrome. J Pediatr, 104: 61-64, 1984.
4. Appel GB, Blum CB, Chien S, Kunis CL, Appel AS: The hyperlipidemia of the nephrotic syndrome. Relation to plasma albumin concentration, oncotic pressure, and viscosity. N Eng J Med, 312: 1544-1548, 1985.
5. Berlyne GM, Mallick NP: Ischemic heart-disease as a complication of nephrotic syndrome. Lancet, ii: 399-400, 1969.
6. Mallick NP, Short CD: The nephrotic syndrome and ischemic heart disease. Nephron, 27: 54-57, 1981.
7. De Mendoza SG, Kashyap ML, Chen CY, Lutmer RF: High density lipoproteinuria in nephrotic syndrome. Metabolism, 25: 1143-1149, 1976.
8. Baxter JH, Goodman HC, Allen JC: Effects of infusions of serum albumin on serum lipids and lipoproteins in nephrosis. J Clin Invest, 40: 490-498, 1961.
9. Marsh JB, Drabkin DL: Experimental reconstruction of metabolic pattern of lipid nephrosis: Key role of hepatic protein synthesis in hyperlipemia. Metabolism, 9: 946-955, 1960.
10. Marsh JB, Sparks CE: Hepatic secretion of lipoproteins in the rat and the effect of experimental nephrosis. J Clin Invest, 64: 1229-1237, 1979.
11. Marsh JB: Lipoprotein metabolism in experimental nephrosis. J Lipid Res, 25: 1619-1623, 1984.
12. Marsh JB, Drabkin DL: Metabolic channeling in experimental nephrosis. V. Lipid metabolism in the early stages of the disease. J Biol Chem, 230: 1083-1091, 1958.
13. Shafrir E, Brenner T: Lipoprotein lipid and protein synthesis in experimental nephrosis and plasmapheresis. I. Studies in rat *in vivo*. Lipids, 14: 695-702, 1979.
14. Davis RA, Engelhorn SC, Weinstein DB, Steinberg D: Very low density lipoprotein secretion by cultured rat hepatocytes: Inhibition by albumin and other macromolecules. J Biol Chem, 255: 2039-2045, 1980.
15. Yedgar S, Weinstein DB, Patch W, Schonfeld G, Casandra FE, Steinberg D: Viscosity of culture medium as a regulator of synthesis and secretion of very low density lipoproteins by cultured hepatocytes. J Biol Chem, 257: 2188-2192, 1982.
16. Goldstein JL, Brown MS: Familial hypercholesterolemia. In: "Metabolic Basis of Inherited Disease", JB Stanbury, JB Wyngaarden, DS Fredrickson, JL Goldstein, MS Brown (Eds), McGraw-Hill, New York, 1983, pp 672-713.
17. Goldstein JL, Brown MS: The low density lipoprotein pathway and its relation to atherosclerosis. Ann Rev Biochem, 46: 897-930, 1977.
18. Vega GL, Grundy SM: Lovastatin therapy in nephrotic hyperlipidemia: Effects on lipoprotein metabolism. Kidney Int, 33: 1160-1168, 1988.
19. Kashyap ML, De Mendoza SG, Cambell M, Chen CY, Lutmer RF, Glueck CJ: Lipoprotein lipase activator deficiency in very low density lipoproteins in rat nephrotic syndrome. Experientia, 34: 1044-1045, 1978.
20. Gherardi E, Vecchia L, Calandra S: Experimental nephrotic syndrome in the rat induced by puromycin aminoglicoside. Plasma and urinary lipoproteins. Exp Mol Pathol, 32: 128-142, 1980.
21. Ohta T, Matsuda I: Lipid and apolipoprotein levels in patients with nephrotic syndrome. Clin Chim Acta, 117: 133-143, 1981.

22. Garber DW, Gottlieb BA, Marsh JB, Sparks CE: Catabolism of very low density lipoproteins in experimental nephrosis. J Clin Invest, 74: 1375-1381, 1984.
23. Yamada M, Matsuda E: Lipoprotein lipase in clinical and experimental nephrosis. Clin Chim Acta, 30: 787-794, 1970.
24. Murase T, Cattram DL, Rubenstein B, Steiner G: Inhibition of lipoprotein lipase by uremic plasma. A possible cause of hypertriglyceridemia. Metabolism, 24: 1279-1286, 1975.
25. The Expert Panel. Report of the National Cholesterol Education Program. Expert Panel on detection, evaluation, and treatment of high blood cholesterol in adults. Arch Intern Med, 148: 36-69, 1988.
26. Grundy SM: Bile acid resins. Mechanisms of action. In: "Pharmacological Control of Hyperlipidemia" JA Prous Science Publishers, SA, Barcelona, 1986, pp 3-19.
27. Brown MS, Goldstein JL: Lipoprotein receptors in the liver: Control signals for plasma cholesterol traffic. J Clin Invest, 72: 743-747, 1983.
28. Lipid Research Clinics Program. The Lipid Research Clinics Primary Prevention Trial Results. II. The relationship of reduction in incidence of coronary heart disease to cholesterol lowering. JAMA, 251: 365-374, 1984.
29. Beil U, Crouse JR, Einarsson K, Grundy SM: Effects of interruption of the enterohepatic circulation of bile acids on the transport of very low density-lipoprotein triglycerides. Metabolism, 31: 438-444, 1982.
30. Crouse JR: Hypertrygliceridemia - A contraindication to the use of bile acid binding resins. Am J Med, 83: 243-248, 1987.
31. Lipid Research Clinics Program. The Lipid Research Clinics Coronary Primary Prevention Trial Results. I. Reduction in incidence of coronary heart disease. JAMA, 251: 351-364, 1964.
32. Valeri A, Gelfand J, Blum C, Appel GB: Treatment of the hyperlipidemia of the nephrotic syndrome: a controlled trial. Am J Kidney Dis, 8: 388-396, 1986.
33. Rabelink AJ, Erkelens DW, Hene RJ, Joles JA, Koomans HA: Effects of simvastatin and cholestyramine on lipoprotein profile in hyperlipidemia of nephrotic syndrome. Lancet, ii: 1335-1338, 1988.
34. Grundy SM, Mok HYI, Zech L, Berman M: Influence of nicotinic acid on metabolism of cholesterol and triglycerides in man. J Lipid Res, 22: 24-36, 1981.
35. The Coronary Drug Project Research Group. Clofibrate and niacin in coronary heart disease (The Coronary Drug Project). JAMA, 231: 360-381, 1975.
36. Canner PL, Berge KG, Wenger NK, Stamler J, Friedman L, Prineas RJ, Friendewald W, et al: Fifteen year mortality in coronary drug project patients: Long-term benefit with niacin. J Am Coll Cardiol, 8: 1245-1255, 1986.
37. Grundy SM: HMG-CoA reductase inhibitors for treatment of hypercholesterolemia. N Eng J Med, 319: 24-33, 1988.
38. Ma PTS, Gil G, Sudhof TC, Bilheimer DW, Goldstein JL, Brown MS: Mevinolin, an inhibitor of cholesterol synthesis, induces mRNA for low density lipoprotein in livers of hamsters and rabbits. Proc Natl Acad Sci USA, 83: 8370-8374, 1986.
39. Kovanen PT, Bilheimer DW, Goldstein JL, Jaramillo JJ, Brown MS: Regulatory role for hepatic low density lipoprotein receptors *in vivo* in the dog. Proc Natl Acad Sci USA, 78: 1194-1198, 1981.
40. Bilheimer DW, Grundy SM, Brown MS, Goldstein JL: Mevinolin and colestipol stimulate receptor-mediated clearance of LDL from plasma in familial hypercholesterolemia heterozygotes. Proc Natl Acad Sci USA, 80: 4124-4128, 1983.
41. Uauy R, Vega GL, Grundy SM, Bilheimer DW: Lovastatin therapy in receptor-negative homozygous familial hypercholesterolemia: Lack of effect on low density lipoprotein concentrations or turnover. J Pediatr, 113: 387-392, 1988.
42. Yamamoto A, Sudo H, Endo A: Therapeutic effects of ML-236B in primary hypercholesterolemia. Atherosclerosis, 35: 259-266, 1980.
43. Garg A, Grundy SM: Gemfibrozil alone and in combination with lovastatin for treatment of hypertriglyceridemia in NIDDM. Diabetes, 38: 364-372, 1989.
44. Grundy SM, Vega GL: Influence of mevinolin on metabolism of low density lipoproteins in primary moderate hypercholesterolemia. J Lipid Res, 26: 1464-1475, 1985.
45. Ginsberg HN, Le NA, Short MP, Ramakrishnan R, Desnick RJ: Suppression of apolipoprotein B production during treatment of cholesterol ester storage disease with lovastatin. Implication for regulation of apolipoprotein B. J Clin Invest, 80: 1692-1698, 1987.

46. Grundy SM, Gotto AMJ, Bierman EL, et al: American Heart Association's Recommendations for Treatment of Hyperlipidemia in Adults. Circulation, 69: 1067A-1090A, 1984.
47. Kesaniemi YA, Beltz WF, Grundy SM: Comparisons of metabolism of apo B in normal subjects, obese patients, and patients with coronary heart disease. J Clin Invest, 76: 586-595, 1985.
48. Beltz WF, Kesaniemi YA, Howard BV, Grundy SM: Development of an integrated model for analysis of kinetics of apolipoprotein B in plasma very low density lipoproteins, intermediate density lipoproteins, and low density lipoproteins. J Clin Invest, 76: 575-585, 1985.
49. East C, Alivizatos PA, Grundy SM, Jones PH, Farmer JA: Rhabdomyolysis in patients receiving lovastatin after cardiac transplantation. N Eng J Med, 318: 47-48, 1988.
50. Grundy SM, Vega GL: Fibric acids: Effects on lipids and lipoprotein metabolism. Am J Med, 83: 9-20, 1987.
51. Stewart JM, Packard JC, Lorimer AR, Boag DE, Shepherd J: Effects of bezafibrate on receptor-mediated and receptor-independent low density lipoprotein catabolism in type II hyperlipoproteinemic subjects. Atherosclerosis, 44: 355-365, 1982.
52. Frick MH, Elo O, Haapa K, Heinonen OP, Heinsalmi P, Helo P, Huttunen JK, et al: Helsinki Heart Study: Primary-prevention trial with gemfibrozil in middle-aged men with dyslipidemia. N Eng J Med, 317: 1237-1245, 1987.
53. Bridgeman JF, Rosen SM, Thorp JM: Complications during clofibrate treatment of nephrotic syndrome hyperlipoproteinemia. Lancet ii: 506-509, 1972.
54. Kesaniemi YA, Grundy SM: Influence of probucol on cholesterol and lipoprotein metabolism in man. J Lipid Res, 25: 780-790, 1984.
55. Kita T, Nagano Y, Yokode M, et al: Probucol prevents the progression of atherosclerosis in Watanabe heritable hyperlipidemic rabbit, an animal model for familial hypercholesterolemia. Proc Natl Acad Sci USA, 84: 5928-5931, 1987.
56. Iida H, Izumino K, Asaka M, Fujita M, Nishino A, Sasayama S: Effect of probucol on hyperlipidemia in patients with nephrotic syndrome. Nephron, 47: 280-283, 1987.

INFECTIONS

5

RENAL COMPLICATIONS OF HUMAN IMMUNODEFICIENCY VIRUS-TYPE I

JACQUES J. BOURGOIGNIE, CARMEN ORTIZ-INTERIAN, DOLLIE F. GREEN, DAVID J. JAFFE, DAVID ROTH AND VICTORIANO PARDO

Division of Nephrology, Departments of Medicine and Pathology,
University of Miami School of Medicine, Miami, Florida 33101, USA

More than 87,000 patients with acquired immunodeficiency syndrome (AIDS) were reported to the Centers for Disease Control in the United States, of whom more than half died through January 1989. When the AIDS epidemic is considered worldwide, these numbers probably should be doubled (1). This review examines the electrolyte disorders and renal complications observed in patients with human immunodeficiency virus (HIV-1) (formerly called HTLV-III) infection.

Infections and neoplasms are the dominant clinical manifestations of AIDS. It is not surprising, therefore, that renal complications have been increasingly recognized. Reasons for the nephrologist to intervene in the care of a patient with HIV-1 infection include: (i) electrolyte and acid-base disorders; (ii) azotemia related to acute or chronic renal failure, and (iii) proteinuria or hematuria.

Typically, electrolyte and acid-base disorders and acute renal failure occur in patients with AIDS whereas the nephrotic syndrome and chronic azotemia are often seen in patients with AIDS-related complex (ARC) or in otherwise asymptomatic HIV-1 carriers, i.e., before the development of opportunistic infections and/or neoplasms typical of AIDS.

ELECTROLYTE AND ACID-BASE DISTURBANCES

Simple and mixed (double or triple) acid-base disturbances and virtually all types of electrolyte disorders can be observed in AIDS patients with gastrointestinal disorders (vomiting, diarrhea, malabsorption, malnutrition), hemodynamic instability (volume depletion, hypotension, sepsis), respiratory, central nervous system and/or renal failure. In contrast to AIDS patients, the frequency and severity of electrolyte abnormalities in patients with ARC is very low (2). Common electrolyte disorders are listed in Table 1.

Table 1. Common electrolyte disorders in patients with AIDS.

Hyponatremia
Hyperkalemia
Hypo-, hypercalcemia
Hypouricemia

Hyponatremia

With a prevalence of 31 to 52% in large series of patients, hyponatremia is the most common electrolyte abnormality encountered (3-5). In the majority of patients (up to 88%), it is associated with volume depletion and is corrected by administration of saline. In the absence of an evident source of fluid loss, volume depletion is usually related to renal salt wasting with an inappropriately high urinary sodium concentration. Adrenal insufficiency may be the cause in a minority of patients (hyperkalemic patients with low ACTH stimulation test); whereas defect(s) in tubular sodium reabsorptive capacity have been postulated in the majority (normo- or hypokalemic patients with normal ACTH stimulation test) (3-5a).

In euvolemic patients with a high urinary sodium concentration, hyponatremia is compatible with non-osmolar inappropriate stimulation of antidiuretic hormone (3-6) as might be anticipated in patients with pulmonary or central nervous system pathology. Hyponatremia in hypervolemic patients is dilutional in origin as a result of excess free water intake in patients with renal insufficiency (3).

The potential for adrenal insufficiency and Addison's disease in patients with AIDS was recognized early on in the AIDS epidemic because of frequent autopsy findings of adrenal necrosis related to cytomegalovirus, mycobacterium, or cryptococcal infection (7-9). As indicated above, however, overt adrenal insufficiency is relatively rare when compared to the frequent autopsy findings of adrenalitis and adrenal necrosis in this patient population. This discrepancy has been ascribed to the fact that cortical necrosis in AIDS patients usually involves less than 70% of the adrenal glands allowing for adequate production of cortisol by the uninvolved tissue.

Nevertheless, even though overt adrenal insufficiency is infrequent, selective partial hypopituitarism (subnormal ACTH release) and/or hypoadrenalism (subnormal cortisol response to ACTH stimulation) may be common in patients with AIDS (10, 11). While adrenal function is normal under baseline condition, a state of limited functional reserve capacity exists and adrenal insufficiency may become clinically evident only under stressful situations.

In vitro, ketoconazole has been shown to inhibit steroid production. *In vivo*, however, ketoconazole has rarely been demonstrated to result in glucocorticoid insufficiency in patients with AIDS. On the other hand, ketoconazole has a greater selectivity for inhibiting androgen production and may induce gynecomastia in patients receiving high-dose prolonged treatment (12).

Hyperkalemia

Hyperkalemia has been reported to occur in 16% of AIDS patients (5). The increased serum potassium may be an expression of Addison's disease, or result from selective hypoaldesteronism with Type IV renal tubular acidosis (13).

Hypocalcemia

Mild to moderate hypocalcemia is found in a majority of AIDS patients (2, 5). It is generally associated with hypoalbuminemia. The latter, however, may not fully account for the hypocalcemia (2, 5).

Hypercalcemia

Conversely, hypercalcemia has been reported in association with granulomatous diseases, disseminated cytomegalovirus infection or with human T-cell leukemia associated with HTLV-1 infection. A parathyroid hormone-like substance has been implicated in the pathogenesis of some hypercalcemia (14). The hypercalcemia may resolve with administration of mithramycin (15) or calcitonin (16). The parathyroid-vitamin D axis remains to be carefully evaluated in patients with AIDS.

Hypouricemia

Hypouricemia was observed in 22% of 96 consecutive patients with AIDS (17). It was associated with a high fractional excretion of uric acid even in volume depleted patients suggesting abnormal renal tubular handling of uric acid.

Thus, electrolyte disorders encountered in AIDS patients may be multiple and variable in their pathogenesis. Some may be the result of renal tubular functional defects while others may be the result of hormonal imbalances.

NEPHROPATHOLOGY IN PATIENTS WITH HIV-1 INFECTION

The nephropathology reported in patients with HIV-1 infection varies depending upon whether autopsy or biopsy specimens were examined (Table 2).

Table 2. Nephropathology in patients with HIV-1 infection.

	Autopsy	Biopsy	Unknown	Total
Acute tubular necrosis	21	-	-	21
Interstitial nephritis	33	3	1	37
Nephrocalcinosis	46	-	-	46
Minimal change	-	5	-	5
Mesangial hyperplasia	79	13	15	107
FSGS	57	138	32	227
Other glomerulonephritides	4	10	-	14

* Focal segmental glomerulosclerosis

In autopsy specimens, the renal lesions most commonly observed are acute tubular necrosis, interstitial nephritis, nephrocalcinosis, mesangial hyperplasia and focal and segmental glomerulosclerosis (FSGS) (5, 18-26). Renal invasion by a variety of pathogens (cytomegalovirus, candida, cryptococcus, pneumocystis, nocardia, mycobacterium) or neoplasms (carcinoma, lymphoma, Kaposi's sarcoma, multiple myeloma) has also been reported.

In contrast, in published series where the sampling process was not specified (27-30) or renal biopsies (18-20, 23-26, 31-39) were reviewed, the predominant histologic abnormalities involved the glomeruli. FSGS was present in 81% of these cases, mesangial hyperplasia in 8%, minimal change disease in 5% and other glomerulonephritides [including diabetic glomerulosclerosis, poststreptococcal glomerulonephritis (GN), membranous or proliferative GN] in 6%. This difference likely reflects the greater probability of biopsying patients with unexplained proteinuria.

Overall, FSGS accounted for 64% and mesangial hyperplasia for 30% of the glomerular pathology encountered in patients with HIV-1 infection. The other glomerulonephritides, including minimal change disease, may represent incidental findings. The greater frequency of mesangial hyperplasia at autopsy and of FSGS at biopsy stems from the fact that mesangial hyperplasia is rarely clinically expressed by more than modest proteinuria and is usually not associated with a progressive decline in renal function (40, 41). As this pathologic survey suggests, the nephrologic presentation of the patient with HIV-1 infection includes acute renal failure, progressive renal insufficiency and/or proteinuria.

ACUTE RENAL FAILURE (ARF)

All forms of ARF have been observed in patients with AIDS (Table 3). ARF is coincidental and related to the underlying complications of AIDS and/or associated with diagnostic or therapeutic interventions. Its clinical manifestations and course are similar to those observed in acutely ill patients who do not have AIDS.

Table 3. Causes of acute renal failure in patients with AIDS

1. Prerenal azotemia
2. Acute tubular necrosis
3. Acute interstitial nephritis
4. Renal interstitial edema
5. Systemic illnesses
6. Acute glomerulonephritis
7. Obstructive uropathy
8. Rapidly progressive FSGS

ARF (including prerenal azotemia) occurred in 55% of 449 AIDS patients admitted to Bellevue Hospital in New York (42). Causes: were volume depletion, 38%; pentamidine, 17%; amphotericin B, 11%; trimethoprim-sulfamethoxazole (TMP/sulfa), 9%; sepsis, 8%; radiocontrast, 4%; aminoglycoside antibiotics, 2%; others, 4%; and unknown, 7%.

Prerenal azotemia is the commonest cause of an increase in serum creatinine and is usually due to dehydration and intravascular volume depletion. If prolonged, however, it can lead to oligo-anuric renal failure with acute tubular necrosis.

ARF may develop in patients with massive proteinuria and severe hypoalbuminemia, presumably secondary to renal interstitial edema (43).

Systemic illnesses may cause ARF in patients with AIDS. There is one reported case of hemolytic uremic syndrome (44), and another of thrombotic thrombocytopenic purpura (43). Multiple myeloma with IgA kappa deposits has been reported (45). Immune complex glomerulonephritis secondary to infection and other acute glomerulonephritides can also be expected in this patient population.

Obstructive uropathy may lead to ARF in patients with AIDS in several clinical settings:

(i) Patients receiving sulfadiazine may develop crystalluria and acute urinary tract obstruction (46-47);

(ii) Patients with lymphoma and retroperitoneal fibrosis (48) or uretero-pelvic lymphomatous infiltration may develop obstructive uropathy. The latter may not be accompanied by hydronephrosis on ultrasonographic examination and may require retrograde urography for diagnosis;

(iii) Tumor chemotherapy in patients with AIDS-related lymphoma may lead to urinary outflow obstruction secondary to hyperuricosuria.

Finally, azotemia often may be the mode of presentation of patients with nephrotic syndrome and a rapidly progressive form of FSGS, characteristic of HIV-1 associated nephropathy (vide infra).

Nephrotoxic agents may be directly responsible for ARF or add insult to injury (Table 4).

Table 4. Commonly used nephrotoxic agents.

1. Radiocontrast dyes
2. NSAID's
3. Pentamidine
4. Sulfonamides
5. Other antibiotics
6. Antifungal agents
7. Antiviral drugs

Radiocontrast dyes and various antimicrobial agents used in AIDS patients can cause acute tubular necrosis or acute interstitial nephritis. Non-steroidal anti-inflammatory drugs (NSAID's) in the context of intravascular volume depletion may decrease glomerular filtration rate dramatically (43).

Pentamidine is nephrotoxic particularly when it induces hypoglycemia (49). Its dosage must be adjusted at creatinine clearance less than 35 ml/min (50, 51). The mechanism of pentamidine nephrotoxicity is not defined. One case report describes ARF resulting from myoglobinuria associated with pentamidine administration (52). TMP/sulfa may increase the serum concentration of creatinine by inhibiting the tubular secretion of creatinine or it may induce severe ARF as a result of acute interstitial nephritis with eosinophiluria. Overall, TMP/sulfa appears to be less nephrotoxic than pentamidine (53, 54). The potential nephrotoxicity of various antibiotics, such as penicillins, cephalosporins, aminoglycosides or antituberculous agents must be closely monitored when treating patients with AIDS exposed to other nephrotoxic events or with preexisting renal insufficiency.

The development of renal insufficiency is anticipated with the use of amphotericin B. It may also cause distal renal tubular acidosis, hypokalemia and nephrocalcinosis. Ketoconazole, another antifungal drug, has no known nephrotoxicity. Foscarnet, a new antiviral agent, may induce ARF (55). While acyclovir and gancyclovir may increase serum creatinine, azidothymidine is not directly nephrotoxic. The prolonged use of azidothymidine, however, may lead to rhabdomyolysis (M. Fischl, personal communication), but ARF has not been reported. Dosage adjustments of these various drugs are recommended for patients with decreased renal function (56).

In most patients, ARF is mild and may be self-limited if the nephrotoxic agent is identified and discontinued. Unless ARF is a terminal event associated with overwhelming infections, respiratory or other organ system failure, recovery of renal function should be expected in patients with AIDS. Supportive dialytic therapy may be temporarily needed before renal function recovers (20, 57).

HIV-ASSOCIATED NEPHROPATHY (HIVN)

The definition of HIVN has been limited to patients with heavy proteinuria (>2 g/24 hr), or the nephrotic syndrome. Patients with HIV-1 infection, modest proteinuria (<2 g/24 hr), and normal or minimally decreased renal function may represent an early stage of the nephropathy. Thus, HIVN is a non-specific glomerulopathy and tubulopathy with a spectrum of clinical manifestations ranging from modest proteinuria with normal or minimally decreased renal function to a full blown nephrotic syndrome with chronic renal insufficiency or failure.

HIVN is not confined to terminally ill patients with AIDS. Indeed, 42 to 85% of patients with HIVN may be otherwise asymptomatic HIV-1 carriers or patients with ARC (33, 57-60). Thus, the nephropathy may develop in early stages of HIV-1 infection and is, therefore, HIV- rather than AIDS-associated.

Clinical Spectrum

The incidence of HIVN (i.e., proteinuria > 2 gm/24 hr and/or FSGS) has been estimated at 6 to 10% of the general patient population with AIDS (20, 25, 57, 61). Modest proteinuria, however, may be one of the first manifestations of HIVN and is of much greater prevalence than indicated above. In a prospective evaluation of 75 consecutive outpatients with AIDS, 32 (43%) excreted more than 0.5 g of protein per 24 hr and 76 (9%) had proteinuria in excess of 3 g/24 hr (62).

Patients with HIVN may present several ways. In our first 100 consultations on patients with HIV-1 infection, we found patients with: (A) Modest proteinuria (27%) and normal or slightly increased serum concentration of creatinine; (B) Nephrotic syndrome (52%) usually with increased serum creatinine concentration; (C) Azotemia (67%); (D) Macroscopic hematuria (3%) associated with renal tuberculosis or glomerular disease (57). These observations have generally been confirmed (20, 32, 33, 59, 61, 63) with the exception of medical centers where white homosexuals are the predominant population with HIV-1 infection (26).

HIVN was initially described in clusters of blacks in New York and in Miami (18, 61, 62, 64). Most reported patients originate from large metropolitan areas in the eastern United States, including New York (18, 20, 32, 59-61), Boston (38), Newark (28), Washington DC (30) and Miami (25, 57). Additional patients were identified from other cities such as Cincinnati (65), San Francisco (26), Los Angeles (37), Detroit (19), Dallas (5) or other countries like Canada (27), Senegal (36), Haiti, the West Indies (31, 34), Trinidad (35), Mexico (22) and Brazil (21). Only one patient reported in the literature is from Africa (36). In the United States, most patients with AIDS are white; nevertheless, most patients with HIVN are black. Although there is a 3 to 1 ratio in the numbers of white vs black patients with AIDS in the United States, the ratio of whites vs blacks reported with HIVN is 1 to 10 (66). The reason for this racial predilection is unknown.

All groups at risk may be affected. The prevalence of HIVN, however, is distinctively lower in white homosexuals than in other groups at risk (57), which probably explains the low incidence of HIVN reported from some areas of the United States and from Europe.

Table 5. Race in HIV-1 Patients with FSGS.

I.v. drug use	Black	White
Present	107	12
Excluded	76	7

It has been argued that the abuse of intravenous (i.v.) drugs is a major etiological factor in the development of HIVN (67). It is clear, however, that HIVN need not be related to i.v. drug use: (i) In large series reported, i.v. drug use was not a risk factor for the majority of patients; (ii) The occurrence of HIVN in children with perinatal AIDS strongly argues against i.v. drug use as a necessary risk factor (25, 27-29); (iii) Even after exclusion of i.v. drug users, a 10 to 1 ratio of HIVN in blacks vs whites remains among published cases (66) (Table 5).

Evidence of peripheral edema may be conspicuously absent in AIDS patients with nephrotic range proteinuria, and hypoalbuminemia (33, 41, 46, 61). Dehydration and low blood pressure as a result of constitutional symptoms, chronic diarrhea, and/or malnutrition/malabsorption may result in intravascular volume depletion and may prevent accumulation of fluid in interstitial tissue. Proteinuria or the nephrotic syndrome, in a patient at risk should alert the physician to the possibility of underlying HIVN (41). Hypertension also is often absent even in patients with advanced uremia (19, 33, 57, 59, 61, 63).

The diagnosis of HIVN relies on a high degree of clinical suspicion, evaluation of possible risk factor(s), negative assessment of other causes of proteinuria and/or renal insufficiency, confirmation of HIV-1 infection and, ultimately, renal biopsy. Ultrasonographic examination of the kidneys is useful in the differential diagnosis. Typically, the echogenicity of HIVN kidneys exceeds that of the liver. The increased echogenicity has been correlated with the increased nephrocalcinosis (68) and/or tubular abnormalities (69) present HIVN. Kidneys with HIVN are normal-sized or frankly enlarged, a useful finding for differential diagnosis (40, 70). Renal size did not correlate with the degree of proteinuria (57).

In most patients with nephrotic range proteinuria, the clinical course of HIVN is one of rapid progression towards end stage renal disease, within weeks to months (20, 32, 33, 57, 59). Rapid progression of renal disease, however, is not a universal finding (26, 62).

Pathology of HIVN

The pathology of HIVN is glomerular and tubulo-interstitial. The typical glomerular lesion of HIVN is FSGS. It is unclear, however, whether FSGS develops *de novo* or whether it may be preceded by another stage of lesser glomerular involvement such as mesangial hyperplasia or minimal change disease. This possibility is suggested by the inordinately high frequency with which mesangial hyperplasia is observed in AIDS patients (Table 2). Thus, one may envision the sequence of renal manifestations of HIVN to include patients with modest proteinuria, normal-sized kidneys and mesangial hyperplasia evolving ultimately into a nephrotic syndrome, typically rapidly progressive toward irreversible renal failure, with enlarged kidneys and FSGS.

In support of this hypothesis, we have observed one patient in whom initially diffuse mesangial hyperplasia on renal biopsy progressed to FSGS at autopsy (23). This two-tiered clinicopathologic separation is not absolute. A continuum of lesions may be present in different segments of the kidney. Patients with nephrotic proteinuria, particularly children (25, 28, 29), may exhibit only mesangial hyperplasia at autopsy. Conversely, FSGS has been found in biopsies or autopsies of patients with only modest proteinuria and normal renal function (22). Finally, macaques inoculated with simian immunodeficiency virus develop with equal frequency glomerular mesangial hyperplasia or a sclerosing glomerulopathy (71).

There is a consensus among nephropathologists on the occurrence of FSGS in AIDS patients with HIV-1 infection. On the other hand, the occurrence of mesangial hyperplasia has been variably reported. Diffuse mesangial hyperplasia, defined by an increase in cells represented by more than 3 nuclei in mesangial stalks of more than 50% of glomeruli, was originally described by Pardo et al (62). This observation has been confirmed by others in adults (5, 18, 20-22, 40) and in children (25, 28, 29). In contrast, mesangial hyperplasia is not a feature of HIV-1 infection in adults for some nephropathologists (24, 37, 60). Rather, Chander et al (60) describe the glomerular mesangium as hypocellular in adults with HIV-1 infection. Such finding may represent a later stage of the nephropathy.

Minimal change disease has also been associated with HIV-1 infection (24, 25, 31). As indicated in Table 2, these instances are rare and may be coincidental although progression from minimal change to FSGS in the same patient has been reported (24). The pathogenesis and the link between minimal change disease or mesangial hyperplasia and FSGS in HIV-1 infection must await further observations.

The characteristic features of FSGS in HIVN are qualitatively similar to those observed in other forms of FSGS including the idiopathic variety and that associated with heroin abuse. Quantitatively, however, FSGS in HIVN appears histologically much more aggressive and virulent in its glomerular and tubulo-interstitial manifestations (23, 24, 37, 60). At autopsy, kidneys from patients with HIV-1 infection are usually enlarged, weighing 50 to 100 % more than normal kidneys or kidneys with mesangial hyperplasia (40).

Lesions of variable severity can be identified by light microscopy in the same biopsy. Early, diffuse mesangial hyperplasia predominates with minor changes of FSGS (40). As indicated above, this is not a universal observation (24, 39, 60). The interstitium usually exhibits an obvious infiltrate of lymphocytes and plasmocytes (24, 40). In established lesions, the visceral epithelial glomerular cells appear hyperplastic and hypertrophic, and contain conspicuous vacuoles of protein droplets (24, 37, 40, 60). Capillary lumina in affected areas are narrowed by "foam cells" with (37) or without (24) segmental increase in mesangial matrix. In advanced lesions, the glomerular capillary obliteration is diffuse and global. Glomeruli are "collapsed", reduced to stumps crowned by a row of hypertrophic visceral epithelial cells (24, 37, 40, 60). Bowman's space frequently appears dilated and filled with proteinaceous material (24, 37, 40, 60) (Figure 1). The infiltrate may now be scanty in an interstitium that frequently appears edematous and replaced by a homogenous acidophilic substance (40, 60). Tubulo-interstitial changes are uniformly prominent. Focal tubular degenerative changes or necrosis at various stages of evolution may be seen in the absence of identifiable nephrotoxic or hemodynamic insult. Epithelial cells may be flattened, "simplified" with loss of nuclei and brush border (24, 37, 60). Tubules are often markedly dilated or microcystic filled with giant variegated casts (24, 37, 40, 60) (Figure 1).

By immunofluorescence, deposits of IgM and C_3 (24, 37, 40, 60) and C_1 (24, 37) are identified in the mesangium and peripheral capillary wall. The same deposits can be identified in HIV-1 patients with normal glomeruli on light microscopic examination (40, 62). Visceral epithelial cells stain for immunoglobulin, and/or albumin in areas corresponding to the intracellular droplets identified by light microscopy (24, 37). The large tubular casts have not been reported in urinary sediment. They may be occlusive and responsible for kidney enlargement. They contain immunoglobulins, light chain protein, albumin and fibrin but not Tamm-Horsfall protein (37).

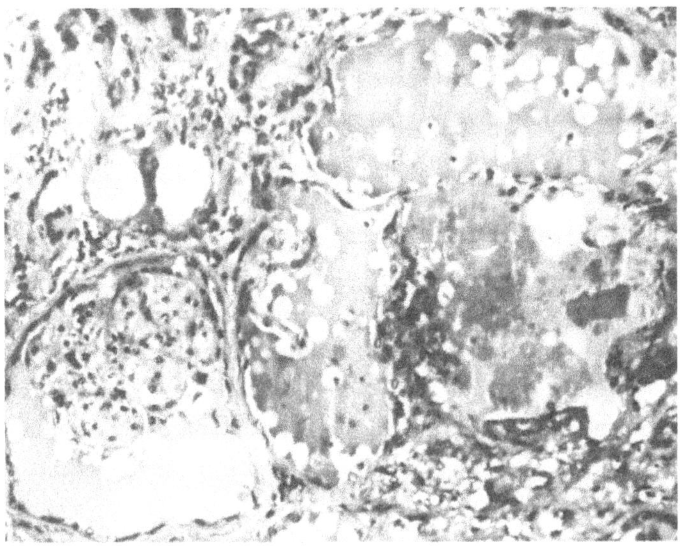

Figure 1. Advanced lesion of HIVN. The glomerulus shows global sclerosis and collapse associated with dilatation of Bowman's space. Microcystic tubules filled with variegated casts are prominent (reprinted with permission from Kidney Int, 31: 1167-1173, 1987).

Ultrastructural changes in HIVN include pronounced foot process effacement (24, 37, 60), wrinkling and folding of the glomerular basement membrane, collapsed glomerular segments and dense deposits in the mesangium (24, 37, 40, 60) and, more rarely, in subendothelial and/or subepithelial areas (24). Numerous tubulo-reticular inclusions involving the glomerular endothelium and interstitial leukocytes are found (24, 37-39, 60, 71), as well as nuclear bodies and granular degeneration of tubular and interstitial cell nuclear chromatin (24, 60). Specific HIV-1 particles or virions have not been identified in kidneys of HIV-1 patients.

None of the above renal manifestations is specific for HIVN. Their combined presence, however, is highly characteristic (24, 37, 40, 60). We have been impressed by our nephropathologist's ability to make a presumptive diagnosis of HIV-1 infection which proved ultimately correct in patients not suspected of having retroviral infection. The same experience has appeared in the literature (37).

Several studies have compared the FSGS of HIVN with that of heroin-associated nephropathy (24, 37, 60, 71). The consensus is that distinctive pathologic features of HIVN include: (A) The "collapsing" and predominantly global pattern of glomerular sclerosis; (B) The severity of visceral epithelial cell hypertrophy and droplet formation; (C) The prominent tubular microcysts and focal tubular degenerative features; (D) The numerous tubulo-reticular inclusions in renal endothelium and infiltrating leukocytes. This ultrastructural marker of HIVN can be seen before the development of AIDS (24, 72) as well as in HIV-1 infected patients without HIVN. Tubulo-reticular inclusions, therefore, are a general feature of HIV-1 infection and are not specific for HIVN per se (24); (E) An increased number of type III (24, 60) and type V (39) nuclear bodies and an increased fibrillo-glomerular transformation of the nuclear chromatin in tubulo-interstitial cells (39, 60) are characteristic for some but not other (37, 72) nephropathologists.

Treatment of HIVN

There is no effective therapy for FSGS in general or for HIVN. Several patients with nephrotic syndrome, particularly children, were administered corticosteroids without success (25). Azidothymidine has not been tried prospectively in patients with HIVN. In our experience, however, its administration to patients with Pneumocystis carinii did not prevent the subsequent development of HIVN in some of those patients.

Supportive dialytic therapy has been applied to patients with HIVN and renal failure. As indicated previously, temporary hemodialysis may permit patient survival and recovery of renal function in the setting of acute renal failure (20, 57). In patients with irreversible renal failure, chronic hemodialysis provides long-term survival of HIV-1 carriers and patients with AIDS-related complex (73). In contrast, chronic hemodialysis does not rehabilitate the patient with AIDS. In general, once AIDS is diagnosed, survival despite hemodialysis is dismal, rarely exceeding one month despite the continuation of hemodialysis (20, 43, 73).

REFERENCES

1. Mann JM, Chin J: AIDS: A global perspective. N Eng J Med, 319: 302-303, 1988
2. Vaziri ND, Barbari A, Licorish K, Cesario T, Gupta S: Spectrum of renal abnormalities in acquired immune-deficiency syndrome. J Nat Med Ass, 77: 369-375, 1985
3. Tang WW, Feinstein EI, Massry SG: Hyponatremia in patients with acquired immune deficiency syndrome and the AIDS related complex. Kidney Int, 33: 211, 1988

4. Cusano AJ, Siegal FP, Maesaka JK: Hyponatremia in AIDS and ARC. Kidney Int, 35: 208, 1989
5. Seney FD Jr, Burns DK, Silva FG, Baker B: Renal and electrolyte disorders in 50 patients with AIDS in Dallas. Kidney Int, 35: 212, 1989
5a. Maesaka JK, Cusano AJ, Siegal FP, Thies HL: Renal salt wasting in AIDS. Kidney Int, 35: 217, 1989
6. Vitting KE, Gardenswartz MH, Zabetakis PM, Tapper ML, Gleim GW, Agarwal MK, Robinson AG, Michelis MF: Frequency of hyponatremia (HN) hypoadrenalism, and nonosmolar vasopressin release in the acquired immunodeficiency syndrome. Kidney Int, 31: 221, 1987
7. Tapper ML, Rotterdam HZ, Lerner CW, Al'Khafaji J, Seitzman PA: Adrenal necrosis in the acquired immunodeficiency syndrome. Ann Intern Med, 100: 239-241, 1984
8. Greene LW, Cole W, Greene JB, Levy B, Louie E, Raphael B, Waitkevicz HJ, Blum M: Adrenal insufficiency as a complication of the acquired immunodeficiency syndrome. Ann Intern Med, 101: 497-498, 1984
9. Guenthner EE, Rabinowe SL, Van Niel A, Naftilan A, Dluhy RG: Primary Addison's disease in a patient with the acquired immunodeficiency syndrome. Ann Intern Med, 100: 847-848, 1984.
10. Membreno L, Irony I, Dere W, Klein R, Biglieri EG, Cobb E: Adrenocortical function in acquired immunodeficiency syndrome. J Clin Endocrinol Metab, 65: 482-487, 1987
11. Biglieri EG: Adrenocortical function in the acquired immunodeficiency syndrome (AIDS). West J Med, 148: 70-73, 1988
12. Somino N: The use of ketoconazole as an inhibitor of steroid production. N Eng J Med, 317: 812-818, 1987
13. Kalin ME, Poretsky L, Seras DS, Zumoff B: Hyporeninemic hypoaldosteronism associated with the acquired immune deficiency syndrome. Am J Med, 82: 1035-1038, 1987
14. Zikos D, Bloch RD, Cheng JC, Skopicki HA, Peterson DR, Fisher KA: AIDS-related hypercalcemic crisis: A potential mechanism. Kidney Int, 35: 388, 1989
15. Jacobs MB: The acquired immunodeficiency syndrome and hypercalcemia. Western J Med, 144: 469-471, 1986
16. Zaloga GP, Chernow B, Eil C: Hypercalcemia and disseminated cytomegalovirus infection in the acquired immunodeficiency syndrome. Ann Intern Med, 102: 331-333, 1985
17. Cusano AJ, Thies HL, Siegal FP, Maesaka JK: Hypouricemia (HU) in AIDS. Kidney Int, 35: 208, 1989
18. Gardenswartz MH, Lerner CW, Seligson GR, Zabetakis PM, Rotterdam H, Tapper ML, Michelis MF, Bruno MS: Renal disease in patients with AIDS: A clinicopathologic study. Clin Nephrol, 21: 197-204, 1984
19. Provenzano R, Kupin W, Santiage GC: Renal involvement in the acquired immunodeficiency syndrome: Presentation, clinical course and therapy. Henry Ford Med J, 35: 38-41, 1987
20. Rao TK, Friedman EA, Nicastri AD: The types of renal disease in the acquired immunodeficiency syndrome. N Eng J Med, 316: 1062-1068, 1987
21. Santos OR, Lopes GS, Vieira LMSF, Oliviera CA, Gonzaga B, Bonecker CW: Acquired immunodeficiency syndrome associated nephropathy. 10th Int Cong Nephrology, London, 1987, p 91
22. Heredia JB, Angeles AA, Gutierrez ER, Correa-Rotter R, Saldiyar S, Pena JC: Nephropatia associada al sindrome di immunodeficiencia acquirida. Rev Invest Clin, 39: 105-115, 1987
23. Pardo V, Bell M, Ortiz C, Strauss J, Bourgoignie JJ: The spectrum of glomerular lesions in patients with HIV infection. Fed Proc, 3: A1281,1989
24. D'Agati V, Cheng JI, Carbone L, Cheng JT, Appel G: The pathology of HIV-Nephropathy: A detailed morphologic and comparative study. Kidney Int (in press).
25. Strauss J, Pardo V, Scott G, Zilleruelo G, Abitbol C, Paredes A, Parks W, Mitchell C: A spectrum of histological changes in children with ARC/AIDS and nephrotic syndrome. Kidney Int, 33: 210, 1988
26. Mazbar SA, Schoenfeld PY, Humphreys MH: Renal involvement in patients infected with HIV: Experience at San Francisco General Hospital (Personal communication).
27. Rousseau E, Russo P, Lapointe N, O'Regan S: Renal complications of acquired immunodeficiency syndrome in children, Am J Kidney Dis, 11: 48-50, 1988
28. Connor E, Gupta S, Joshi V, Di Carlo F, Offenberger J, Minnefor A, Uy C, Oleske J, Ende N: Acquired immunodeficiency syndrome-associated renal disease in children. J Pediatrics, 113: 39-44, 1988
29. Chander P, Sagel I, Weiss R, Pimentel C, Gupta A, Bamji M, Treser G: Renal disease in human immunodeficiency virus infected children. Kidney Int, 35: 368, 1989

30. Cantor ES, Kimmel PL, Bosch JP: Impact of race on renal disease in patients with AIDS. Kidney Int, 35: 222, 1989
31. Singer DR, Jenkins AP, Gupta S, Evans DJ: Minimal change nephropathy in the acquired immune deficiency syndrome. Br Med J, 291: 868, 1985
32. Kaplan MS, Wechsler M, Benson MC: Urologic manifestations of AIDS. Urology, 30: 441-443, 1987
33. Langs, C, Gallo GR, Schacht RG, Baldwin DF: Rapid renal failure in AIDS nephropathy. Kidney Int, 33: 198, 1988
34. Dosquet P, Haddoum F, Viron B, Mougenot B, Mayaud C, Ronco P, Mignon F: Focal and segmental glomerulosclerosis (FSG) during acquired immunodeficiency syndrome (AIDS): Two observations. Kidney Int, 33: 1041-1042, 1988
35. Patrick AL, Roberts LA, Burton EN, Jankey N, Shah DH: Focal and segmental glomerulosclerosis in the acquired immunodeficiency syndrome. W I Med J, 35: 200-202, 1986
36. Hory B, Bresson C, Lorge JF, Perol C: Associated focal and segmental glomerulosclerosis in the acquired immunodeficiency syndrome. Am J Kidney Dis, 12: 169, 1988
37. Cohen AH, Nast CC: HIV-associated nephropathy: A unique combined glomerular, tubular and interstitial lesion. Mod Pathol, 1: 87-97, 1988
38. Alpers CE, Harawi S, Rennke HG: Focal glomerulosclerosis with tubuloreticular inclusions: Possible predictive value for acquired immunodeficiency syndrome (AIDS). Am J Kidney Dis, 12: 240-242, 1988
39. Chander P, Agarwal A, Soni A, Kim K, Treser G: Renal cytomembranous inclusions in idiopathic renal disease as predictive markers for the acquired immunodeficiency syndrome. Hum Pathol, 19: 1060-1064, 1988
40. Pardo V, Meneses R, Ossa L, Jaffe DJ, Strauss J, Roth D, Bourgoignie JJ: AIDS-related glomerulopathy: Occurrence in specific risk groups. Kidney Int, 31: 1167-1173, 1987.
41. Bourgoignie JJ, Meneses R, Pardo V: The nephropathy related to acquired immune deficiency syndrome. Adv Nephrol, 17: 113-126, 1988
42. Valeri AM, Neusy AJ: Acute renal failure in AIDS patients. Kidney Int, 35: 235, 1989
43. Rao TKS: Renal complications in patients with AIDS. Kidney failure is potentially manageable and reversible. J Crit Illness, 3: 55-74, 1988
44. Boccia RV, Gelmann EP, Baker CC, Marti G, Longo DL: A hemolytic-uremic syndrome with the acquired immunodeficiency syndrome. Ann Intern Med, 101: 716-717, 1984
45. Thomas MA, Ibels LS, Wells JV, Isbister JP, Cooper DA, McMahon C: IgA kappa multiple myeloma and lymphadenopathy syndrome associated with AIDS virus infection. Aust NZ J Med, 16: 402-404, ç 1986
46. Carbone LG, Bendixen B, Appel GB: Sulfadiazine-associated obstructive nephropathy occurring in a patient with the acquired immunodeficiency syndrome. Am J Kidney Dis, 12: 72-75,1988
47. Goadsby, PJ, Donaghy AJ, Lloyd AR, Wakefield D: Acquired immunodeficiency syndrome (AIDS) and sulfadiazine-associated acute renal failure. Ann Intern Med, 107: 783-784, 1987
48. Mohler JL, Jarow JP, Marshall FF: Unusual urological presentations of acquired immune deficiency syndrome: Large cell lymphoma. J Urol, 138: 627-629, 1987
49. Stahl-Bayliss CM, Kalman CM, Laskin OL: Pentamidine-induced hypoglycemia in patients with the acquired immune deficiency syndrome. Clin J Pharm Ther, 39: 271-275, 1986
50. Andersen R, Boedicker M, Ma M, Goldstein EJ: Adverse †reactions associated with pentamidine isethionate in AIDS patients: Recommendations for monitoring therapy. Drug Intell Clin Pharm, 20: 862-868, 1986
51. Conte JE Jr, Upton RA, Lin ET: Pentamidine pharmacokinetics in patients with AIDS with impaired renal function. J Infect Dis, 156: 885-890, 1987
52. Sensakovic JW, Suarez M, Perez G, Johnson ES, Smith LG: Pentamidine treatment of Pneumocystis carinii pneumonia in the acquired immunodeficiency syndrome. Association with acute renal failure and myoglobinuria. Arch Intern Med, 145: 2247, 1985
53. Gordin FM, Simon GL, Wofsky CB, Mills J: Adverse reactions to trimethoprim-sulfamethoxazole in patients with the acquired immunodeficiency syndrome. Ann Intern Med, 100: 495-499, 1985
54. Sattler FR, Cowan R, Nielsen DM, Ruskin J: Trimethoprim-sulfamethoxazole compared with pentamidine for treatment of Pneumocystis carinii pneumonia in the acquired immunodeficiency syndrome. A prospective noncrossover study. Ann Intern Med, 109: 208-287, 1988

55. Cacoub O, Deray G, Baumelou A, Le Hoang P, Rozenbaum W, Gentilini M, Soubrie C, Rousselie R, Jacobs C: Acute †renal failure induced by foscarnet: 4 cases. Clin Nephrol, 29: 315-318, 1988
56. Van Scoy RE, Wilson WR: Antimicrobial agents in adult patients with renal insufficiency: Initial dosage and general recommendations. Mayo Clin Proc, 62: 1142-1145, 1987
57. Bourgoignie JJ, Meneses R, Ortiz C, Jaffe D, Pardo V: The clinical spectrum of renal disease associated with human immunodeficiency virus. Am J Kidney Dis, 12: 131-137, 1988
58. Rao TKS, Mallis LR, Friedman EA: Nephropathy as the initial manifestation of human immunodeficiency virus disease. Kidney Int, 33: 205, 1988
59. Carbone L, D'Agati V, Cheng JT, Appel GB: The course and prognosis of HIV-associated nephropathy. Am J Med (in press)
60. Chander P, Soni A, Suri A, Bhagwat R, Yoo K, Treser G: Renal ultrastructural markers in AIDS-associated nephropathy. Am J Pathol, 126: 513-526, 1987
61. Valeri AM, Neusy AJ: Clinical features of AIDS-associated nephropathy. Kidney Int, 35: 234, 1989
62. Pardo V, Aldana M, Colton RM, Fischl MA, Jaffe D, Moskowitz L, Hensley GT, Bourgoignie JJ: Glomerular lesions in the acquired immunodeficiency syndrome. Ann Intern Med, 101: 429-434, 1984
63. Soni A, Agarwal A, Chander P, Treser G: Evidence for an HIV-related nephropathy: A clinicopathological study. Kidney Int, 35: 213, 1989
64. Rao TK, Filippone EJ, Nicastri AD, Landesman SH, Frean E, Chen CK, Friedman EA: Associated focal and segmental glomerulosclerosis in the acquired immunodeficiency syndrome. N Eng J Med, 310: 669-673, 1984
65. Weiss MA, Daquioag E, Margolin EG, Pollak VE: Nephrotic syndrome, progressive irreversible renal failure, and glomerular "collapse": A new clinicopathologic entity? Am J Kidney Dis, 7: 20-28, 1986
66. Bourgoignie JJ, Ortiz-Interian C, Green DF, Roth D: Race, a co-factor in HIV-1 associated nephropathy. Transpl Proc (in press)
67. Humphreys MH, Schoenfeld PY: Renal complications in patient with the acquired immune deficiency syndrome. Am J Nephrol, 7: 1-7, 1988
68. Falkoff GE, Rigsby CM, Rosenfield AT: Partial, combined cortical and medullary nephrocalcinosis: US and CT patterns in AIDS-associated MAI infection. Radiology, 162: 343-344, 1987
69. Hamper UM, Goldblum LE, Hutchins GM, Sheth S, Dahnert WF, Bartlett JG, Sanders RC: Renal involvement in AIDS: Sonographic-pathologic correlation. Am J Roentg, 150: 1321-1325, 1988
70. Schaffer RM, Schwartz GE, Becker JA, Rao TK, Shih YH: Renal ultrasound in acquired immune deficiency syndrome. Radiology, 153: 511-513, 1984
71. Alpers CE, Baskin GB: Sclerosing glomerulopathy in rhesus monkeys with simian AIDS. Kidney Int, 35: 339, 1989
72. Pardo V, Ortiz C, Strauss J, Bourgoignie JJ: Histologic and ultrastructural specificity of HIV-associated focal and segmental sclerosis (FSS). Kidney Int, 33: 330, 1988
73. Ortiz Meneses R, Jaffe D, Fernandez JA, Perez G, Bourgoignie J: Outcome of patients with human immunodeficiency virus on maintenance hemodialysis. Kidney Int, 34: 248-254, 1988

RENAL STONE DISEASE

6

THE TREATMENT OF RENAL STONES BY LITHOTRIPSY: INDICATIONS, LIMITS, RESULTS, COMPLICATIONS

MALACHY J. GLEESON AND DONALD P. GRIFFITH

Scott Department of Urology, Baylor College of Medicine, Houston, Texas 77030, USA

Extracorporeal shockwave lithotripsy (ESWL) was introduced clinically in 1980, eight years after renal calculi were successfully destroyed *in vitro* using shock waves (1, 2). To date, more than 500,000 patients have been treated worldwide and ESWL, either alone or in conjunction with percutaneous nephrolithotomy (PCNL), has replaced open surgery as the ideal mode of treatment for the vast majority of symptomatic renal calculi. Herein, we have reviewed the treatment results, the complications and the limits of ESWL therapy with the Dornier HM3 lithotriptor. This task is complicated by the lack of uniformity between different published series and the absence of substratification of patient populations with regards to stone site, size and multiplicity. We have also briefly outlined the characteristics of the various "second generation lithotriptors" which are available worldwide.

TREATMENT INDICATION

The indications for treating renal calculi are (a) pain, (b) hematuria, (c) infection, (d) obstruction and (e) increasing stone size.

The morbidity associated with ESWL is perceived to be less than with open surgery, but should not act as a stimulus to treat all asymptomatic renal calculi.

TREATMENT RESULTS

In 1984, Chaussy and Schmiedt reported that 90% of their first 896 patients with renal calculi became stone free (3). However, most published series have now reported that 72% to 74% of their patients become stone-free (4-6). Unfortunately, in an effort to reproduce Chaussy's results, many papers in the urological literature started citing their "successful" treatment rates which included kidneys which became stone-free or contained "clinically insignificant fragments", less than 5 mm in size (7, 8). Prior to the era of ESWL, conservative management of patients with renal colic showed that ureteric calculi <4 mm in diameter passed spontaneously in 80% of cases compared to one-quarter of calculi 5-8 mm in size (9, 10). Larger calculi rarely passed spontaneously. However, although it may have seemed reasonable to expect that these small fragments would pass spontaneously after ESWL, this does not invariably occur (5). Most residual calculi remain in the dependent part of the renal collecting system (lower calyces) which may be partly due to the diminished urinary flow there which Schulz et al have demonstrated *in vitro* and in patients with calcium oxalate urolithiasis (11). Each series consists of a heterogeneous collection of calculi which make accurate prediction of a true stone-free outcome difficult. In an effort to substratify stone populations, Griffith and Valiquette proposed the PICA/Burden staging system, which stratifies upper urinary tract stones by their complexity, location and burden (the sum of the longest axial diameter of all stones) (12).

Table 1 Percentage of kidneys with solitary calculi rendered stone-free three months after ESWL.

	Site	Original Stone Burden		
Baylor College of Medicine, Houston (4)		≤15mm	16-29mm	≥30mm
	Pelvis	87	72	70
	Upper calix	88	64	83
	Middle calix	73	70	-
	Lower calix	69	64	33
Methodist Hospital, Indianapolis (13)		0-10mm	11-20mm	21-30mm
	Pelvis	90	83	81
	Upper calix	77	75	67
	Middle calix	80	71	50
	Lower calix	80	58	32
American Study Group (14)			All Burdens	
	Pelvis		83.8	
	Upper calix		64.1	
	Middle calix		75.7	
	Lower calix		71.1	
University of Bochum, Herne (5)*			All Burdens	
	Pelvis		83.8	
	Upper calix		78.6	
	Middle calix		75.5	
	Lower calix		57.8	

* % stone-free at 19 months

This staging system has aided interpretation of some of the many factors which influence the treatment outcome. A stone-free outcome is dependent on stone site, size, multiplicity, and composition, as well as the presence or absence of obstruction or renal anomalies.

For descriptive purposes, treatment results will be discussed separately for solitary, multiple and staghorn calculi.

The stone-free results of solitary calculi treated at Baylor College of Medicine, Houston, USA, are outlined in Table 1 and compared to those from other institutions who have attempted to substratify their stone populations.

The general trend is that better stone-free results are achieved with smaller calculi and with those calculi which are situated in the renal pelvis or upper calyx. Sofras et al also reported decreasing stone-free rates when larger stone burdens were treated but did not substratify their calculi according to site (15).

The stone-free results of multiple calculi are outlined in Table 2.

As with solitary calculi, the stone-free rates decrease as the stone burdens increase. The stone-free rates also decrease as the actual number of calculi increase.

Table 2. Percentage stone-free rates of multiple calculi three months post-ESWL.

	Site	Original Stone Burden		
Baylor College of Medicine, Houston (16)		≤15mm	16-29mm	≥30mm
	Pelvic	100	75	25
	Calyceal	67	45	35
	Infundibular	-	-	35
	Pelvic+calyceal	81	61	51
	Pelvic+infundibular	-	50	39
	Calyceal+infundibular	-	0	26
	Pelvic+calyceal+ infundibular	-	-	38
Methodist Hospital, Indianapolis (13)		Number of Calculi		All Burdens
		2		60
		3		45
		4		33
American Study Group (14)		2		54
		3		49.3
		4		29

The treatment of patients with staghorn calculi attempts to render them stone-free in an effort to prevent stone recurrence and associated urinary tract infections. Nonoperative management was reported in 1976 to result in a 28% mortality during 20 years of follow-up with all survivors having persistent pain and urinary tract infections (17). The incidence of residual calculi following a variety of open surgical procedures has ranged from 0% to 29% (18, 19).

Percutaneous nephrostolithotomy (PCNL) was described in 1976 by Fernstrom and Johansson and had largely replaced open surgery as the treatment of choice for most staghorn calculi by 1985 (20).

Table 3. Treatment results of staghorn calculi.

Procedure	Authors	Kidneys	Treatments per Kidney	Average Hospitalization Days	Stone-Free at 3 Months
PCNL					
	Adams et al (21)	11	2.2	18	63%
	Kerlan et al (22)	20	1.8		90%
	Young et al (23)	25	2.9	10.3[a]	68%
	Snyder and Smith (18)	75	1.24	13.3	85%
	Lee et al (24)	124	1.3	12.5	85%
	Eisenberger et al (25)	42	1.3	13	69%
	Gleeson et al (26)	30	1.43		60%
ESWL					
	Eisenberger et al (25)	31	1.5	11	50%[b]
	Rocco et al (27)	84	1.5		63%[c]
	Wirth and Frohmuller (28)	174			54%
	Harada et al (29)	47			51%
	Sohn et al (30)	20			30%
	Pode et al (31)	41	2.6	20	44%
	Gleeson et al (26)	18	1.28		66%
PCNL-ESWL					
	Eisenberger et al (25)	78	2.7	20	60%
	Kahnoski et al (32)	36	2.6[d]	14.2	85%[d]
	Segura et al (33)	16			23%[e]
	Lingeman (34)	313			91%-92%
	Schulze et al (35)	87[f]	2.8	19	58%
	Gleeson et al (26)	23	2.44	10.3	52%

[a] Hospitalization time after first procedure.
[b] Stone-free rate after 18 months.
[c] Rocco EXL catheter used in 20 cases.
[d] Includes cases treated with ESWL and PCNL monotherapy.
[e] Six months follow-up.
[f] 77 calculi were partial or complete staghorns.

Since its clinical introduction, ESWL has also been used to treat staghorn calculi both as monotherapy and in combination with PCNL. The results of PCNL monotherapy, ESWL monotherapy and combination PCNL-ESWL therapy for staghorn calculi are outlined in Table 3.

Interpretation of published world data is complicated by varying definitions of staghorn calculi and the fact that all renal collecting systems are different.

The stone-free results of PCNL monotherapy are 60%-90% which compares favorably with those of open surgery. Moreover, comparative studies have shown that PCNL is less expensive, is associated with a smaller need for blood transfusion, requires a shorter hospital stay and allows a more rapid return to work than open surgery (9, 18). The cost of ESWL and PCNL are comparable (36).

ESWL monotherapy has generally resulted in lower stone-free results, ranging from 30% to 66%. Many series preselected these staghorn patients on the basis of lack of associated hydronephrosis and relative radiolucency of calculi so that the results may be higher than in non-selected patients (26). In spite of this, stone-free results are less than those achieved with PCNL monotherapy.

Combination PCNL-ESWL therapy has reportedly resulted in stone-free rates of between 23% and 92%. The excellent results achieved in Indianapolis are the result of repeated PCNL and ESWL procedures during one long hospital stay which are supplemented by flexible PCNL with lavage of residual debris (34). The stone-free rate with struvite staghorn calculi from the Mayo Clinic was significantly less than their PCNL monotherapy stone-free results. This drop in stone-free efficacy was attributed to a less aggressive effort at initial PCNL when follow-up ESWL was planned (33).

In conjunction with the previously cited factors (stone size, site and multiplicity), the presence of hydronephrosis or renal anomalies (e.g., horseshoe kidney) and the stone composition also influence the treatment outcome of ESWL (26, 34). Dretler has demonstrated *in vitro* that the fragmentation characteristics of renal calculi are dependent on their compositions, with calcium oxalate dihydrate and uric acid stones being the most easily fragmented, whereas calcium oxalate monohydrate and cystine calculi are the least easily fragmented (37). This has also been confirmed clinically with ESWL (7, 13).

However, the problem remains that the pre-ESWL differentiation of the various stone compositions with standard investigations is inaccurate and is made more difficult by the fact that the majority of renal calculi are of mixed composition. Following ESWL, most of the residual stone burdens are in the form of sand in the dependent calyces. Initially some doubt existed as to what the eventual outcome of this might be, but Graff et al have reported a regrowth rate of 58.4% in their series with follow-up of 12-26 months (7).

The treatment of symptomatic calyceal diverticular calculi with ESWL remains controversial. Although the majority of patients will become asymptomatic (follow-up = 6 months), only 20% will be rendered stone-free (38, 39).

Our practice in Baylor College of Medicine is to treat most symptomatic calculi <3 cm in size with ESWL monotherapy. Ureteric stents are inserted prophylactically prior to ESWL with calculi >2 cm in size, to reduce the incidence of steinstrasse. All patients with calculi >3 cm in size are encouraged to undergo PCNL. After one procedure, if a large residual stone burden (>3 cm) remains, a secondary PCNL is performed. Residual fragments ≥5 mm may be treated with PCNL or ESWL depending on social and anatomical factors. Occasionally, patients with massive staghorn calculi (>10 cm) are offered open surgery as the best treatment alternative to render them stone-free after a single procedure.

COMPLICATIONS

The most common complications which may occur following ESWL are outlined in Table 4.

Table 4. Complications of ESWL·

Complication	% of ESWL cases
Renal colic (7, 40, 41)	18-27
Steinstrasse (6, 8, 15, 16, 40)	1.9-7.6
Urosepsis (6, 8, 15, 16, 40, 41)	0.3-4.1
Perirenal Hematomas (6-8, 15, 16, 40, 41)	0.2-0.66
Arrhythmias (6-8, 15, 16, 40, 41)	0.1-1.0
Hypertension (42-45)	3.1-8.2

In the majority of patients with renal colic, symptomatic relief can be provided as outpatients. Steinstrasse (stone streets) are aggregations of particles which are seen in the ureter on plain x-rays. They can be classified as type I (sand only), type II (sand proximal to one large fragment) or type III (impacted large fragments)(46). In many cases they are asymptomatic and resolve spontaneously.

Type I will pass eventually, although it may take several weeks. If associated with obstruction and pain, a percutaneous nephrostomy tube is indicated. This wait-and-see policy with a partially obstructed kidney should have no detrimental effect on the long-term renal function if total relief of the obstruction is realized within two weeks (47). Type II requires initial decompression of the kidney and contact lithotripsy of the leading fragment through a ureteroscope. Type III requires renal decompression and either repeated ESWL or a combination of antegrade and retrograde contact lithotripsy. Coptcoat et al (46) reported the need to perform an open ureterolithotomy on their one case of a type III lower ureteric steinstrasse. The incidence of steinstrasse increases as the treated stone burden increases, but can be reduced with prophylactic insertion of ureteric stents prior to ESWL (48).

The incidence of urosepsis has been reported to be directly proportional to the stone size and to be more common with staghorn calculi (49). All patients with staghorn calculi should be given culture-specific antimicrobials parentally prior to ESWL. Post-ESWL pyrexias may occur in up to 30% of patients (40). In many cases no identifiable source of infection is found and it is thought to be partly due to a transient endotoxemia secondary to breakdown of the cell walls of bacteria residing within the calculi (50).

Subcapsular or perirenal hematomas are more common in patients with hypertension, urinary tract infections, and those who have simultaneous bilateral treatment (51). The incidence in controlled hypertensives is 2.5%, but increases to 3.8% if the hypertension is poorly controlled (51). The stone size or the number of shocks administered are unrelated to their development. Clinically, the diagnosis can be suspected if there is post-ESWL pain and a decrease of >2 grams in the hemoglobin level, but the diagnosis must be confirmed with ultrasonography or computed tomography. The majority of patients can be managed conservatively with resuscitation and observation of their hemodynamic status, but they should be followed carefully with computed tomography (CT) scans to monitor hematoma resolution and blood pressure determination to detect the possible development of hypertension secondary to a Page kidney (52).

In the majority of cases, shock wave induced extrasystoles are prevented by ECG controlled triggering of the electrode discharges. However, occasionally antiarrhythmias occur. Many uneventful ESWL procedures have now been performed on patients with pacemakers. Liedl et al (42) reported a 3.1% incidence of post-ESWL hypertension in their 487 patients which were followed for an average of 40 months. This compares favorably with a 2.8% incidence in an age matched control group. However, the results were based on a telephone follow-up of the patients which suggests that the data is questionable. Peterson and Finlayson (43) reported sustained hypertension which required treatment in 3 of 79 patients (4%), whereas Williams et al (44) and Lingeman and Kulb (45) reported 8% hypertension rates in their series of 91 and 295 patients respectively. The theoretical cause for this hypertension is postulated to be the Page kidney effect (52). The sequence of events is trauma $\rightarrow$ perirenal hemorrhage $\rightarrow$ fibrosis $\rightarrow$ increased interstitial pressure $\rightarrow$ decreased renal perfusion $\rightarrow$ increased renin production $\rightarrow$ hypertension secondary to angiotensin II production. The actual cause of the hypertension is probably multifactorial because the incidence in the Indianapolis series (8.2%) is far greater than their incidence of ultrasound detected perirenal hematomas (0.66%) (45, 51). Other complications which have been reported infrequently include pancreatitis, ileus, hemophtysis, pneumonitis, pleural effusion, cutaneous bruising and renal failure (4, 6, 15, 16, 40).

There are also numerous reports of subclinical acute renal damage in the world literature. Radiological studies have demonstrated renal enlargement secondary to edema (53, 54), intrarenal hematomas (54), loss of corticomedullary demarcation (51), decreased effective renal plasma flow (44) and an increased parenchymal transit time index following treatment (55). Biochemical estimations have detected elevations in serum bilirubin (6), lactic dehydrogenase (6, 56), N-acetyl-beta-glucosamidase (NAG) (56, 57), betagalactosidase (BGAL) (57), glutamic transaminase (6), gamma-glutamyl transferase (57) and creatinine phosphokinase (6). The majority of these changes revert to normal within the first month post-ESWL.

RADIATION

The Dornier HM3 (SD050) lithotriptor utilizes radiographic and fluoroscopic imaging systems for stone localization.

Table 5. Comparative data of patients' radiation doses.

Series	Procedure	Skin Surface Dose (Roentgen)
Laws and Rosenstein (58)	Abdomen (KUB)	1.7
	Intravenous Pyelogram	5.5
Pavlicek et al (59)	Carotid angiography	23
McCrohan et al (60)	CT head	2.4-7.6
McCullough and Payne (61)	CT body	2.2-11
Stacey et al (62)	Cardiac catheterization	33
Van Husen et al (63)	Endoscopic retrograde cholangiopancreatography	23
Bush et al (64)	Percutaneous stone removal	27.8
Griffith et al (65)	ESWL	15.2 (9.5)*
Bush et al (66)	ESWL	17.2
Van Swearingen (67)	ESWL	22.4
Lin and Hrejsa (68)	ESWL	26
Saunders and Coleman (69)	ESWL	13.3

* Patient exposure after physician awareness education.

Dornier originally suggested that patient radiation exposure was approximately equivalent to an intravenous urogram, but published reports have demonstrated greater radiation exposure (Table 5).

The time/dose ratio of radiographic "snapshots" compared to fluoroscopic "stills" is 15:1 (65). Griffith et al demonstrated the effectiveness of a physician radiation awareness program which reduced patient radiation exposure by 37.5%, primarily by diminishing the number of radiographic "snapshots" (65). Radiation exposure to the medical personnel involved has been shown to be acceptably low, although some doubt remains concerning the need for protective aprons (66, 69, 70).

NOISE LEVEL

During treatment, the patient and medical staff are exposed to noise levels of 80-95 dB (69). Each acoustic pulse lasts about 150 msec and although there is no general agreement about safety levels for pulsed sound, ear protection for patients and staff has been recommended.

SECOND GENERATION LITHOTRIPTORS

The characteristics of all currently available lithotriptors are outlined in Table 6. All second generation lithotriptors have only been operational for a limited time period so that published data with regard to treatment stone-free results is sparse. The principal differences between the different machines from a clinical point of view are whether or not lithotripsy can be performed without analgesia and whether fluoroscopy or ultrasonography is preferable for stone localization.

Pain related to ESWL is a result of the shock-wave pressure produced by the energy source, the size of the focal point (F_2) and the area of skin through which the shock-wave enters. Presently the Wolf Piezolith 2300 and the EDAP LT01 lithotriptors require no analgesia during treatment whereas the Lithostar (Siemens), Sonolith 2000 (Technomed), Medstone 1050 and Dornier HM4 and MFL 5000 generally require moderate degrees of intravenous sedation and analgesics. The Dornier HM3 and the Tripter X_7 (Direx) require general or spinal anesthesia.

Lithotriptors that utilize fluoroscopic imaging can localize stones in all locations of the upper urinary tract. Ultrasonography, on the other hand, images most pelvic and calyceal stones satisfactorily but is of limited or no value in localizing ureteral stones (by most operators) except for stones in the distal juxtavesical ureter. Stones located at the ureteropelvic junction in extrarenal pelves may also be difficult or impossible to localize with ultrasonography. Thus, systems that utilize fluoroscopic imaging generally embrace a wider patient population than do systems that utilize only sonographic imaging.

Table 6. Characteristics of Lithotriptors.

Company	Machine	Energy Source	Coupling	Imaging System	F_2 (mm)
Dornier	HM3	Spark gap	Water bath	F+Fluoro	12x50
	HM4	Spark gap	Water cushion	F+Fluoro	12x50
	MPL 9000	Spark gap	Water cushion	US	3x20
	MFL 5000	Spark gap	Water cushion	F+Fluoro	
Technomed	Sonolith 2000	Spark gap	Partial water bath	US	15x30
Siemens	Lithostar	Electro-magnetic	Water cushion	F+Fluoro	10x60
Wolf	Piezolith 2300	Piezo-electric	Partial water bath	US	4x12
EDAP	LT01	Piezo-electric	Water cushion	US	5x15
Northgate	SD-3	Spark gap	Water cushion	US	
Yashiyoda	Azide disintegrator	Lead azide	Water bath	F+Fluoro	
Medstone	1050	Spark gap	Water cushion	Fluoro	
Nitech		Spark gap	Water cushion	US	41x19
Diasonics		Piezo-electric	Water cushion	F+Fluoro +US	
John Hopkins		Spark gap	Water cushion	US	
Direx	Tripter X_7	Spark gap	Water cushion	F+Fluoro +US	5x15
International Biomedics	1B1-ELC	Spark gap	Water cushion	Fluoro	

F = Film; Fluoro = Fluoroscopy; US = Ultrasound

The principal disadvantage of the piezoelectric lithotriptors is that several treatment sessions may be required to fully fragment calculi, whereas one treatment is usually adequate with the spark-gap lithotriptors (71-74).

In conclusion, the treatment results of extracorporeal shock-wave lithotripsy are dependent on the stone size, site, multiplicity, and composition and whether or not obstruction is present. Stone fragmentation can be achieved by all available machines but at a price. Machines with a spark gap energy source generally require analgesia or anesthesia but will achieve stone fragmentation with fewer treatment sessions than the truly analgesia free piezoelectric lithotriptors.

REFERENCES

1. Chaussy C, Brendel W, Schmiedt E: Extracorporeal induced destruction of kidney stones by shock waves. Lancet, 2: 1265-1268, 1980.
2. Hepp W: Varversuche zur Zerkleinerung von nierensteinen durch Stobwellen. Dornier System, Versuchsbericht 638, 1972.
3. Chaussy C, Schmiedt E: Extracorporeal shock wave lithotripsy (ESWL) for kidney stones. An alternative to surgery? Urol Radiol, 6: 80-87, 1984.
4. Politis G, Griffith DP: ESWL: stone-free efficacy based upon stone size and location. World J Urol, 5: 255-258, 1987.
5. Graff J, Diederichs W, Schulze H: Long-term follow-up in 1,003 extracorporeal shock wave lithotripsy patients. J Urol, 140: 479-483, 1988.
6. Lingeman JE, Newman D, Mertz JHO, Mosbaugh PG, Steele RE, Kahnoski RJ, Coury TA, Woods JR: Extracorporeal shock wave lithotripsy: The Methodist Hospital of Indiana experience. J Urol, 135: 1134-1137, 1986.
7. Charig CR, Webb DR, Payne SR, Wickham JEA: Comparison of treatment of renal calculi by open surgery, percutaneous nephrolithotomy and extracorporeal shockwave lithotripsy. Br Med J, 292: 879-882, 1986.
8. Eisenberger F, Fuchs G, Miller K, Bub P, Rassweiler J: Extracorporeal shock wave lithotripsy and endourology: an ideal combination for the treatment of kidney stones. World J Urol, 3: 412-47, 1985.
9. Cartensen HE, Hausen TS: Stones in the ureter. Acta Chir Scand, Suppl, 433: 66-71, 1973.
10. Ueno A, Kawamura T, Ogawa A, Takayasu H: Urology 10: 544-546, 1977.
11. Schulz E, Hengst E, Brundig P, Haerting R, Pirlich W, Gunther H: Disturbed urinary transport in the pelvi-calyceal system in calcium-oxalate stone patients. Urol Res, 15: 109-112, 1987.
12. Griffith DP, Valiquette L: PICA/Burden: a staging system for upper tract urinary stones. J Urol, 138: 253-257, 1987.
13. Newman DM, Scott JW, Lingeman JE: Two-year follow-up of patients treated with extracorporeal shock-wave lithotripsy. J Endourol, 2: 163-171, 1988.
14. Drach GW, Dretler S, Fair W, Finlayson B, Gillenwater J, Griffith D, Lingeman J, Newman D: Report of the United States Cooperative Study of extracorporeal shock-wave lithotripsy. J Urol, 135: 1127-1133, 1986.
15. Sofras F, Karayannis A, Kostakopoulos A, Delakas D, Kastriotis J, Dimopoulos C: Methodology, results and complications in 2,000 extracorporeal shock-wave lithotripsy procedures. Br J Urol, 61: 9-13, 1988.
16. Gleeson MJ, Shabsigh R, Griffith DP: Outcome of ESWL in patients with multiple renal calculi based on stone burden and location. I Endourol, 2: 145-149, 1988.
17. Blandy JP, Singh M: The case of more aggressive approach to staghorn stones. J Urol, 115: 505-506, 1976.
18. Snyder JA, Smith AD: Staghorn calculi: Percutaneous extraction versus anatrophic nephrolithotomy. J Urol, 136: 351-354, 1986.
19. Moores WK, O'Boyle PJ: Staghorn calculi of the kidneys. A clinical review. Eur Urol, 2: 216-220, 1976.
20. Fernstrom I, Johanson B: Percutaneous pyelolithotomy: a new extraction technique. Scand J Urol Nephrol, 10: 257-259, 1976.
21. Adams GW, Oke EJ, Dunnick NR, Carson CC: Percutaneous lithotripsy of staghorn calculi. Am J Radiol, 145: 803-807, 1985.
22. Kerlan RK, Kahn RK, Laberge JM, Pogany AC, Ring EJ: Percutaneous removal of renal staghorn calculi. Am J Radiol, 145: 797-801, 1985.
23. Young AT, Hulbert JC, Cardella JF, Hunter DW, Castaneda-Zuniga WR, Reddy P, Amplatz K: Percutaneous nephrolithotomy: application to staghorn calculi. Am J Radiol, 145: 1265-1269, 1985.
24. Lee WJ, Smith AD, Cubelli V, Vernace FM: Percutaneous nephrolithotomy: analysis of 500 consecutive cases. Urol Radiol, 8: 61-66, 1986.

25. Eisenberger F, Rassweiler J, Bub P, Kallert B, Miller K: Differentiated approach to staghorn calculi using extracorporeal shock-wave lithotripsy and percutaneous nephrolithotomy: an analysis of 151 consecutive cases. World J Urol, 5: 248-254, 1987.
26. Gleeson MJ, Lerner SP, Griffith DP: Treatment of staghorn calculi with extracorporeal shock-wave lithotripsy and percutaneous nephrolithotomy. Urology, 1989 (in press).
27. Rocco F, Larcher P, Caimi D, Decobelli O, Musci R, Meroni T: Treatment of renal staghorn calculi with ESWL monotherapy using the Rocco EXL catheter. Presented at 4th Symposium on Shock-Wave Lithotripsy: State-of-the-Art, Indianapolis, USA (March 5-6, 1988).
28. Wirth MP, Frohmuller HGW: Results of primary treatment of staghorn calculi with extracorporeal shock-wave lithotripsy. Presented at 4th Symposium on Shock-Wave Lithotripsy: State-of-the-Art, Indianapolis, USA (March 5-6, 1988).
29. Harada M, Okuda H, Maeda H, Fusjisawa M, Fujii A, Goji K, Kamidona S: ESWL treatment of staghorn calculi and large stones. Presented at 4th Symposium on Shock-Wave Lithotripsy: State-of-the-Art, Indianapolis, USA (March 5-6, 1988).
30. Sohn M, Deutz FJ, Rohrmann D, Fischer N, Rubben H: Anesthesia-free ESWL monotherapy with Double J stents versus PCNL/ESWL combined approach in staghorn disease. A prospective randomized study. Presented at 4th Symposium on Shock-Wave Lithotripsy: State-of-the-Art, Indianapolis, USA (March 5-6, 1988).
31. Pode D, Verstandig A, Shapiro A, Katz G, Caine M: Treatment of complete staghorn calculi by extracorporeal shock-wave lithotripsy monotherapy with special reference to internal stending. J Urol, 140: 260-265, 1988.
32. Kahnoski RJ, Lingeman JE, Coury TA, Steele RE, Mosbaugh PG: Combined percutaneous and extracorporeal shock-wave lithotripsy for staghorn calculi: An alternative to anatrophic nephrolithotomy. J Urol, 135: 679-681, 1986.
33. Segura JW, Patterson DE, Le Roy AJ: Combined percutaneous ultrasonic lithotripsy and extracorporeal shock-wave lithotripsy for struvite staghorn calculi. Word J Urol, 5: 245-247, 1987.
34. Lingeman JE: Results of 313 staghorn treatments. Presented at 4th Symposium on Shock-Wave Lithotripsy: State-of-the-Art, Indianapolis, USA (March 5-6, 1988).
35. Schulze H, Hertle L, Graff J, Funke PJ, Senge T: Combined treatment of branched calculi by percutaneous nephrolithotomy and extracorporeal shock-wave lithotripsy. J Urol, 135: 1138-1141, 1986.
36. Lingeman JE, Saywell RM Jr, Woods JR, Newman DM: Cost analysis of extracorporeal shock wave lithotripsy relative to other surgical and nonsurgical treatment alternative for urolithiasis. Med Care, 24: 1151-1160, 1986.
37. Dretler SP: Stone fragility - a new therapeutic distinction. J Urol, 139: 1124-1127, 1988.
38. Psihramis KE, Dretler SP: Extracorporeal shock wave lithotripsy of caliceal diverticula calculi. J Urol, 138: 707-711, 1987.
39. Wilbert DM, Jenny E, Stoeckle M, Riedmiller H, Jacobi G: Calyceal diverticular stones: is ESWL worthwhile? J Urol, 135: 183A, 1986.
40. Coptcoat MJ, Webb DR, Kellet MJ, Fletcher MS, McNicholas TA, Dickinson IK, Whitfield HN, Wickham JEA: The complications of extracorporeal shockwave lithotripsy: management and prevention. Br J Urol, 58: 578-580, 1986.
41. Palfrey ELH, Bultitude MI, Challa S, Pemberton J, Shuttleworth KED: Report of the first 1000 patients treated at St. Thomas' Hospital by extracorporeal shockwave lithotripsy. Br J Urol, 58: 573-577, 1986.
42. Liedl B, Jochum D, Lunz C, Schuster C, Schmiedt E: Five-year follow-up of urinary stone patients treated with extracorporeal shockwave lithotripsy. J Endourol, 2: 157-162, 1988.
43. Peterson JC, Finlayson B: Effects of ESWL on blood pressure. In "Extracorporeal shockwave lithotripsy for renal stone disease" (Eds J Gravenstein, K Peter), Butterworth, Boston, 1986, pp. 145-150.
44. Williams CM, Kaude JV, Newman RC, Peterson JC, Thomas WC: Extracorporeal shockwave lithotripsy: long-term complications. Am J Radiol, 150: 311-315, 1988.
45. Lingeman JE, Kulb TB: Hypertension following extracorporeal shockwave lithotripsy. J Urol, 137: 142A, 1987.
46. Coptcoat MJ, Webb DR, Kellett MJ, Whitfield HN, Wickham JEA: The steinstrasse: a legacy of extracorporeal lithotripsy. Eur Urol, 14: 93-95, 1988.
47. Leahy AL, Ryan PC, McEntee GM, Dervan PA, Fitzpatrick JM: Renal functional recovery and microvascular damage after partial ureteric obstruction in the dog. J Urol, 139: 249A, 1988.
48. Libby JM, Meacham RB, Griffith DP: The role of silicone ureteral stents in extracorporeal shockwave lithotripsy of large renal calculi. J Urol, 139: 15-17, 1988.

49. Michaels EK, Fowler JE Jr, Mariano M: Bacteriuria following extracorporeal shockwave lithotripsy of infection stones. J Urol, 140: 254-259, 1988.
50. Tanaka M, Matsumoto T, Kitada S, Kumazawa J, Hara S, Yamaguchi A: Endotoxemia in patients who underwent ultrasonic lithotripsy and extracorporeal shockwave lithotripsy. Eur Urol, 14: 173-177, 1988.
51. Knapp PM, Kulb TB, Lingeman JE, Newman DM, Mertz JHO, Mosbaugh PG, Steele RE: Extracorporeal shockwave lithotripsy-induced perirenal hematomas. J Urol, 139: 700-703, 1988.
52. Sufrin G: The Page kidney: a correctable form of arterial hypertension. J Urol, 113: 450-454, 1975.
53. Grantham JR, Millner MR, Kaude JV, Finlayson B, Hunter PT, Newman RC: Renal stone disease treated with extracorporeal shockwave lithotripsy: short term observations in 100 patients. Radiology, 158: 203-206, 1986.
54. Rubin JI, Arger PH, Pollack HM, Banner MP, Coleman BG, Mintz MC, Van Arsdalen KN: Kidney changes after extracorporeal shockwave lithotripsy: CT evaluation. Radiology, 162: 21-24, 1987.
55. Bomanji J, Boddy SAM, Britton KE, Nimmon CC, Whitfield HN: Radionuclide evaluation pre- and postextracorporeal shockwave lithotripsy for renal calculi. J Nucl Med, 28: 1284-1289, 1987.
56. Marcellan FJR, Servio LI: Evaluation of renal damage in extracorporeal lithotripsy by shock waves. Eur Urol, 12: 73-75, 1986.
57. Assimos DG, Boyce WH, Furr EG, Espeland MA, Harrison LH, Kroovand RL: Urinary enzyme levels after extracorporeal shockwave lithotripsy (ESWL). J Urol, 137: 143A, 1987.
58. Laws PW, Rosenstein M: A somatic dose index for diagnostic radiology. Health Phys, 35: 629-642, 1978.
59. Pavlicek W, Weinstein MA, Modic MT, Buonocore E, Duchesneau PM: Patient doses during digital subtractive angiography of the carotid arteries: comparison with conventional angiography. Radiology, 145: 683-685, 1982.
60. McCrohan JL, Patterson JF, Gagne RM, Goldtein HA: Average radiation doses in a standard head examination for 250 CT systems. Radiology, 163: 263-268, 1987.
61. McCullough EC, Payne JT: Patient dosage in computed tomography. Radiology, 129: 457-463, 1978.
62. Stacey AJ, Davis R, Kerr IH: Personnel protection during cardiac catheterization with a comparison of the hazards of undercouch and overcouch x-ray tube mountings. Br J Radiol, 47: 16-23, 1974.
63. Van Husen N, Hogeman B, Egen V, Mehnert C: Radiation exposure in endoscopic retrograde cholangiopancreatography. Endoscopy, 16: 112-114, 1984.
64. Bush WH, Brannen GE, Gibbons RP, Correa RJ Jr, Elder JS: Radiation exposure of patient and urologist during percutaneous nephrostolithotomy. J Urol, 132: 1148-1152, 1984.
65. Griffith DP, Gleeson MJ, Politis G, Glaze S: Effectiveness of radiation control program for Dornier HM3 lithotriptor. Urology, 33: 20-25, 1989.
66. Bush WH, Jones D, Gibbons RP: Radiation dose to patient and personnel during extracorporeal shock wave lithotripsy. J Urol 138: 716-719, 1987.
67. Van Swearingen FL, McCullough DL, Dyer R, Appel B: Radiation exposure to patients during extracorporeal shockwave lithotripsy. J Urol, 138: 18-20, 1987.
68. Lin P-JP, Hrejsa AF: Patient exposure and radiation environment of an extracorporeal shock wave lithotriptor system. J Urol, 138: 712-715, 1987.
69. Saunders JE, Coleman AJ: Physical characteristics of Dornier extracorporeal shockwave lithotriptor. Urology, 29: 506-509, 1987.
70. Glaze S, Le Blanc AD, Bushong SC, Griffith DP: Patient and personnel exposure during extracorporeal lithotripsy. Health Phys, 53: 623-629, 1987.
71. Marberger M, Turk C, Steinkogler I: Painless piezoelectric extracorporeal lithotripsy. J Urol, 139: 695-699, 1988.
72. Vallancien G, Aviles J, Munoz R, Veillon B, Charton M, Brisset JM: Piezoelectric extracorporeal lithotripsy by ultrashort waves with the EDAP LT01 device. J Urol, 139: 689-694, 1988.
73. Ziegler M, Mast G, Neisius D, Zwergel T, Kopper B, Zwergel U, Wurster H, Reidlinger R: Results in the use of extracorporeal piezoelectric lithotripsy (EPL) for treatment of urinary calculi. Urol Int, 43: 35-41, 1988.
74. Rassweiler J, Gumpinger R, Bub P, Kohl H, Mayer A, Eisenberger F: Wolf Piezolith 2200 versus the modified Dornier HM3. Efficacy and range of indications. Eur Urol, 16: 1-6, 1989.

HYPERTENSION

7

HAS TRANSLUMINAL ANGIOPLASTY PROVED TO BE EFFICACIOUS IN TREATMENT OF ATHEROSCLEROTIC RENAL ARTERY STENOSIS ?

ALBERT STEINER, PETER GREMINGER AND WILHELM VETTER

Department of Internal Medicine, University Hospital, 8091 Zürich, Switzerland

INTRODUCTION

Renal artery stenosis is the most frequent form of curable hypertension. For years, the only causative treatment was nephrectomy. Once antihypertensive drugs were available, it soon became apparent that patients with renovascular hypertension often required high dosages of antihypertensive drugs and multiple drug regimens. With rapid advances in cardiovascular and transplantation surgery, operative procedures in renovascular hypertension became more and more sophisticated. In recent years, surgical results have been excellent, and even patients with rather complex forms of renovascular hypertension have been successfully operated upon. Antihypertensive treatment was optimized by introducing a new class of blood pressure lowering agents: the angiotensin-converting enzyme inhibitors. Unfortunately, their effectiveness is also cause for their major complication, i.e. decreased renal function. Finally, a fascinating technique, the percutaneous transluminal angioplasty, has rapidly advanced to become one of the most popular methods in the treatment of hypertension secondary to renal artery stenosis. Percutaneous transluminal angioplasty, originally developed for large peripheral vascular lesions, was refined and substantially improved by miniaturization by A. Grüntzig and then successfully used to dilate coronary and renal artery stenoses (1).

HISTORY

Percutaneous transluminal angioplasty (PTA) of lower extremity arteries was first described in 1964 by Dotter and Judkins (2). The second major advance in the development of PTA occurred in 1974, when A. Grüntzig devised a double-lumen, polyvinyl balloon catheter with unique expansion characteristics. The Grüntzig catheter was sufficiently flexible to provide access to various arteries. Grüntzig used it for peripheral and coronary dilatations, as well as for renal occlusive disease. The application of PTA to the renal arteries was first reported in 1978 (3). Subsequent early reports evoked widespread interest, and renal PTA is now being instituted in many centers for the treatment of renovascular hypertension due to renal artery stenosis.

PTA, SURGERY OR MEDICAL TREATMENT?

Up to now, prospective randomized studies to compare the effectiveness of PTA, surgery or medical treatment in renovascular hypertension have never be undertaken. While there is universal agreement that severe hypertension requires some form of treatment, the choice of therapy is less clear.

In a retrospective study by our group, the effect of various therapeutic procedures such as surgery, PTA and medical treatment was analyzed in 202 patients with renovascular hypertension (4). Surgically treated patients were significantly younger and showed a shorter duration of hypertension, a lower serum creatinine, a lower incidence of bilateral stenoses and a higher blood pressure than dilated or medically treated cases. The two latter groups exhibited only minor and statistically insignificant differences in ages, duration of hypertension and creatinine. However, patients who underwent PTA had a significantly lower blood pressure and a markedly lower incidence of bilateral stenoses than cases who were treated with antihypertensive drugs (Table 1).

Under standard medical therapy (according to a stepped-care program: diuretic, antiadrenergic, vasodilatator) both in patients with atherosclerotic stenosis (AS) and in those with fibromuscular dysplasia (FMD) a highly significant fall in mean mean blood pressure to values within the normal range could be observed. In dilated patients, post treatment values were 153/89 mm Hg in cases with AS and 136/89 mm Hg in those with FMD. In operated patients the corresponding values were 148/90 mm Hg and 135/85 mm Hg respectively. However, pretreatment values were significantly higher in surgically treated (208/125 mm Hg) than in dilated (189/110 mm Hg) patients.

Table 1. Clinical and laboratory data in patients with renovascular hypertension treated either with surgery (n = 68), PTA (n = 59) or antihypertensive drugs (n = 75)

	Surgery	PTA	Drugs
Age, years	41.0	47.6	48.6
Duration of hypertension, years	2.9	4.7	5.0
Creatinine, mg%	1.19	1.37	1.35
Bilateral stenoses, %	12	20	31
Blood pressure, mm Hg	208/125	189/110	206/119

Under standard medical therapy 51% of patients with AS and 60% of those with FMD showed blood pressure values of 160/95 mm Hg or less. Surgically treated cases exhibited a slightly lower incidence of unimproved patients than cases who underwent PTA.

These data show that regardless of whether patients with renal artery stenosis are operated, dilated percutaneously or medically treated, in general a good effect can be expected. In conclusion, these results document that each of the three described methods (surgery, dilatation, antihypertensive drugs) effectively lowers blood pressure in patients with renovascular hypertension. Since our findings also indicate that certain patient characteristics had influenced the choice of treatment, a direct comparison between the described procedures is not possible. A certain advantage of PTA over surgery may be that it can be undertaken in patients who would be turned down for surgery because of associated conditions such as coronary artery disease or cerebrovascular disease, both of which are common in patients with atheromatous renovascular hypertension.

INDICATIONS AND CONTRAINDICATIONS FOR PTA

Patients with renovascular hypertension resulting from an accessible renal artery stenosis and a functional or potentially functional kidney are candidates for PTA. Stenoses are considered accessible when they involve the main renal artery or its primary branches. Occlusion of the main renal artery is also an indication for PTA if angiographic evidence of retrograde filling and distal reconstitution of the renal artery from collateral perfusion is present. A small number of patients with hypertension, compromised renal function, and either bilateral atherosclerotic renovascular stenoses or occlusive disease in a solitary functioning kidney have undergone PTA of the renal arteries aiming primarily at the preservation of renal function. Finally, a few instances of transplant anastomotic stenoses associated with severe hypertension have been treated with PTA.

When hypersensitivity to contrast media and a bleeding diathesis are excluded, the contraindications to renal PTA are only mechanical. Severe calcification of the renal arterial wall is a contraindication because of the risk of vascular cracking. Further severe tortuosity of the renal artery and angled origin may be important technical obstacles to the procedure (5).

RESULTS OF TREATMENT WITH PTA

Since the introduction in the management of renovascular hypertension in 1978 PTA for renal artery stenosis has proven its efficacy and simplicity. Various studies on the effect of PTA on renovascular hypertension report cures and improved the hypertension in 30-75% of patients with atherosclerotic stenosis (6-10). Therefore, PTA has become the favored method for treating renal artery stenosis in the majority of cases with renovascular hypertension.

A recently published study of our group determined the long-term effect of PTA on blood pressure and renal function with special regard toward patients which were classified as improved after the procedure (11). In 48 patients with atherosclerotic renal artery stenosis (AS) who had underwent successful PTA (stenosis in postdilatation angiography was less than 50%) a follow-up of at least 6 month after PTA was obtained. The most important baseline data from these 48 patients are given in Table 2.

Table 2. Clinical data in 48 patients with renovascular hypertension

Mean age, years	56±8
Sex (%m, %f)	67/33
Mean duration of hypertension, years	5.9±7.2
Mean blood pressure, mm Hg	195±30/110±14
Mean creatinine, mg%	1.93±0.72
Bilateral stenosis, %	29

After a mean observation period of 26 months the patients were classified as cured, improved or unimproved according the following criteria: (1) cured: decrease in blood pressure to 160/95 mm Hg or less without antihypertensive therapy, (2) improved: decrease in blood pressure to 160/90 mm Hg or less with additional antihypertensive therapy, and (3) unimproved: blood pressure of more than 160/95 mm Hg despite antihypertensive therapy.

Mean Blood Pressure

The effect of PTA on mean blood pressure is shown in Figure 1. A significant fall in systolic and diastolic blood pressure was observed. Mean blood pressure before PTA was 195±30 /110±14 mm Hg and after a period of 26 month 155±24/91±8 mm Hg.

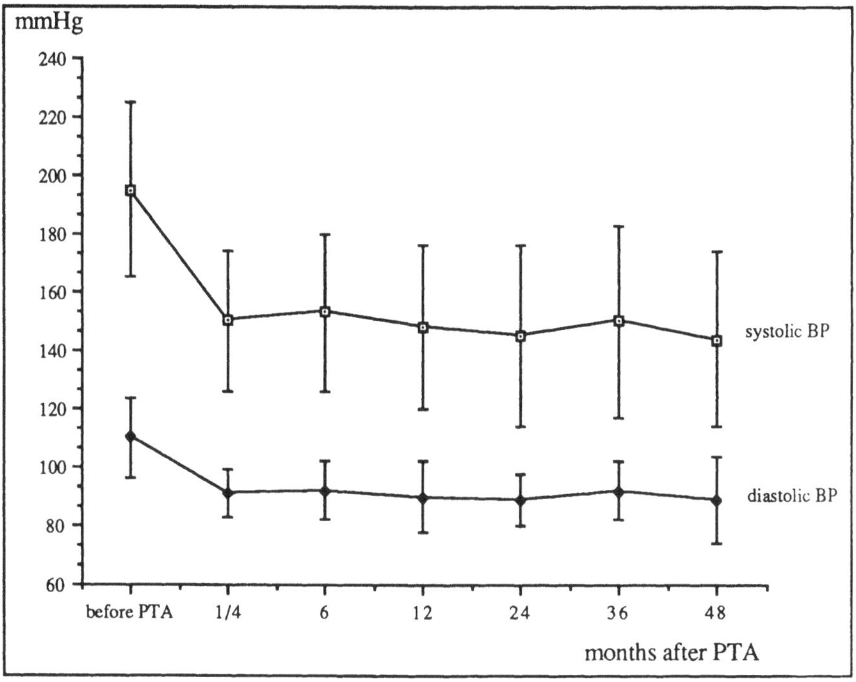

Figure 1. Systolic and diastolic blood pressure (BP) before and 1 week and 6, 12, 24, 36 and 48 months after PTA of renal artery stenosis due to AS. Indicated are mean values and standard deviation.

Cure Rate

The cure rate after an observation period of 26 month was 23%. A reduction to a diastolic blood pressure value of 90 mm Hg or less without antihypertensive medication was seen in 8 of the 48 patients with AS (17%).

54% of the patients showed an improvement of hypertension after PTA. Furthermore, in these patients with improved blood pressure values a reduction of antihypertensive agents was possible since after PTA 83% of patients needed one or two drugs and only 17% three or four drugs for blood pressure control whereas the corresponding rates before PTA were 52% and 48% respectively. These results are similar to those reported by other authors as shown in Table 3.

Kidney Function

For the total group no significant change in serum creatinine level before and 26 months after PTA could be observed. Analysis of the creatinine values in the subgroups with cure, improvement or no improvement after PTA revealed a different pattern since cured cases showed a slight decrease whereas unimproved cases had a slight but significant increase in serum creatinine. Patients who were classified as improved after PTA exhibited a statistically insignificant decrease in creatinine.

Table 3. Results of PTA series for treatment of renovascular hypertension

Author	n	Cured (%)	Improved (%)	Failed (%)	References
Geyskes(12)	44	9	43	48	42
Greminger	48	23	54	23	11
Grim(13)	25	4	36	60	43
Sos	20	25	45	30	10
Schwarten	52	44	48	84	41
Total	189	28	45	34	

Patients with cure of hypertension after PTA obviously reflect the true benefit of the procedure. Improvement rates, however, were questioned recently (14) since comparable improvement of hypertension in medically treated patients with PTA of renal artery stenosis (36%) compared with medically treated essential hypertensives without any other intervention (32%) has been observed. It was therefore suggested that the reported improvement of blood pressure after PTA might be inconsistent. However, in those patients with renovascular hypertension, in whom correction of renal artery stenosis by PTA was not possible, improvement of blood pressure was seen in only 13% of cases during follow-up (14). Therefore the question arises, whether essential hypertensives represent a valid 'control' group in evaluating the effect of PTA in patients with renovascular hypertension.

Although various authors (6-10) used differing criteria for definition of cure, improvement or failure, in most studies 'improvement' was characterized by the fact that after angioplasty patients showed blood pressure values within the normal range but still required antihypertensive medication. Comparison of blood pressure values in these patients is difficult since in a substantial part of cases classified as improved or unimproved antihypertensive therapy was changed during follow-up. Furthermore, it has to be considered that the intervention itself might have improved patient compliance with drug therapy.

The natural history of renal artery stenosis whether medically treated or untreated is characterized by progression of stenosis with eventual total occlusion and by progressive deterioration of kidney function (15, 16). A retrospective study in 85 patients with renal artery sclerosis who underwent one or more repeated renal angiogram showed in 37 patients (44%) a progressive renal artery sclerosis. Progression to complete occlusion of the involved renal artery occurred in 14 cases (16%). Half of the patients with progressive stenosis showed an increase in serum creatinine values (17). An earlier study with a smaller number of patients has shown a deterioration of renal function (15% or greater decreases in clearance studies) in 4 out of 21 patients (19%) with AS after a mean observation period of 40 months (18). Therefore, our observation of a slight, though statistically insignificant, decrease in serum creatinine after a mean observation period of 26 months in patients with improvement of blood pressure may indicate that the effect of PTA in this group is not spurious.

In summary, these results and those in the literature document a good long term effect of PTA in renovascular hypertension due to AS. In a few patients blood pressure was reduced to normal or significantly decreased for a period of more than 7 years. Furthermore, it has to be considered that in cases classified as cured or improved after the intervention serum creatinine levels decreased or remained stable whereas the natural history of renal artery stenosis is characterized by a progressive deterioration of kidney function. We therefore recommend PTA as the treatment of choice in hypertensive patients with AS of renal artery.

RESTENOSIS

Recently it has been demonstrated that balloon dilatation produces "controlled injury" to the vessel wall which results in longitudinal fissures in the intima and complete or partial concentric tears and separation between the media and the adventitia (19-22). The outer wall of the artery is slightly dilated and the atheromatous material is displaced and compressed into it. The lesion becomes "turned inside out" and heals in the dilated state.

It is probably that the approximately 20% restenosis rate widely reported in the renal artery (23, 24) is due to under-dilation and the resultant incomplete "cracking" of the atheromatous core and incomplete dilatation of the very resistant adventitia. Stenoses after PTA may recur for at least two principal reasons. First, the dilated vessel can gradually return to its predilated state due to its elasticity. The second is the continued progression and build up of atheromatous material at the site of the residual stenosis due to turbulent flow (25). In PTA a satisfactory post-dilatation lumen greater than 70% has a higher correlation with the long-term relief of hypertension than the decrease in pressure gradient. For these reasons it has been proposed balloons one or two millimeters greater in diameter than that of the vessel on the arteriogram should be used routinely. Under such conditions restenosis rate of only 10% has been reported (25). Other investigators showed a recurrence of stenosis after PTA of 42% in patients with AS (26). They also have shown that it is not possible to predict which AS patients will develop restenosis and which will not. In fact, the presence of generalized atherosclerosis, the severity of the stenosis and the extent to which the stenosis was dilated were not different between patients who developed restenosis and those who did not (27). A higher incidence of recurrent renal artery stenosis after PTA was observed with ostial lesions compared to non-ostial lesions (74% vs 55%) (28).

COMPLICATIONS

Experience suggests that PTA of the renal arteries is a relatively low risk-procedure. Nevertheless, several sources of morbidity have been identified. The reported complication rates for renal PTA range from 6% to 15% (29-33).

A classification of the complications of PTA in renal artery stenosis has been proposed according to their severity and their direct or indirect relationship to PTA (34). "Minor" complications are reversible within the normal recovery period after PTA, while "major" complications are irreversible or reversible but necessitate extended hospitalization or surgery. The following complications are reported in the literature as being directly related to PTA: hemorrhage at the puncture site (31), hemorrhage from renal or access artery perforation or rupture (35), occlusive or non occlusive dissection of the renal or access arteries (9), renal artery thrombosis (36), renal artery spasm or embolism leading to segmental renal infarctation (37), peripheral artery embolisation, and balloon rupture complications (38). The indirectly related complications include transient or irreversible renal insufficiency (39), contrast media hypersensitivity (10), pressure-drop-related cerebral (36) or myocardial ischemia (10), and anticoagulation-related hemorrhage (36, 40) or infections (10) (Table 4).

Table 4. Comparative complication rates (direct, indirect) in renal artery PTA

Author, (Ref.)	Number of patients	Direct % all	Direct % major	Indirect %	Deaths %
Boomsma (35)	80	50	4	3	3
Colapinto (31)	68	-	6	5	0
Löhr (39)	128	12	10	-	-
Mahler (34)	80	10	4	1	1
Martin (42)	31	10	10	-	-
Puijlaert (38)	114	8	3	2	1
Richter (43)	56	6	2	-	0
Schneider (44)	62	-	7	4	0
Schwarten (41)	66	9	6	-	-
Sos (10)	89	11	6	5	0
Tegtmeyer (45)	38	16	8	3	3

PTA FOR PRESERVATION OF KIDNEY FUNCTION

It has been reported that angioplasty can cause a significant improvement in renal function in patients with renal failure. These patients had either a critical stenosis of a solitary kidney, or severe bilateral stenoses. Such cases are difficult to treat with antihypertensive agents, because a reduction of blood pressure is associated with a dramatic deterioration of renal function. This is most common when angiotensin converting enzyme inhibitors are used (46). When PTA can be performed in this situation it is especially beneficial, because it can both improve renal function and make the blood pressure easier to control.

In a series of 57 patients who had serum creatinine levels greater than 2 mg/dl PTA has been attempted (47). The majority of patients had stenoses of both renal arteries, nearly always due to atheroma. In 20% there was complete occlusion of one renal artery. The patients have been divided into two groups according to whether the angioplasty was technically successful or not, that is whether the angioplasty balloon could be passed across the stenosis or not. On this basis, 43 patients were classified as successful, and 14 as unsuccessful. The baseline characteristics of the two groups were similar, the serum creatinine levels in the unsuccessful group were a little higher than in the successful group, but the differences were not significant. Both groups have been followed for about two years. In the successful group 62% showed a decrease of their serum creatinine at 3-6 months after PTA, 12% no change, and 26% an increase. In the unsuccessful group none showed a decrease, 21% no change, and 79% an increase (Figure 2).

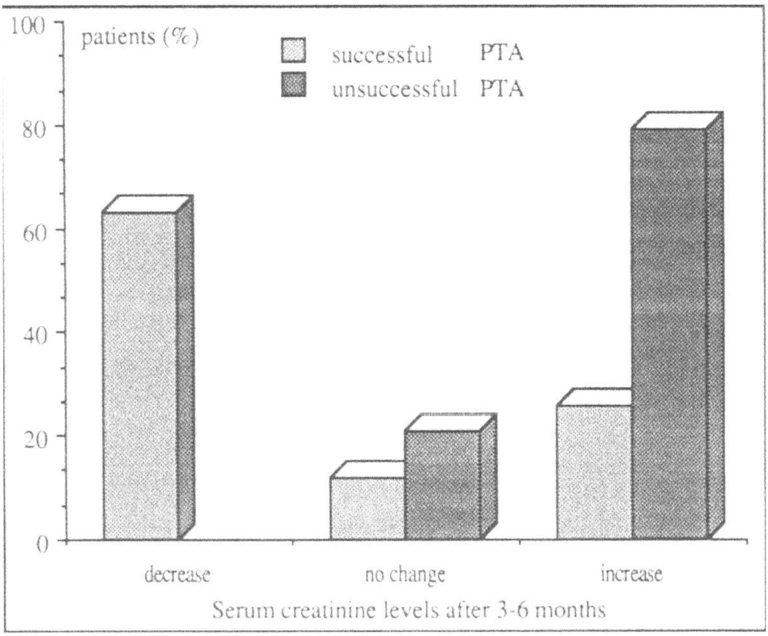

Figure 2. Changes in serum creatinine levels after 3-6 months after successful and unsuccessful PTA. Indicated are % of patients for decrease, no change and increase in serum creatinine levels.

During the two years of follow-up 12% of the successful group died, as compared to 57% of the unsuccessful group; 14% of the successful group eventually needed dialysis, and 43% of the unsuccessful group. These results suggest that, when PTA can be achieved in such patients, a significant number shows a sustained improvement or a delayed decline in their renal function, in contrast to the persistent deterioration in patients in whom the procedure was technically impossible (47). In another study PTA was attempted in 12 azotemic patients with severe hypertension, who had stenoses of both renal arteries or a solitary kidney. Improved renal function was reported in only three patients (48). Further 12 patients had surgery, with improvement in 10. The patients were not randomly allocated to the two forms of treatment, however, so that is probable the PTA patients had more extensive disease.

In conclusion, it is reasonable to suggest that PTA of the renal arteries has emerged as a potent alternative to both, renovascular surgery and pharmacotherapy in the management of renovascular hypertension. PTA has proved repeatedly its long-term efficacy in the treatment of renal artery stenosis and should therefore be the favored procedure in patients with AS of renal artery.

REFERENCES

1. Grüntzig A: Transluminal dilatation of coronary-artery stenosis. Lancet, i: 263, 1978
2. Dotter CT, Judkins MP: Transluminal treatment of arteriosclerotic obstruction: Description of a new technique and a preliminary report of its application. Circulation, 30: 654-670, 1964
3. Grüntzig A, Kuhlmann U, Vetter W, Lütolf U, Meier B, Siegenthaler W: Treatment of renovascular hypertension with percutaneous transluminal dilatation of a renal artery stenosis. Lancet, i: 801-802, 1978
4. Greminger P, Lüscher TF, Zuber J, Kuhlmann U, Schneider E, Siegenthaler W, Largiader F, Vetter W: Surgery, transluminal dilatation and medical therapy in the management of renovascular hypertension. Nephron, 44 (Suppl. 1): 36-39, 1986
5. Madias NE, Millan V: Percutaneous transluminal renal angioplasty in the treatment of renovascular hypertension. In: Breslin DJ et al. (eds), Renovascular hypertension. Williams and Wilkins, Baltimore, 148-165, 1982
6. Geyskes, CG, Puylaert CBAJ, Oei HY, Dorhout Mees EJ: Follow-up study of 70 patients with renal artery stenosis treated by percutaneous transluminal dilatation. Br Med J, 287: 333-336, 1983
7. Greminger P, Knorr M, Schneider E, Kuhlmann U, Siegenthaler W, Vetter W; Long-term results of percutaneous transluminal dilatation in renovascular hypertension. In: Glorioso N, Laragh JH, Rapelli A, Renovascular hypertension: pathophysiology, diagnosis, and treatment. Raven Press, New York, 491-497, 1987
8. Grim CE, Yune HY, Donohue JP, Weinberger MH, Dilley R, Klatte EC: Renal vascular hypertension. Surgery vs. dilatation. Nephron, 44 (Suppl.1): 96-100, 1986
9. Mahler F, Probst P, Haertel M, Weidmann P, Krneta A: Lasting improvement of renovascular hypertension by transluminal dilatation in atherosclerotic and non-atherosclerotic renal artery stenoses. Circulation, 65: 611-617, 1982
10. Sos TA, Pickering TG, Sniderman K, Saddekni S, Case DB, Silane MF, Vaughan ED, Laragh JH: Percutaneous transluminal renal angioplasty in renovascular hypertension due to atheroma or fibromuscular dysplasia. N Engl J Med, 309: 274-279, 1983
11. Greminger P, Steiner A, Schneider E, Kuhlmann U, Steurer J, Siegenthaler W, Vetter W: Cure and improvement of renovascular hypertension after percutaneous transluminal angioplasty of renal artery stenosis. Nephron, 51: 362-366, 1989
12. Geyskes GG: Follow-up study of 70 patients with renal artery stenosis treated by percutaneous transluminal dilatation. In: Schilfgaarde RV et al (eds), Clinical aspects of renovascular hypertension. Martinus Nijhoff, Boston, 225-237, 1983
13. Grim CE, Yune HY, Donahue JP, Weinberger MH, Dilly R, Klatte EC: Treatment of renal vascular hypertension: a comparison of patients treated by surgery or by percutaneous transluminal angioplasty. In: Schilfgaarde RV et al (eds), Clinical aspects of renovascular hypertension. Martinus Nijhoff, Boston, 238-242, 1983
14. Brawn LA, Ramsay LE: Is 'improvement' real with percutaneous transluminal angioplasty in the management of renovascular hypertension? Lancet, ii: 1313-1316, 1987
15. Hunt CJ, Strong CG: Renovascular hypertension. Mechanisms, natural history and treatment. Am J Cardiol, 32: 562-574, 1973
16. Pohl MA, Novick AC: Natural history of atherosclerotic and fibrous renal artery disease: clinical implications. Am J Kidney Dis, 5: A120-A130, 1985
17. Schreiber MJ, Pohl MA, Novick AC: The natural history of atherosclerotic and fibrous renal artery disease. Urol Clins N Am, 11: 383-392, 1984
18. Wollenweber J, Sheps SG, Davies GD: Clinical course of atherosclerotic renovascular disease. Am J Cardiol, 21: 60-71, 1968
19. Höhn P, Wagner R, Zeitler E: Histologische Befunde nach der Katheterbehandlung arterieller Obliterationen nach Dotter und ihre Bedeutung. Herz/Kreisl 7: 13-23, 1975

20. Jester HG, Sinapius D: Morphologic alterations after percutaneous transluminal recanalization of chronic femoral atherosclerosis. In: Zeitler E, Grüntzig A, Schoop W (eds) Percutaneous vascular Recanalization, Springer Verlag, Berlin, 55, 1978
21. Castaneda-Zuniga WR, Formaneck A, Tadavarthy M: The mechanism of balloon angioplasty. Radiology, 135: 565-571, 1980
22. Block PC, Baughman KL, Pasternak RC, Fallon JT: Transluminal angioplasty: correlation of morphologic and angiographic findings in experimental model. Circulation, 61: 778-785, 1980
23. Schwarten DE: Transluminal angioplasty of renal artery stenosis: 70 experiences, Am J Radiol, 135: 969-974, 1980
24. Tegtmeyer CJ, Dyer R, Teates CD: Percutaneous transluminal dilatation of the renal arteries: techniques and results. Radiology, 135: 589-599, 1980
25. Sos TA, Pickering TG, Sniderman KW, Saddekni S, Case DB, Silane MF, Vaughan ED, Laragh JH: Percutaneous transluminal angioplasty in renovascular hypertension due to atheroma or fibromuscular dysplasia. N Engl J Med, 309: 274-279, 1983
26. Kremer TK, Jong PE de, Zeeuw D de, Donker AJM, Schuur KH, Hem GK van der: Restenosis prevalence and long-term effects on renal function after percutaneous transluminal renal angioplasty. Nephron, 44 (Suppl. 1): 64-67, 1986
27. Jong de PE, Zeeuw D de, Smit AJ, Hoorntje SJ, Schuur KH, Donker AJM, Hem GK van der: The effect of transluminal dilatation of stenosed renal arteries on kidney function. Neth J Med, 26: 266, 1983
28. Hayes JM, Risius B, Novick AC, Geisinger M, Zelch M, Gifford RW jr., Vidt DG, Olin JW: Experience with percutaneous transluminal angioplasty for renal artery stenosis at the Cleveland Clinic. J Urol, 139: 488-492, 1988
29. Tegtmeyer CJ, Teates CD, Crigler N: Percutaneous transluminal angioplasty in patients with renal artery stenosis: Follow-up studies. Radiology, 131: 53-58, 1979
30. Oleaga JA, Grossman RA, McLean GK: Arteriovenous fistula of a segmental renal artery branch as a complication of percutaneous angioplasty. Am J Radiol, 136: 988-989, 1981
31. Colapinto RF, Stronell RD, Harries-Jones EP, Gildiner M, Hobbs BB, Farrow GA, Wilson DR, Morrow JD, Logan AG, Birch SJ: Percutaneous transluminal dilatation of the renal artery. Am J Radiol, 139: 727-732, 1982
32. Mills SR, Wertman DE jr., Grossman SH: Renal cortical arteriovenous fistula complicating percutaneous renal angioplasty. Am J Radiol, 137: 1251-1253, 1981
33. Grim CE, Yune HY, Weinberger MH: Balloon dilatation for renal artery stenosis causing hypertension: Criteria, concerns and cautions. Ann Intern Med, 92: 117-119, 1980
34. Mahler F, Triller J, Weidmann P, Nachbur B: Complications in percutaneous transluminal dilatation of renal arteries. Nephron, 44 (Suppl. 1): 60-63, 1986
35. Boomsma H: Percutaneous transluminal dilatation of stenotic renal arteries in hypertension, Drukkerij van Denderen, Grossingen, 1982
36. Kuhlmann U, Vetter W, Grüntzig A, Schneider E, Puouliadis G, Steurer J, Siegenthaler W: Percutaneous transluminal dilatation of renal artery stenosis: 2 year's experience. Clin. Science, 61: 481-483, 1981
37. Beinart C, Sos TA, Saddekni S, Weiner MA, Sniderman KW: Arterial spasm during renal angioplasty. Radiology, 149: 97-99, 1983
38. Puijlaert CBAJ, Geyskes GG, Ruijs JHJ, Wüstenfeld HPJ, Mali WPT: Renal angioplasty in hypertension. Technique, radiological and clinical results, and complications in 134 dilatations. In: Dotter CT, Grüntzig A, Schoop W, Zeitler E (eds), Percutaneous transluminal angioplasty, Springer, Berlin, 279, 1983
39. Löhr E, Weichert HC, Hartjes H, Schrijvers A: Percutaneous transluminal angioplasty of renal arteries. A therapeutic principle. Case report of 128 patients with renovascular hypertension. In: In: Dotter CT, Grüntzig A, Schoop W, Zeitler E (eds), Percutaneous transluminal angioplasty, Springer, Berlin, 281, 1983
40. Madias NE, Ball JT, Milland VG: Percutaneous transluminal renal angioplasty in the treatment of unilateral atherosclerotic renovascular hypertension. A J Med, 70: 1078-1084, 1981
41. Schwarten DE, Yune HY, Klatte EC, Grim CE, Weinberger MH: Clinical experience with percutaneous transluminal angioplasty (PTA) of stenosed renal arteries. Radiology, 135: 601, 1980
42. Martin EC, Mattern RF, Baer L, Fankuchen EI, Casarella WJ: Renal angioplasty for hypertension: Predictive factors for long term success. Am J Roentg, 137: 921-924, 1981
43. Richter EI, Krönert E, Zeitler E: Techiniques, indications, and results of percutaneous transluminal renal artery dilatation. In: Dotter CT, Grüntzig A, Schoop W, Zeitler E (eds), Percutaneous transluminal angioplasty, Springer, Berlin, 286, 1983

44. Schneider E, Vetter W, Pouliadis G, Lüscher T, Grüntzig A, Siegenthaler W: Late results of percutaneous transluminal angioplasty for renovascular hypertension (Personal communication)
45. Tegtmeyer CJ, Teates CD, Crigler N, Gandee RW, Ayers CR, Stoddard M, Wellons HA: Percutaneous transluminal angioplasty in patients with renal artery stenosis. Radiology, 140: 323-330, 1981
46. Hricik DE, Browning PJ, Kopelman R, Goome WR, Madia ME, Dzau VJ: Captopril-induced functional renal insufficiency in patients with bilateral renal-artery stenoses or renal-artery stenosis in a solitary kidney. N Engl J Med, 308:373-376, 1983
47. Pickering TG, Sos TA: Medical aspects of renal angioplasty. In: Renovascular hypertension, Glorioso N, Laragh HJ, Rappelli A (eds), Raven Press, New York, 413-424, 1987
48. Luft FR, Grim CE, Weinberger MH: Intervention in patients with renovascular hypertension and renal insufficiency. J. Urol, 130: 921-924, 1983

THE KIDNEY AND DIABETES

8

EARLY DIAGNOSIS OF DIABETIC NEPHROPATHY.
Twelve assertions on microalbuminuria and early nephropathy.

CARL ERIK MOGENSEN AND SALLY M. MARSHALL

Medical Department M, Second University Clinic of Internal Medicine, Kommunehospitalet, DK-8000 Aarhus C, Denmark

Microalbuminuria in diabetics, particularly insulin-dependent diabetics (IDDM), is now widely accepted as an early laboratory warning of late, clinically-important nephropathy. Microalbuminuria is defined as an elevated urinary albumin excretion rate, but in a range not detectable by currently used laboratory techniques for measuring clinical proteinuria, such as dipstick tests or the acetylsalicylic acid test (1).

IDDM-patients with persistent microalbuminuria are at high risk of developing nephropathy, and the term "incipient diabetic nephropathy" has been proposed. It is also becoming more and more accepted that persistent microalbuminuria is an early sign of renal disease rather than a susceptibility factor. However, it is important to note that intensified intervention in patients with microalbuminuria may reverse this abnormality, which probably reflects an early phase of glomerular pathology (2). Therefore, it may be difficult at the present time to extrapolate from earlier follow-up studies which indicated a poor prognosis in patients with microalbuminuria, simply because the natural course of the disease may have changed radically due to better medical care for diabetic patients with microalbuminuria in the 80s, compared with the situation 10-20 years ago, when the early studies on the long-term consequences of microalbuminuria were initiated (3-7).

This article will review a number of issues regarding early diagnosis of diabetic renal disease by discussing 12 assertions on microalbuminuria, based upon literature from the last few years.

I. MICROALBUMINURIA CAN BE DEFINED AND RELATED TO DIABETIC NEPHROPATHY

Two approaches are being used in the definition of microalbuminuria. The first approach is based on the excretion rate of albumin in normal persons as related to the Albustix® positive level. The upper level of the albumin excretion rate in young healthy persons in the resting position rarely exceeds 15-20 μg/min (Figure 1). In one paper the upper 95% confidence interval in normal healthy persons was found to be 20 μg/min (8). Therefore, a level above this excretion rate, but below the Albustix® positive range (approximately 200 μg/min provided normal urine flow of 1 ml/min), could be used in the definition of microalbuminuria.

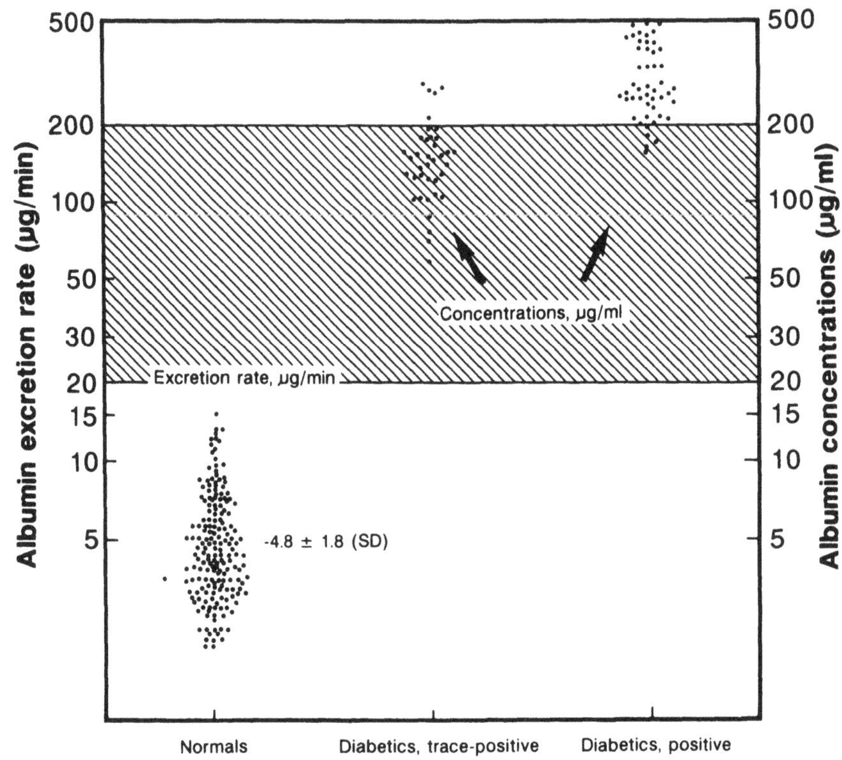

Figure 1. Albumin excretion rate in 179 young normals, and in diabetics with trace-positive Albustix®, and in diabetics with positive Albustix® (morning urines).

Another approach would be to consider the range that is predictive of late diabetic nephropathy. The lower range predictive of diabetic nephropathy varies between 15 and

30 μg/min (3-5), although a very high level of 70 μg/min was reported in one study, using 24 hr collections and only a 6-year follow-up (6). Based upon these studies a lower range of 20 μg/min has been proposed with an upper level of 200 μg/min, i.e. the Albustix® positive level (1). Obviously there is a grey area which may be defined as a level between 15 and 30 μg/min excreted in the resting position. Also, the exact transition to clinical proteinuria is poorly defined, and some workers may therefore prefer to use the urinary albumin excretion rate (UAER) when evaluating patients (9).

However, in clinical practice as well as in clinical research, it is of great importance to have internationally approved ranges, and the level 20-200 μg/min, when persistingly found, is gaining more and more acceptance as the microalbuminuria range, indicative of incipient diabetic nephropathy, and thus to be used when identifying at risk patients (9). This range is, however, quite considerable with a factor of 10 between the lowest and highest level. It now seems clear that patients with rather low levels of microalbuminuria, for instance up to 70 μg/min, still have well-preserved kidney function and intervention may be more effective in these patients, especially with respect to optimised insulin treatment. The level of GFR is certainly higher in this low microalbuminuric range as compared with the high microalbuminuria range. This would suggest that GFR starts to decline during the phase of microalbuminuria. It is certainly not surprising that a patient with an UAER of 30 μg/min (with GFR of 145 ml/min) is different from a patient with an excretion rate of 190 μg/min (and with a GFR of 105 ml/min) (10).

II. MICROALBUMINURIA CAN BE QUANTIFIED RELATIVELY EASILY BY NEW LABORATORY ASSAYS, USING STANDARD PROCEDURES OF URINE COLLECTION

Several procedures for collection of urine have been proposed (11-16). For screening procedures the albumin concentration in an early morning urine may be used. The value of this test may be slightly improved if albumin concentration is related to creatinine concentration as illustrated in Figure 2 (11). A totally random urine sample is not very useful because of the great variability in urine output during the daytime. This is in contrast to the rather well-defined and low urine output during the night, and as a consequence the early morning urine sample must be preferred for screening.

Often a more exact excretion rate is important in the evaluation of patients and therefore a timed urine collection must be used. Many centers prefer the overnight urine collection for several reasons (3). Patients are usually at rest during the night and complete urine collection is not too difficult, although some patients may forget to collect urine when voiding during the night. Therefore, it is advisable to measure creatinine excretion, and to collect urine over several nights. Otherwise, spuriously low excretion rates, due to incomplete urine collection, may be seen with great variability between collection periods. Some centers prefer to use a 24-hour collection, but there are few arguments in favour of such a procedure unless the patients are very accustomed to collect 24-hour urines (8).

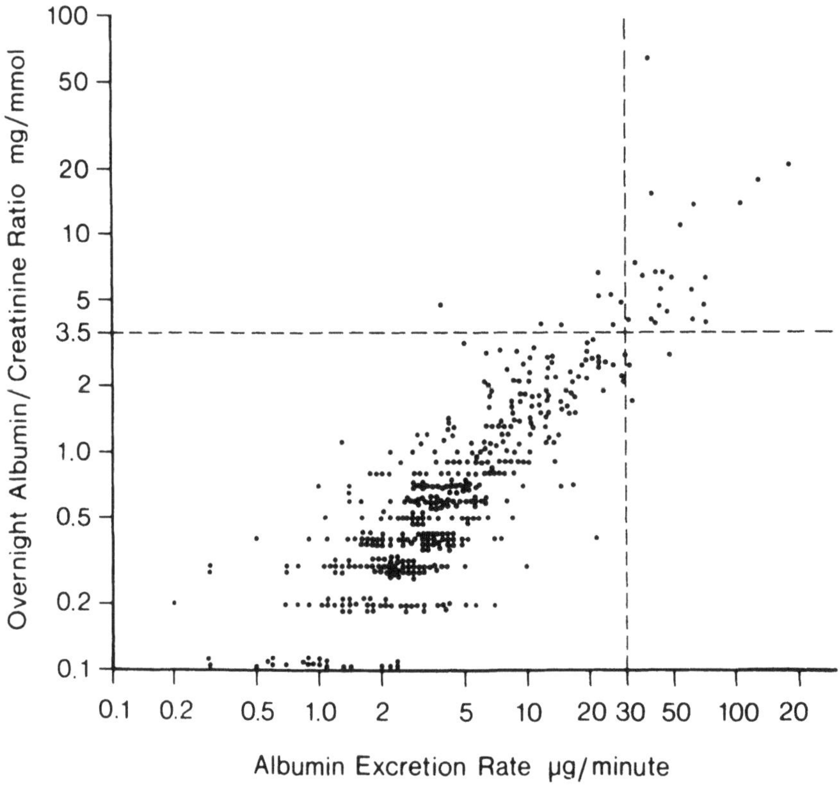

Figure 2. The relationship between the overnight urinary albumin/creatinine ratio (ONA/C) and the overnight albumin excretion rate (AER) in 446 diabetics from the Poole survey. Assessment of screening test: ONA/C > 3.5 mg/mmol predicts AER > 30 μg/min; sensitivity 85%, specificity 98%, and predictive value 74%. (From Gatling W, Rowe DJF, Hill RD: Microalbuminuria: an appraisal of assay techniques and urine collection procedures for measuring urinary albumin at low concentrations. In: "The Kidney and Hypertension in Diabetes Mellitus" (Ed. CE Mogensen), Martinus Nijhoff Publishing, Boston, 1988, pp 41-50).

If clearance studies are performed, the albumin excretion rate can quite easily be measured in the urine samples from the clearance procedure (10). If a constant infusion technique is used, multiple measurements can be performed. Care must be taken to avoid early samples with spuriously high values due to the wash-out phenomenon (15). If a single shot GFR-procedure is performed, urine can be collected as one or two samples during the procedure, which often lasts several hours.

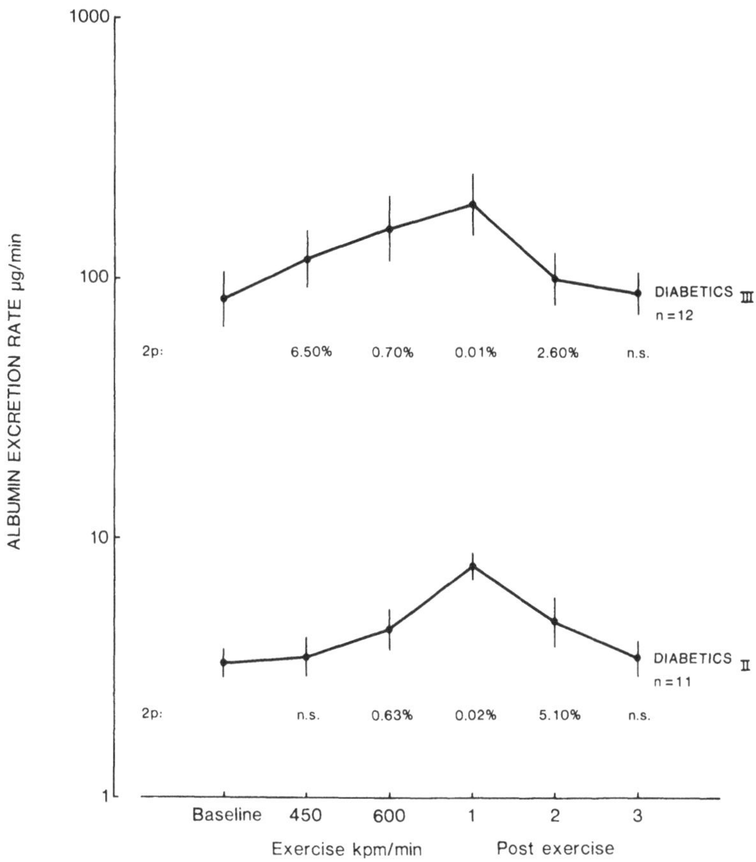

Figure 3. Urinary albumin excretion rate (geometric mean x/+ confidence factor, before, during and after exercise in diabetic patients with incipient diabetic nephropathy ($DIABETICS_{III}$) and comparable diabetic patients with normal baseline albumin excretion ($DIABETICS_{II}$).

Quantitation of microalbuminuria is quite important when evaluating the spontaneous course of early nephropathy, and, in particular, the measurement of excretion rate is very important when evaluating new possibilities of intervention. Clinical laboratories now offer the diabetologists a large number of inexpensive immunoassays for measuring urinary proteins, especially albumin, in small concentration (11, 13). In a clinical or a research laboratory the choice of measurement will depend upon general experience with either radio-immunoassay, turbidometry or nephelometry-immunoassay, fluoroimmunoassays or the popular enzyme-immunoassays. All assays have advantages and disadvantages. Although radioimmunoassay is usually the most sensitive, all procedures are generally sensitive enough for clinical practice. In some situations, e.g. when using diluted urine samples for clearance studies, radio-immunoassay may be an advantage (10). Tablet screening tests or slide agglutination tests are also available and are useful in small laboratories (11).

III. MICROALBUMINURIA VARIES CONSIDERABLY AND IS INFLUENCED BY PHYSICAL EXERCISE

All studies indicate that the day-to-day variation in urinary albumin excretion rate is quite high, both in normal and diabetic patients with normal as well as elevated albumin excretion rates. Usually, the coefficient of variation is around 40%(8). In consequence, it is generally recommended to include at least three urine samples before classifying patients. However, assuming that the relative variance from day to day is 40 per cent, even a single urine sample will usually allow for classification of patients (8). However, there are certainly exceptions, for instance a high excretion rate may rapidly return to normal, and since measurement of excretion rate is quite easy, multiple collections can strongly be recommended.

There are several factors that are known to increase the urinary albumin excretion rate (9, 11, 15). The most important factor relevant to daily life is physical exercise, but very poor metabolic control is also important. Moderate physical exercise increases urinary albumin excretion rate considerably in patients with microalbuminuria, and also in some patients with a normal albumin excretion rate (Figure 3)(17-19). Since excretion rate may increase considerably by exercise, physical exercise should obviously be avoided when collecting urines.

At present the predictive value of exercise-induced microalbuminuria is not known, but preliminary evidence suggests that exercise-induced microalbuminuria is not predictive of nephropathy. Interestingly, a physical exercise test may be used to evaluate the effect of treatment, especially antihypertensive treatment with both beta-blockers and ACE inhibitors (18, 20).

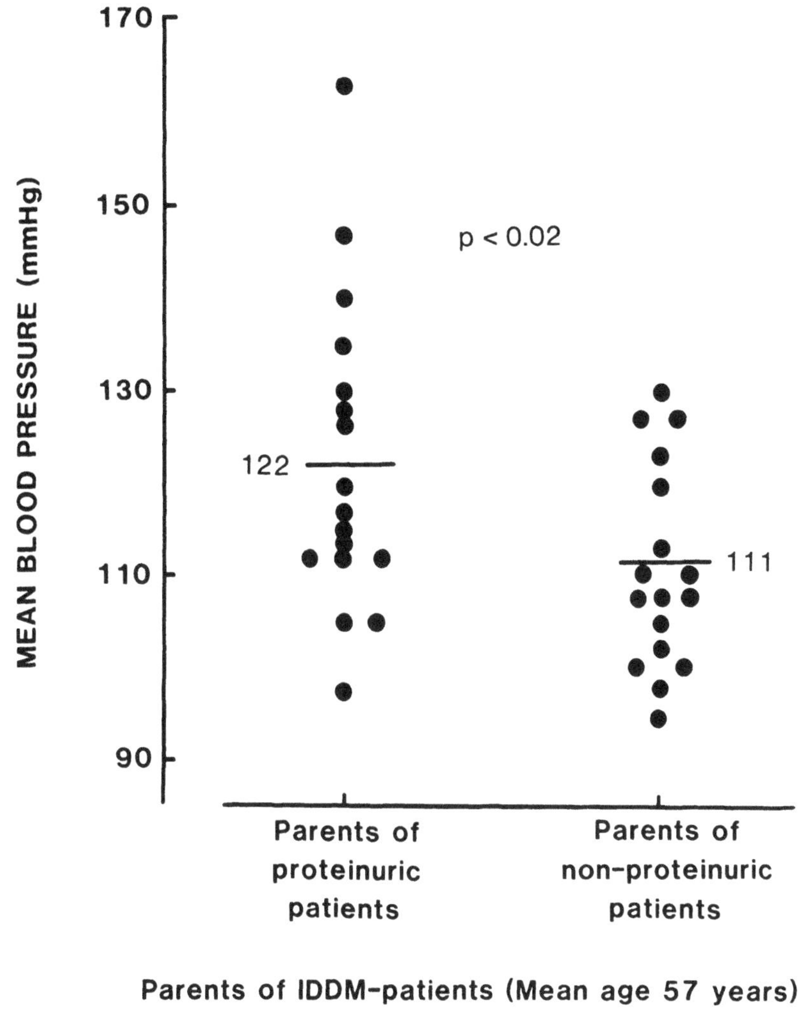

Figure 4. Mean blood pressure in parents with higher arterial pressure of 17 proteinuric (propositi) and 17 non-proteinuric (controls) diabetic patients. Bars are means. Difference between sample means 11 mm Hg (95% confidence interval 1.7 to 20.3 mm Hg; $t = 2.6$, $df = 16$, $p < 0.02$). (From Viberti GC, Keen H, Wiseman MJ: Raised arterial pressure in parents of proteinuric insulin dependent diabetics. Br Med J, 295: 515-517, 1987).

IV. DOES PARENTAL PREDISPOSITION TO HYPERTENSION PREDICT MICROALBUMINURIA AND DIABETIC NEPHROPATHY?

Although development of diabetic nephropathy is to some extent associated with poor metabolic control, there seems to be a considerable overlap in the level of HbA1c in patients with and without microalbuminuria/proteinuria. Therefore, genetic determinants for susceptibility to nephropathy have been suspected. It has been suggested that raised blood pressure may not be a consequence of renal disease, but rather an independent marker which confers susceptibility to renal disease if diabetes is present. This hypothesis was recently tested by Viberti et al. (21) by examining parents of proteinuric diabetics and matched diabetic controls without renal disease. Blood pressure may be significantly elevated in parents of proteinuric diabetics as seen in Figure 4. Krolewski et al. (22) recently published similar findings, and this group reported that having a parent with hypertension tripled the risk of nephropathy and the risk was even higher in patients who also had poor glycemic control during the first decade of diabetes. Mediation of blood pressure increase through familial sharing of environmental factors cannot, of course, be excluded. Both groups (21, 23) also found significantly higher values for maximal velocity of lithium-sodium counter-transport in red cells (a parameter believed to be a marker of essential hypertension, at least in some patients).

New studies from Copenhagen have not, however, confirmed these results (24). The Copenhagen study was very well planned. The number of patients required to document differences, not only with regard to blood pressure elevation in parents of diabetic patients with and without nephropathy, but also the level of sodium lithium counter transport activity in erythrocytes, was determined before start of the prospective study. The reason for discrepancy with previous studies is not clear, but no trend at all was observed in the Copenhagen study. Therefore, widespread clinical consequences should not be drawn from the London and Boston studies at the present time.

V. HIGH BLOOD PRESSURE BEFORE THE ONSET OF DIABETES MAY PREDICT MICROALBUMINURIA AND DIABETIC NEPHROPATHY IN CERTAIN NIDDM PATIENTS

Interesting data have recently been published by Knowler et al. (25) on long-term follow-up studies in Pima Indians. In these special NIDDM patients blood pressure prior to development of diabetes was recorded and subsequently albumin excretion was studied. In these patients (without proteinuria before onset of type II diabetes) pre-diabetic blood pressure appeared to be significantly higher in those who later developed diabetic nephropathy. Patients were followed for a mean of 5 years (range 0-19 years) after diagnosis of diabetes. Abnormal albumin excretion rate (higher than the level of 100 mg albumin per 24 hours) was found in 12%, 26% and 36% of subjects, whose pre-diabetic systolic blood pressure had been <140, 140-159 or ≥ 160 mm Hg (p<0.01). Thus, this study suggests that blood pressure before onset of diabetes (essential hypertension?) predicts an abnormal albumin excretion rate in type II diabetes. This means that elevated blood pressure is not entirely the result of renal disease, at least in this population, but may proceed or even contribute to development of nephropathy.

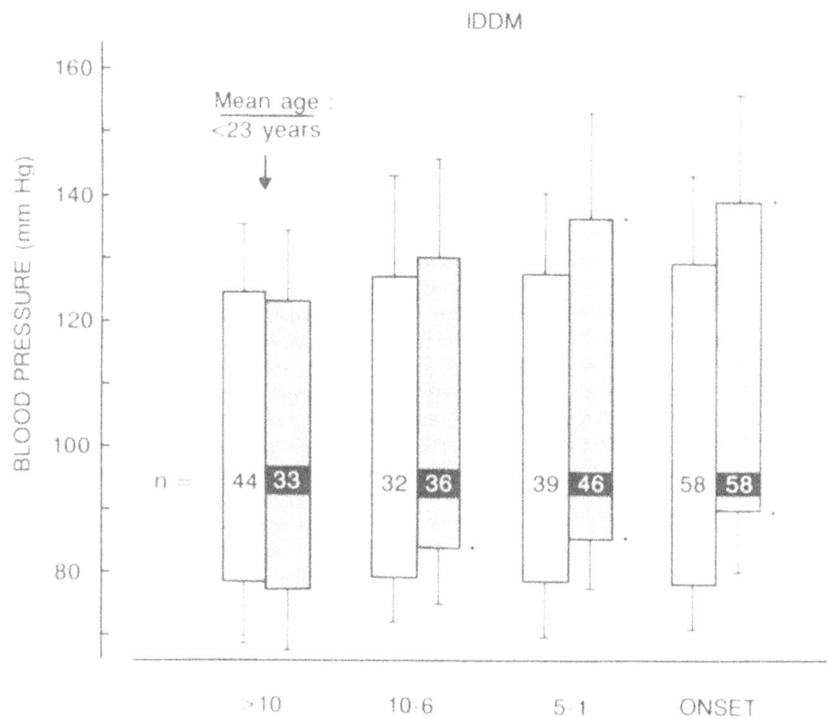

Figure 5. Blood pressure in the years before onset of proteinuria, in patients with diabetic nephropathy (gray columns) and comparable controlled patients (white columns) (* = significant increase). (From Jensen T, Borch-Johnsen K, Deckert T: Changes in blood pressure and renal function in patients with type I (insulin-dependent) diabetes mellitus prior to clinical diabetic nephropathy. Diabetes Res, 4: 159-162, 1987).

Such studies are difficult to conduct in type I diabetes, and no longitudinal follow-up study is available. As shown in Figure 5, it is also clear that blood pressure in diabetic patients prior to nephropathy is quite normal in type I diabetic patients who are later developing this complication (26). The pre-diabetic blood pressure must also have been normal. Thus, important differences seem to exist between the two types of diabetes. This may be related to obesity (and as a consequence higher peripheral insulin levels), which is quite often seen in NIDDM-patients, in particular the Pima Indians. There are no data available on the level of GFR before onset of diabetes. Thus, a possible link between prediabetic hyperfiltration and late nephropathy cannot be evaluated. However, high GFR at the onset of IDDM is not predictive of nephropathy (27).

VI. THE TRANSITION FROM NORMOALBUMINURIA TO MICROALBUMINURIA IN IDDM DEPENDS UPON POOR METABOLIC CONTROL

The transition from normoalbuminuria to microalbuminuria is a very important phase in the course of IDDM.

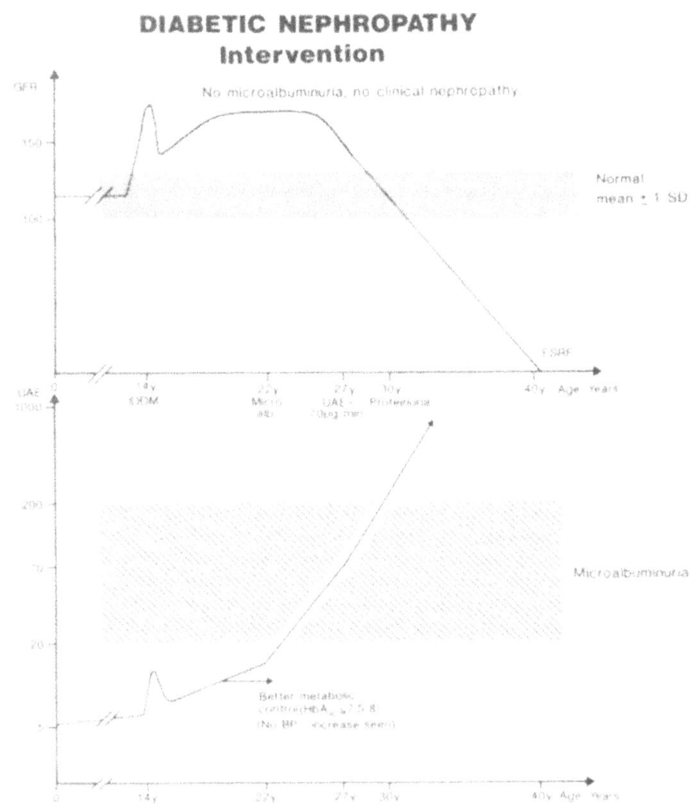

Figure 6. The course of diabetic nephropathy, the spontaneous course and the perspective of better control before the development of microalbuminuria.

Longitudinal studies over 4 years have now revealed that patients who develop microalbuminuria had already had albumin excretion rates in the upper normal range before the microalbuminuric level was reached. Therefore, such patients with "high normal" UAER should be followed carefully. It has also been shown that patients who develop microalbuminuria have a higher level of glycated hemoglobin than persisting normoalbuminuric patients. Indeed, the study by Mathiesen et al. (28) showed that the mean value of glycated hemoglobin in these patients was always above 7.5-8 %, as evaluated by multiple measurements. If glycated hemoglobin is below 8%, the risk of developing microalbuminuria was negligeable in a 4-year follow-up. On the other hand there are patients whose albumin excretion rate remains normal in spite of elevated levels of glycated hemoglobin. The cause of this "protection" is not clear, but low-normal blood pressure (seen in long-term survivors of diabetes) may play a role (29). Blood pressure, on the other hand, appears to be quite normal before the development of microalbuminuria, but rises a few years after microalbuminuria is clearly established. Importantly, this study suggests that the early phase of microalbuminuria is more closely related to poor metabolic control than to blood pressure elevation. Soon after development of microalbuminuria, however, an elevation in blood pressure, albeit small, is clearly established (11, 28). Figure 6 outlines the natural history of renal changes in diabetes and the possibility of early metabolic intervention.

VII. POOR METABOLIC CONTROL AND ELEVATED BLOOD PRESSURE DETERMINE PROGRESSION OF MICROALBUMINURIA IN INCIPIENT DIABETIC NEPHROPATHY

Two main factors have been identified as determinants for the rate of progression in patients with established microalbuminuria: quality of glycemic control as measured by HbA1c and blood pressure level (Figures 7a and 7b). Both factors must be evaluated by multiple measurements. When studying diabetic populations there is usually not a major difference in quality of metabolic control between normoalbuminuric and microalbuminuric patients, although the latter patients always tend to have poorer metabolic control. However, when looking at progression of microalbuminuria, e.g. percentage increase per year, the rate of increase in microalbuminuria is positively correlated with glycemic control as measured by level of HbA1c. This correlation was identified only when intensified metabolic control was introduced in some of the patients in a controlled clinical trial thereby including a rather wide range of quality of metabolic control; a correlation could thus be more easily established. If HbA1c values were below a level of 7.5-8%, progression rate was generally slow and even regression could be observed (30).

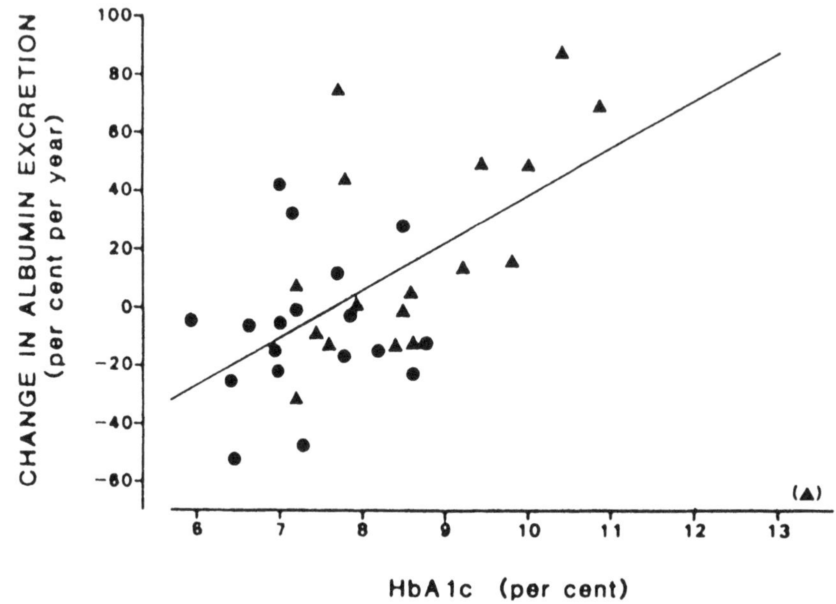

Figure 7a. Correlation between long-term metabolic control (as indicated by mean HbA1C from third month of study) and change in urinary albumin excretion. Closed circles represent patients receiving continuous subcutaneous insulin infusion (n = 18), closed triangles those receiving unchanged conventional treatment (n = 18). Correlation for conventional-treatment group (n = 17, excluding anorexia patient shown in parentheses): $r = 0.61$, $p < 0.005$. Correlation for insulin-infusion group (n = 18): $r = 0.13$, NS. Correlation for both groups (n = 35): $r = 0.57$, $p < 0.001$.

The other important factor is level of blood pressure, or, more importantly, an increase in the blood pressure level during the observation period. If mean arterial blood pressure is below 100 mm Hg (e.g. approximately corresponding to a systolic value of 130 and a diastolic value of 85), progression is usually quite slow (10, 31). The relative importance of the two abnormalities, blood pressure and metabolic control, has not been exactly defined. For instance, will pharmacological blood pressure reduction mean that patients are less susceptible to renal disease, even in spite of poor or semi-poor control of metabolism?

VIII. THE MECHANISMS OF ELEVATED BLOOD PRESSURE IN MICROALBUMINURIC PATIENTS CAN BE DEFINED

The development of arterial hypertension in IDDM-patients is closely related to the time of onset of microalbuminuria and blood pressure is further elevated in the presence of clinical proteinuria. Blood pressure usually starts to rise some years after development of microalbuminuria. The mean increase in mean blood pressure is around 3 per cent per year indicating that progression from normotension to clearly elevated blood pressure usually takes about 5 to 10 years.

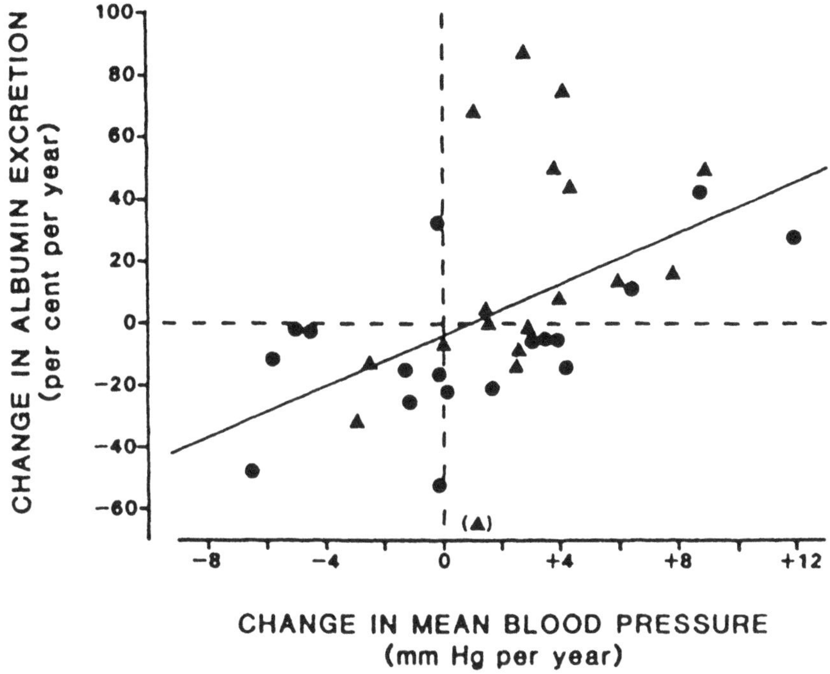

Figure 7b. Correlation between annual change in mean blood pressure and annual change in urinary albumin excretion. Closed circles represent patients receiving continuous subcutaneous insulin infusion ($n = 18$), closed triangles those receiving unchanged conventional treatment ($n = 18$). Both groups: $n = 36$: $r = 0.49$, $p < 0.001$. Conventional-treatment group: $r = 0.45$, $p < 0.05$. Insulin-infusion group: $r = 0.57$, $p < 0.01$.

Some progress has been made regarding the understanding of the pathophysiology of hypertension in diabetic patients. Exchangeable sodium is elevated in diabetic patients, and among microalbuminuric and proteinuric patients a correlation between blood pressure and the degree of exchangeable sodium has been documented (Figure 8) (32).

It has been proposed that blood pressure starts to increase in IDDM patients, if the increased GFR starts to decline. This impaired renal function may cause increased sodium retention.

The decline in GFR may be explained by a number of factors, including mesangial expansion. However, mesangial expansion may in turn be worsened by blood pressure elevation (33).

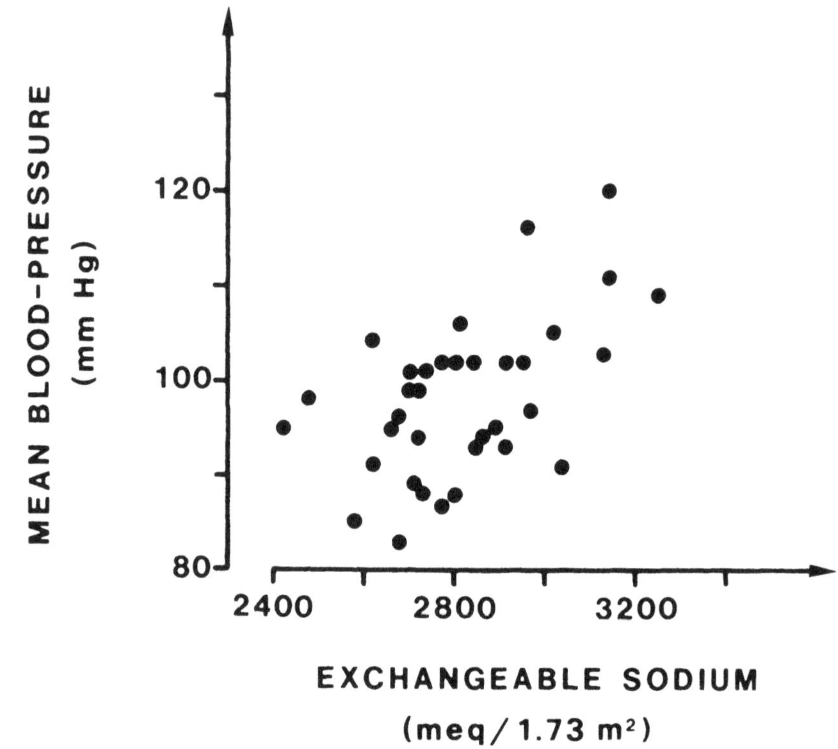

Figure 8. Exchangeable sodium versus mean blood pressure in 35 type 1 (insulin-dependent) diabetic patients with elevated urinary albumin excretion (30-300 mg/24 h, i.e. incipient diabetic nephropathy); $r = 0.54$, $p < 0.001$. (From Feldt-Rasmussen B, Mathiesen ER, Deckert T, Giese J, Christensen NJ, Bent-Hansen L, Nielsen MD: Central role for sodium in the pathogenesis of blood pressure changes independent of angiotensin, aldosterone and catecholamines in type 1 (insulin-dependent) diabetes mellitus. Diabetologia, 30: 610-617, 1987).

IX. MORTALITY AND MICROALBUMINURIA IS ASSOCIATED IN IDDM AND NIDDM PATIENTS

The predictive value of microalbuminuria for nephropathy in insulin-dependent patients was established in several long-term follow-up studies (3-7). Long-term prognosis of these patients is of considerable interest and a 14-year follow-up of 12 patients with increasing microalbuminuria has recently been completed (27). Three of these patients died during the observation period. Only one patient of 27 without microalbuminuria died, due to myocardial infarction. All but two of the microalbuminuric diabetics developed clinical proteinuria and 7 showed decline in renal function as indicated by increase in serum creatinine. Four developed considerably reduced renal function or end-stage renal failure. Two patients showed regression in microalbuminuria but only because of early antihypertensive treatment. Thus IDDM patients with microalbuminuria carry a sinister long-term prognosis, unless early intervention is effective (Table 1).

Table 1. Fourteen-year follow-up on IDDM patients with microalbuminuria. (From Mogensen CE, Schmitz A, Christensen CK: Comparative renal pathophysiology relevant to IDDM and NIDDM patients. Diabetes/Metabolism Reviews, 4: 453-483, 1988).

		Follow-up data				
Patient	Initial UAER µg/min	Years since initial examination	Clinical proteinuria g/l	Serum Creatinine µmol/l	BP mm Hg	Retinopathy degree
1	30,6	14	5,5	98	140/90	simplex
2	22,1	13	no**	77	115/90*	simplex
3	30,6	11	1,4	113	130/90*	prolif.
4	25,6	13	1,2	78	135/85*	prolif.
5	22,2	11	3,6	233	185/105*	prolif.
6	44,0	13	5,8	331	185/110*	blind
7+	15,0	18	6,2	ESRF	160/105*	prolif.
8	22,0	14	no**	75	140/90*	simplex
9	27,3	17	1,7	128	160/100*	prolif.
10	70,1	12	1,9	83	140/85*	prolif.
11+	70,6	17	4,2	133	175/125*	prolif.
12+	96,3	17	+++	ESRF	160/110	prolif.

+ = died; * = on treatment; ** = before treatment; ESRF = end-stage renal failure. (Follow-up of data from N Eng J Med, 311: 89-93, 1984).

In NIDDM-patients the impact on mortality of microalbuminuria as well as other risk factors has also been investigated in a 10-year follow-up study of 503 predominantly NIDDM patients (34). The main purpose of the study was to evaluate mortality according to albumin excretion: 265 patients died. Using Cox regression analysis the prognostic influence of age, sex, age at diagnosis, known diabetes duration, blood pressure, fasting plasma glucose, relative weight, serum creatinine, retinopathy and treatment modality was evaluated in addition to urinary albumin concentration. Morning urinary albumin concentration (UAC) was divided into four categories, i.e. UAC $\leq$ 15 µg/ml (strictly normal), 15-40 µg/ml, 40-200 µg/ml and UAC > 200 µg/ml. Age, UAC, known duration and serum creatinine were the only significant risk factors that could be identified. After correction for the other three independent risk factors, the mortality due to elevated UAC remained highly statistically significant (Figure 9). Fasting plasma glucose was correlated to UAC, but only weakly, and increased UAC was also associated with retinopathy.

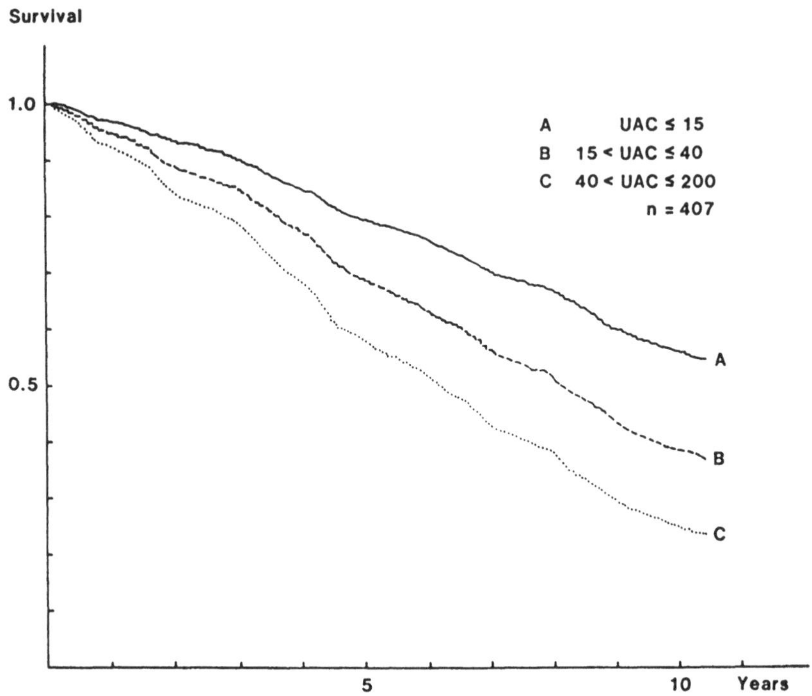

Figure 9. Survival curves for the three UAC groups after correction for age, diabetes duration and serum creatinine; n = 407, subjects with missing value(s) excluded. (From Schmitz A. Microalbuminuria and mortality in non-insulin-dependent diabetes. In: "The Kidney and Hypertension in Diabetes Mellitus" (Ed. CE Mogensen), Martinus Nijhoff Publishing, Boston, 1988, pp 65-70).

A recent prospective 6-year follow-up study has confirmed the predictive power of microalbuminuria with respect to early mortality in NIDDM. Interestingly, an increase in mortality according to albumin excretion could also be seen in non-diabetic controls, although at a lower level (35). Patients with NIDDM generally die from cardiovascular disease, not from uremia.

X. MECHANISM OF RENAL PROTECTION BY TREATMENT. - DOES IT HELP TO EXPLAIN DEVELOPMENT OF NEPHROPATHY?

After the start of antihypertensive treatment a fall in urinary protein or albumin excretion is seen both in incipient (36, 37) and overt nephropathy (38, 39) in IDDM patients. This finding shows that protein excretion is partially pressure-dependent and also seems to suggest that reduction of blood pressure will induce a fall in intraglomerular pressure. Thus glomerular hypertension may be influenced by systemic antihypertensive treatment in these patients, also during exercise (18, 19). A low protein diet is also associated with a fall in protein excretion and hyperfiltration, probably also due to a fall in intraglomerular pressure (40-42). Hyperfiltration can be reduced by a diet lower in protein than the usual protein-rich diabetic diet (41, 42). The effect of optimised insulin treatment is less striking, but still in concert with a reduction of intraglomerular pressure (43).

Table 2. Effects of intervention modalities. (From Mogensen CE: Therapeutic interventions in nephropathy of IDDM. Diabetes Care, 11 (Suppl.1): 10-15, 1988).

Test Parameter	Insulin (pumps)	Antihypertensive: ACE Inhibition	Antihypertensive: Non-ACE Inhibition	Low Protein Diet
Hyperfiltration	Long-term ↓ GFR 5%	↓FF	No studies	↓GFR
Borderline elevated UAER	Normalization	No studies	No studies	No studies
Persistent microalbuminuria	Stabilization	Somewhat ↓	Long-term regression	↓ on a short-term basis
Proteinuria without ↑ BP possibly with ↓ GFR	No studies	Studies ongoing	No studies	↓ fall rate in GFR and proteinuria
Proteinuria, ↑ BP, ↓ GFR	No effect in small series (does not rule out an effect)	May reduce progression	Cardioselective ß-blockers and diuretics reduce decline in GFR	No studies

UAER = urinary albumin excretion rate; BP = blood pressure; GFR = glomerular filtration rate; FF = filtration fraction; ↑ = Increased; ↓ = decreased.

It can be hypothesized that during antihypertensive treatment (and also with a low protein diet) relatively healthy glomeruli survive due to a decrease in glomerular capillary pressure. On the other hand, those glomeruli already in the phase of being destroyed soon become totally occluded and thus do not leak protein. Induction of good metabolic control may operate by similar mechanisms. This hypothetical mechanism explains the long-term beneficial effect of antihypertensive treatment seen in diabetic patients. Proteinuria is reduced and rate of decline in GFR can be lowered from about 1 ml/min/month to 0.35 ml/min/month or less, by reducing blood pressure from a level of 160/95 to 135/85 mm Hg (38, 39). Even more optimistic results are obtained in incipient diabetic nephropathy where antihypertensive treatment produces a short-term and a long-term reduction in UAER, while GFR on a long-term basis is well preserved (36, 37). Table 2 outline results of a clinical trial carried out during the last few years (44).

XI. MANY VASCULAR ABNORMALITIES ARE ASSOCIATED WITH MICROALBUMINURIA IN INCIPIENT DIABETIC NEPHROPATHY

Many studies suggest that patients with microalbuminuria are in the process of developing multiple vascular lesions (Table 3), and microalbuminuria or increased rate of microalbuminuria are easily measurable indicators of disease activity. Several studies have shown a 5 to 10 per cent elevation of blood pressure in patients with microalbuminuria compared to normoalbuminuric patients (10, 16-19, 30, 45-48), although there is a considerable overlap between groups. Blood pressure has been found to correlate significantly with rising UAER, also expressed as per cent per year (10, 30). Diastolic elevation is in particular characteristic of patients with rising UAER. Because hypertension parallels the rise in UAER, it is difficult to determine which abnormality is primary, although early rise in UAER seems to be the initial abnormality. A recent study from Japan (2) reported that glomerular lesions, diffuse and nodular, as well as arteriolar hyalinosis are found more commonly in patients with microalbuminuria, but not to the extent seen in macroproteinuric patients.

Table 3. Abnormalities associated with microalbuminuria in incipient diabetic nephropathy (IDDM). (From Mogensen CE, Schmitz A, Christensen CK: Comparative renal pathophysiology relevant to IDDM and NIDDM patients. Diabetes/Metabolism Reviews, 4: 453-483, 1988).

1. Renal structural damage already present (degree of abnormality between normo- and macroalbuminuria).
2. Still well-preserved renal function, early in incipient diabetic nephropathy still some hyperfiltration.
3. Without intervention about 80% will develop overt diabetic nephropathy.
4. More advanced retinopathy, predicted to worsen.
5. Increased blood pressure, increasing by about 3-4% per year (without intervention).
6. More advanced neuropathy.
7. Evidence of increased general vascular damage, i.g., increased transcapillary escape of albumin.
8. Decreased aerobic working capacity.
9. Unfavorable lipid profiles.
10. Glycemic control poorer than in normoalbuminuria, but with considerable overlap.

Although microalbuminuria also predicts proliferative diabetic retinopathy (49), there is a somewhat inconsistent relationship between retinopathy and nephropathy (50). Patients with a normal UAER may show rather advanced retinal lesions, although there is most often a good correlation between retinopathy and UAER.

It has recently been shown that patients with slight degrees of microalbuminuria show increased left ventricular contractility as measured by ultrasound technique (51). Thereafter, with increasing albumin excretion and overt nephropathy, contractility decreases, probably because of advancing cardiac disease in patients with nephropathy and hypertension.

Patients with microalbuminuria and associated increases in blood pressure exhibit more generalized vascular disease and leakage of albumin (52), impaired aerobic work capacity (53), and new studies suggest adverse lipid abnormalities, not only in overt, but also in incipient nephropathy (54). Diabetic patients with incipient nephropathy characteristically exhibit sodium retention, perhaps related to peripheral hyperinsulinism (32).

XII. MICROALBUMINURIA IS OF DIFFERENT NATURE IN IDDM AND NIDDM PATIENTS

As pointed out earlier, microalbuminuria is predictive of renal disease and to some extent increased mortality in IDDM patients. In NIDDM patients microalbuminuria clearly predicts early mortality whereas relatively few patients develop end-stage renal disease, instead patients die from cardiovascular disease (34). Therefore, it might be anticipated that microalbuminuria is of a different nature in the two types of diabetes, and there are certain indications that this is indeed the case although, of course, a number of similarities exist (55).

Microalbuminuria is very rarely seen in IDDM patients during the first five years of diabetes, whereas microalbuminuria is observed with all durations in NIDDM patients, probably because of the long silent phase of IDDM before clinical diagnosis, when renal and vascular damage may already have occurred (55). In IDDM patients microalbuminuria is to some extent associated with poor metabolic control, although overlap is great. However, in some studies the level of glycemic control seems to be approximately at the same in the two types of diabetes. Early in the course of microalbuminuria hyperfiltration may be found, in some patients even quite striking hyperfiltration with GFR values above 150 ml/min (reference values mean 114±14 ml/min ±SD) (10). No such hyperfiltration has been found in NIDDM patients (27).

This difference may be due to an age effect suggesting that hyperfiltration may not develop readily in elderly persons. However, renal hypertrophy has been established both in IDDM and NIDDM patients, particularily in microalbuminuric patients although there is a great overlap between normoalbuminuria and microalbuminuria with respect to renal size in the two types of diabetes (56).

Progression of microalbuminuria is rather well defined in IDDM patients. The mean increase in the albumin excretion rate per year is usually around 15-20%, depending upon blood pressure and metabolic control (10, 30). Follow-up studies have been carried out in NIDDM-patients only to a limited extent and the natural history of microalbuminuria is far less established in this type of diabetes.

Table 4. Differences in advanced nephropathy or ESRF between IDDM and NIDDM patients in the Western World. (From Mogensen CE, Schmitz A, Christensen CK: Comparative renal pathophysiology relevant to IDDM and NIDDM patients. Diabetes/Metabolism Reviews, 4: 453-483, 1988).

	IDDM	NIDDM
Age	40-50	60-70
Sex	M > F (1.7:1)	M = F
Race	European	Afro, Caribbean, or Asian*
Known diabetes duration	Long (e.g. > 20 yr)	May develop ESRF within first 5 years of known disease
Decline in renal function	10 ml/min/yr (without treatment)	May be slower, but not studied
% of death from renal failure	25%	3-5% (in Europe)
Associated diabetic complications	Often retinopathy, neuropathy, and cardiovascular diseases	Similar to IDDM

* Nonwhites develop NIDDM at an earlier age.

There also seem to be considerable differences with respect to intervention. Antihypertensive treatment is able to reduce microalbuminuria in IDDM patients, not only on a short-term but also a long-term basis, when patients are followed for one or several years (36, 37). Such long-term studies have not been published in NIDDM-patients (57), and the long-term beneficial effect of antihypertensive treatment is less clear in these patients.

Also, the role of better metabolic control in ameliorating progression of microalbuminuria is suggested in IDDM-patients, but so far there is no such evidence in NIDDM-patients, although early normalization of metabolic derangement at the clinical diagnosis results in a clear reduction in microalbuminuria, also in NIDDM-patients (58).

As mentioned earlier, microalbuminuria is a clear predictor of early mortality in NIDDM patients, mainly due to cardiovascular disease, rather than to renal disease. The microalbuminuria in NIDDM-patients may reflect a generalized increase in the permeability of the vessels, not only in the kidney, but also in the heart and the arterial system, conferring a risk towards increased arteriosclerosis. This abnormality is also be seen in IDDM-patients (52), but it can be anticipated that these rather young patients develop end-stage renal disease before fatal cardiovascular disease. Table 4 outlines difference in advanced nephropathy between the two types of diabetes (27).

FINAL REMARKS

Microalbuminuria is now a well-established indicator of early renal disease, and is at present used in many clinics throughout Europe. In the US the test is also becoming increasingly popular (16). When classifying patients both in the clinical and in the research situation, stratification according to albumin excretion rate is clearly important. Microalbuminuria is interesting not only with respect to the diagnosis of renal involvement, but also with respect to cardiovascular disease, in particular in NIDDM-patients. Regarding intervention microalbuminuria is an easy marker for the efficacy of therapy, e.g. antihypertensive treatment, better metabolic control, or the protein reduced diet. The number of papers on microalbuminuria is rapidly increasing, and probably we are only in the beginning of an era, where we will achieve better and better understanding of the main complications of diabetes of both types.

ACKNOWLEDGEMENT

Sally M. Marshall is a British medical research council travelling fellow.

REFERENCES

1. Mogensen CE, Chachati A, Christensen CK, Close CF, Deckert T, Hommel E, Kastrup J, Lefebvre P, Mathiesen ER, Feldt-Rasmussen B, Schmitz A, and Viberti GC: Microalbuminuria: an early marker of renal involvement in diabetes. Uremia Invest, 9: 85-95, 1985-86.
2. Inomata S, Oosawa Y, Itoh M, Inoue M, Masamune O: Analysis of urinary proteins in diabetes mellitus - with reference to the relationship between microalbuminuria and diabetic renal lesions. J Japan Diab Soc, 30: 429-435, 1987.
3. Viberti GC, Jarrett RJ, Mahmud U, Hill RD, Argyropoulos A, Keen H: Microalbuminuria as a predictor of clinical nephropathy in insulin-dependent diabetes mellitus. Lancet, I: 1430-1434, 1982.
4. Mogensen CE: Microalbuminuria predicts clinical proteinuria and early mortality in maturity-onset diabetes. N Engl J Med, 310: 356-360, 1984.
5. Mogensen CE, Christensen CK: Predicting diabetic nephropathy in insulin-dependent patients. N Engl J Med, 311: 89-93, 1984.
6. Mathiesen ER, Oxenbøll B, Johansen K, Svendsen PA, Deckert T: Incipient nephropathy in type I (insulin-dependent) diabetes. Diabetologia, 26: 406-410, 1984.
7. Parving H-H, Oxenbøll B, Svendsen PA, Christensen JS, Andersen AR: Early detection of patients at risk of developing diabetic nephropathy. A longitudinal study of urinary albumin excretion. Acta Endocrinol (Copenh), 100: 550-555, 1982.
8. Feldt-Rasmussen B. Microalbuminuria and clinical nephropathy in type 1 (insulin-dependent) diabetes mellitus: Pathophysiological mechanisms and intervention studies. Dan Med Bull, 1989 (in press).
9. Mogensen CE: Microalbuminuria as a predictor of clinical diabetic nephropathy. Kidney Int, 31: 673-689, 1987.
10. Christensen CK, Mogensen CE: The course of incipient diabetic nephropathy: Studies of albumin excretion and blood pressure. Diab Med, 2: 97-102, 1985.
11. Mogensen CE: Diabetic renal involvement and disease in patients with insulin-dependent diabetes. In: "The Diabetes Annual/4" (Eds. KGMM Alberti, LP Krall), Elsevier Science Publishers, B.V., 1988, pp 411-448.
12. Gatling W, Rowe DJF, Hill RD: Microalbuminuria: an appraisal of assay techniques and urine collection procedures for measuring urinary albumin at low concentrations. In: "The Kidney and Hypertension in Diabetes Mellitus" (Ed. CE Mogensen), Martinus Nijhoff Publishing, Boston, 1988, pp 41-50.
13. Hutchinson AS, Paterson KR: Collecting urine for microalbumin assay. Diab Med, 5: 527-532, 1988.
14. Hutchinson AS, O'Reilly DStJ: Albumin excretion rate, albumin concentration, and albumin/creatinine ratio compared for screening diabetics for slight albuminuria. Clin Chem, 34: 2019-2021, 1988.
15. Mogensen CE: Microalbuminuria and kidney function. Notes on methods, interpretation, and classification. In: "Methods in Diabetes Research, Volume II: Clinical Methods" (Eds. WL Clarke, J Larner, SL Pohl), John Wiley & Sons, New York, Chichester, Brisbane, Toronto, Singapore, 1986, pp. 611-622.
16. Consensus Statement. Am J Kidney Dis, 13: 2-6, 1989.
17. Feldt-Rasmussen B, Baker L, Deckert T: Exercise as a provocative test in early renal disease in type 1 (insulin-dependent) diabetes: albuminuric, systemic and renal hemodynamic responses. Diabetologia, 28: 389-396, 1985.
18. Romanelli G, Giustina A, Cimino A, Valentini U, Agabiti-Rosei E, Muiesan G, Giustina G: Short term effect of captopril on microalbuminuria induced by exercise in normotensive diabetics. Br Med J, 298: 284-288, 1989.
19. Christensen CK: Abnormal albuminuria and blood pressure rise in incipient diabetic nephropathy induced by exercise. Kidney Int, 25: 819-823, 1984.
20. Christensen CK, Mogensen CE: Acute and long-term effect of antihypertensive treatment on exercise-induced albuminuria in incipient diabetic nephropathy. Scand J Clin Lab Invest, 46: 553-559, 1986.

21. Viberti GC, Keen H, Wiseman MJ: Raised arterial pressure in parents of proteinuric insulin dependent diabetics. Br Med J, 295: 515-517, 1987.
22. Krolewski AS, Canessa M, Warram JH, Laffel LMB, Christlieb AR, Knowler WC, Rand LI: Predisposition to hypertension and susceptibility to renal disease in insulin-dependent diabetes mellitus. N Eng J Med, 318: 140-145, 1988.
23. Mangili R, Bending JJ, Scott G, Li LK, Gupta A, Viberti GC: Increased sodium-lithium countertransport activity in red cells of patients with insulin-dependent diabetes and nephropathy. N Eng J Med, 318: 146-150, 1988.
24. Nørgaard K, Jensen JS, Mathiesen ER, Hommel E, Borch-Johnsen K, Funder J, Brahm J, Parving H-H, Deckert T. Increased blood pressure and red cell sodium/lithium countertransport activity are not inherited in diabetic nephropathy. Second Meeting of the European Diabetic Nephropathy Study Group. Workshop on renal pharmacology and factors affecting the renal vascular barrier. May 12-13, 1989, Aarhus, Denmark, 1989 (Abstract).
25. Knowler WC, Bennett PH, Nelson RG, Saad MF, Pettitt DJ: Blood pressure before the onset of diabetes predicts albuminuria in Type 2 (non-insulin-dependent) diabetes (Abstract). Diabetologia, 31: 509A, 1988.
26. Jensen T, Borch-Johnsen K, Deckert T: Changes in blood pressure and renal function in patients with type I (insulin-dependent) diabetes mellitus prior to clinical diabetic nephropathy. Diabetes Res, 4: 159-162, 1987
27. Mogensen CE, Schmitz A, Christensen CK: Comparative renal pathophysiology relevant to IDDM and NIDDM patients. Diabetes/Metabolism Reviews, 4: 453-483, 1988.
28. Mathiesen ER, Rønn B, Jensen T, Storm B, Deckert T: Microalbuminuria is prior to elevation in blood pressure in diabetic nephropathy. In 1st Workshop on Blood Pressure and Diabetic Nephropathy: Pathogenesis and Treatment. EDNSG, Pisa, 1988 (Abstract).
29. Borch-Johnsen K, Nissen H, Henriksen E, Kreiner S, Salling N, Deckert T, Nerup J: The natural history of insulin-dependent diabetes mellitus in Denmark: 1. long-term survival with and without late diabetic complications. Diab Med, 47: 363-370, 1987.
30. Feldt-Rasmussen B, Mathiesen E, Deckert T: Effect of two years of strict metabolic control on the progression of incipient nephropathy in insulin-dependent diabetes. Lancet, II: 1300-1304, 1986.
31. Christensen CK, Mogensen CE: Antihypertensive treatment: long-term reversal of progression of albuminuria in incipient diabetic nephropathy. A longitudinal study of renal function. J Diab Compl, 1: 45-52, 1987.
32. Feldt-Rasmussen B, Mathiesen ER, Deckert T, Giese J, Christensen NJ, Bent-Hansen L, Damkjær Nielsen M: Central role for sodium in the pathogenesis of blood pressure changes independent of angiotensin, aldosterone and catecholamines in type 1 (insulin-dependent) diabetes mellitus. Diabetologia, 30: 610-617, 1987.
33. Mauer SM, Steffes MW, Ellis EN, Sutherland DER, Brown DM, Goetz FC: Structural-functional relationships in diabetic nephropathy. J Clin Invest, 74: 1143-1155, 1984.
34. Schmitz A, Væth M: Microalbuminuria - a major risk factor in non-insulin-dependent diabetes. A 10-year follow-up study of 503 patients. Diab Med, 5: 126-134, 1988.
35. Damsgaard EM, Frøland A, Mogensen CE: Microalbuminuria is a strong predictor of 6 year mortality of elderly non-insulin dependent diabetics and non-diabetics. A prospective study. Diabetologia, 31: 483A, 1988.
36. Christensen CK, Mogensen CE: Antihypertensive treatment: long-term reversal of progression of albuminuria in incipient diabetic nephropathy. A longitudinal study of renal function. J Diab Compl, 1: 45-52, 1987.
37. Marre M, Chatellier G, Leblanc H, Guyenne T-T, Ménard J, Passa P: Prevention of diabetic nephropathy with enalapril in normotensive diabetics with microalbuminuria. Br Med J, 297: 1092-1095, 1988.
38. Mogensen CE: Long-term antihypertensive treatment inhibiting progression of diabetic nephropathy. Br Med J, 285: 685-688, 1982.
39. Parving H-H, Andersen AR, Smidt UM, Hommel E, Mathiesen ER, Svendsen PA: Effect of antihypertensive treatment on kidney function in diabetic nephropathy. Br Med J, 294: 1443-1447, 1987.

40. Viberti GC, Dodds RA, Bending JJ, Bognetti E: Non glycemic intervention in diabetic nephropathy: the role of dietary protein intake. In: "The Kidney and Hypertension in Diabetes Mellitus" (Ed. CE Mogensen). Martinus Nijhoff Publishing, Boston, 1988, pp 205-216.

41. Kupin WL, Cortes P, Dumler F, Feldkamp CS, Kilates MC, Levin NW: Effect on renal function of a change from high to moderate protein intake in type I diabetic patients. Diabetes, 36: 73-79, 1987.

42. Pedersen O, Jørgensen FS, Pedersen MM, Møller B, Lykke G, Mogensen CE: The effect of moderate protein restriction on kidney function in normoalbuminuric type 1 diabetic patients. Diabetologia, 31: 530A, 1988.

43. Christensen CK, Christiansen JS, Schmitz A, Christensen T, Hermansen K, Mogensen CE: Effect of continuous subcutaneous insulin infusion on kidney function and size in IDDM patients: A 2 year controlled study. J Diab Compl, 1: 91-95, 1987.

44. Mogensen CE: Therapeutic interventions in nephropathy of IDDM. Diabetes Care, 11 (Suppl.1): 10-15, 1988.

45. Berglund J, Lins P-E, Adamson U, Lins L-E: Microalbuminuria in long-term insulin-dependent diabetes mellitus. Prevalence and clinical characteristics in a normotensive population. Acta Med Scand, 222: 333-338, 1987.

46. Niazy S, Feldt-Rasmussen B, and Deckert T: Microalbuminuria in insulin-dependent diabetes: Prevalence and practical consequences. J Diab Compl, 1: 76-80, 1987.

47. Parving H-H, Hommel E, Mathiesen E, Skøtt P, Edsberg B, Bahnsen M, Lauritzen M, Hougaard P, and Lauritzen E: Prevalence of microalbuminuria, arterial hypertension, retinopathy, and neuropathy in patients with insulin-dependent diabetes. Br Med J, 296: 156-160, 1988.

48. Wiseman M, Viberti G, MacKintosh D, Jarrett RJ, and Keen H: Glycaemia, arterial pressure and micro-albuminuria in type 1 (insulin-dependent) diabetes mellitus. Diabetologia, 26: 401-405, 1984.

49. Vigstrup J, Mogensen CE: Proliferative diabetic retinopathy: At risk patients identified by early detection of microalbuminuria. Acta Ophthalmol, 63: 530-534, 1985.

50. Agardh E, Tallroth G, Bauer B, Cavallin-Sjöberg U, Agardh C-D: Retinopathy and nephropathy in insulin-dependent diabetics: An inconsistent relationship? Diab Med, 4: 248-250, 1987.

51. Thuesen L, Christiansen JS, Mogensen CE, Henningsen: Cardiac hyperfunction in insulin-dependent diabetic patients developing microvascular complications. Diabetes, 37: 851-856, 1988.

52. Feldt-Rasmussen B: Increased transcapillary escape rate of albumin in type 1 (insulin-dependent) diabetic patients with microalbuminuria. Diabetologia, 29: 282-286, 1986.

53. Jensen T, Richter EA, Feldt-Rasmussen B, Kelbæk H, Deckert T: Impaired aerobic work capacity in type I (insulin-dependent) diabetic patients with increased urinary albumin excretion. Br Med J, 1988 (in press).

54. Jensen T, Stender S, Deckert T: Abnormalities in plasma concentrations of lipoproteins and fibrinogen in type 1 (insulin-dependent) diabetic patients with increased urinary albumin excretion. Diabetologia, 31: 142-145, 1988.

55. Marshall SM, Alberti KGMM: Comparison of the prevalence and associated features of abnormal albumin excretion in insulin-dependent and non-insulin-dependent diabetes. Quart J Med, New Series, 70: 61-71, 1989.

56. Schmitz A, Møller A, Christensen T, Mogensen CE: Kidney function and cardiovascular risk factors in non-insulin-dependent diabetics (NIDDM) with microalbuminuria. (submitted for publication), 1989.

57. Schmitz A, Pedersen MM, Mogensen CE: Effects of felodipine on urinary albumin excretion and metabolic control in hypertensive non-insulin-dependent diabetics. (submitted for publication), 1989.

58. Schmitz A, Christensen T: Kidney function in newly diagnosed type 2 diabetic patients before and during treatment. Diabetologia,1989 (in press).

PEDIATRIC NEPHROLOGY

9

MANAGEMENT OF GROWTH RETARDATION IN CHILDREN WITH CHRONIC RENAL DISEASE

THOMAS E. NEVINS AND S. MICHAEL MAUER

Department of Pediatrics, Variety Club Children's Hospital, University of Minnesota, Minneapolis, Minnesota, 55455, USA

INTRODUCTION

Normal growth is the end product of a complex set of cellular, hormonal, and nutritional processes. Disruption of normal growth may result from a wide variety of causes thus, growth velocity represents an exquisitely sensitive barometer of a child's health and well-being. Slow growth is a consistent and pervasive feature of significant uremia in childhood. As such, the correction of impaired growth is both a goal and a critical measure of the adequacy of any approach to conservative or renal replacement therapy.

In general, the extent of uremic growth failure is related to the patient's age at disease onset, as well as to the duration and severity of the renal impairment. When chronic renal failure (CRF) originates in the perinatal period, the adverse impact on growth is particularly profound (1). In addition to the effect on general somatic growth, CRF early in life may also produce devastating deficits of central nervous system growth (acquired microcephaly) and development (2-4).

Given the intricate and delicate process of normal growth, the pathogenesis of uremic growth failure is an extremely complex problem to dissect and correct. Genetic background, nutrition, hormonal influences, osteodystrophy, the nature of the renal disease itself and the age at onset, all play a role in determining the final extent of growth impairment. This review will specifically focus on management strategies directed toward pediatric CRF treated conservatively, by dialysis, or with renal transplantation and concentrate primarily on work published in the last 5 years.

GROWTH MEASUREMENTS

Discussions of growth are incomplete unless major emphasis is accorded to the techniques for documenting growth and analyzing the resultant data. Fortunately, background work on the general topic of human auxology (5) and in the more specific area of children with CRF (6, 7) has already been well done.

Standard measurements which should be recorded include: chronologic age, to two decimal places; height or length, measured with a stable stadiometer or length table; weight; occipital-frontal head circumference, using a non-stretch tape measure; mid-arm circumference; skinfold thickness, using a calibrated skinfold caliper; and pubertal stage (8). Radiologic evaluation of skeletal maturation is obtained on a regular schedule as required (9). The height of both parents should be documented, to allow prediction of the child's adult height and to assist in evaluating the child's present growth curve (9).

Needless to say, any measurements are useless if they are not carefully taken by a trained observer. More reliability is likely if the same individual obtains the sequential measurements. When properly determined, measurements of height or length are reproducible to within 2-3 mm, however, casual measurements may vary by as much as 15 mm (10). The transition from the measurement of recumbent length to standing height should occur at a standard time between 2 and 3 years of age. Similarly care must be exercised to weigh children using the same equipment and while they are comparably clothed. Head circumference should be the maximum value obtained from three attempts. Again care needs to be taken to minimize artifacts resulting from hairstyle. Once measurements are available, it is important to have appropriate comparison standards drawn from the same pediatric population. Fortunately again, contemporary standards are now widely available (11-14).

The mode of data presentation is critical for correct interpretation. The most useful data sets will include: (a) the individual values; (b) those values expressed as the standard deviation (SD) score (or Z-score) for the measurement (height, weight, etc.); (c) actual, calculated growth velocity (for one calendar year); (d) the standard deviation score for the growth velocity derived for each measurement. Growth velocity index (7), growth increment, "actual/expected" ratios and similar presentations are too frail and imprecise to allow an adequate evaluation of patient growth. Moreover, use of the SD scores permits comparisons of normally distributed data, simultaneously factoring out variations arising solely from differences in age and sex. This allows individuals presenting at different ages to be grouped and described by population statistics.

However, the actual dimension of the height SD increases with increasing age through puberty and then decreases. Since this is the case, a stable growth velocity in the normal range will result in a modest improvement in prepubertal SD score, giving the appearance of "catch-up" growth. Furthermore, although very sensitive, growth velocity itself is a somewhat less robust estimate since it sums the inherent errors of two measurements and then projects that value over an interval (usually one year), perhaps ignoring seasonal variations in velocity (10). These problems maybe minimized by obtaining more frequent, reliable measurements prospectively over periods of at least one year or longer. Thus, the most complete patient picture is available if the actual growth data, the derived growth velocity, and the SD scores for each are presented together.

The concept of "catch-up" growth deserves further mention. Each normally growing individual seems to follow a predetermined "channel" on the growth curve, deviations above or below this path will result in a corresponding decrease or increase in growth velocity restoring growth to the "correct" channel. When children are sick for an interval and their growth diminishes, recovery is regularly associated with a period of increased growth leading to true "catch-up" growth (15, 16). Therefore, documentation of actual catch-up growth requires that the individual have an increase in growth velocity above the mean for age (i.e. growth velocity SD > 0.0) and that this increase is sustained long enough to bring the SD score significantly closer to the mean.

DIAGNOSIS

Selecting the most appropriate therapeutic strategy for a child with CRF requires a specific diagnosis. When the uremic patient's course is complicated by growth failure, it is critical to investigate and exclude other causes of poor growth and to not simply assume that the observed growth delay is a secondary consequence of CRF. Specifically, infantile forms of congenital nephrotic syndrome (17), cystinosis (18), the fetal alcohol syndrome (19), some cases of primary oxalosis (20), Lowe's syndrome (21), Jeune's syndrome (22), and XY gonadal dysgenesis (23) are all systemic diseases capable of producing remarkable growth retardation, frequently out of proportion to that seen with the attendant CRF alone. Similarly, infants born prematurely or small for their gestational age, with primary or secondary CRF may have their course further complicated by nonuremic growth delay. In these special cases, growth retardation may persist in the face of very aggressive and otherwise successful CRF therapy. Finally, in individual children with CRF and growth failure, endocrine dysfunction, including hypothyroidism (e.g. cystinosis) or growth hormone deficiency (history of a profound hypotensive episode, cerebral edema {24} or marked hypoglycemia{25}), may warrant further investigation.

CONSERVATIVE (PRE-RENAL REPLACEMENT) THERAPY

As noted by several reviewers (26-29) the management of growth failure in children with significant but moderate CRF is vexing. Although therapeutic approaches have generally emphasized the correction of fluid and electrolyte abnormalities especially acidosis, adequacy of diet, plus supplemental vitamin D, none have been uniformly successful.

The dietary therapy of renal insufficiency has a long history (30, 31). More recent work (32, 33) has refocused on the role of diet in the progression of renal disease and has emphasized the potential importance of reduced dietary protein intake in slowing the rate of decline in renal function in adult patients. However, presently there are no published trials in childhood CRF to provide guidelines for such dietary protein modification while attempting to maintain normal growth. Pediatricians, on the other hand, have generally been more interested in promoting optimal nutritional intake leading to maximal growth (34-38), than in extending the duration of CRF prior to end stage uremia requiring dialysis or transplantation.

In addition to dietary or fluid restrictions a number of other barriers to adequate nutrition may arise. Many children with CRF experience anorexia, the etiology of which is unknown. Especially in younger children, gastroesophageal reflux with vomiting is common and may significantly complicate the struggle to maximize oral intake. In congenital nephrotic syndrome, pyloric stenosis may further hamper feeding efforts. Previously, efforts directed at supplementing children's daily caloric intake to the level of 100% of the RDA for calories (39) have resulted in improvements in serum protein values but less regularly resulted in improved growth.

Studies of children with uremia early in life (40, 41), tend to confirm earlier work (1) suggesting that, after an initial period of lost growth potential, many adequately nourished uremic children will grow at a near normal velocity for age, but do not experience significant "catch-up" growth. However, the question still remains as to whether aggressive medical management without dialysis might be more effective if initiated earlier in infancy when there is maximal growth potential.

A study of infants managed with meticulous attention to nutritional therapy, before dialysis becomes necessary, indicates that some continued growth is possible but this depends upon an adequate diet, maintenance of near normal fluid and electrolyte balance, and the residual endogenous renal function (42). Growth velocity was confirmed as the most sensitive monitor of adequate growth and reinforced the observations of Betts and Magrath (1), that growth was best in those patients maintaining a calculated creatinine clearance (43) greater than 25 ml/min/1.73 m^2. Others (44) have made similar observations but speculated that the uremic infant may represent an especially difficult challenge since normal growth is so rapid and the inherent problems of maintaining salt and water balance, as well as caloric intake are often enormous. In older, nondialyzed children with significant CRF, the common experience is that conservative management, with careful attention to detail (45), can yield and sustain reasonable growth, although the rates are regularly low or below the normal range and lead to a steady decline in SD scores.

It is tempting to speculate that vitamin D, which is activated by renal metabolism and is critical to bone growth might play a major role in the growth failure which is seen in uremic children. In fact, some patients were reported to have benefited from treatment with vitamin D analogs (46). However longer term studies by the same group of investigators did not show substantial growth gains in those patients treated with vitamin D (47). Nonetheless, since bone mineralization and growth without rachitic deformities all depend on adequate vitamin D, appropriate supplementation with calcium and vitamin D analogs, while avoiding hypercalcemia remains an appropriate intervention with all pediatric CRF patients (38).

A core question in this instance is whether either infants or older children with CRF might experience any growth benefit from the earlier initiation of dialysis or renal transplantation. Useful data regarding this question will only arise from carefully controlled prospective intervention trials.

DIALYSIS TREATMENT

Presently, acute hemodialysis or peritoneal dialysis (PD) are available to children of virtually any age or size. In theory, chronic dialysis is also an option for every uremic child. Therefore questions regarding the mode of therapy, when to begin, and the relative risk-benefit ratio arise for each new child presenting with CRF.

Hemodialysis

Chronic hemodialysis has been available to children for approximately 15-20 yrs (48-51). Early reports indicated that chronic hemodialysis could be technically successful either in a medical center (52, 53) or a home setting (54). However these same early reports did not provide encouraging growth data for chronically hemodialyzed children.

More recently, a large, single center study followed 76 children on hemodialysis for at least 1 and for up to 9 yrs (55). Growth was generally discouraging, with children on dialysis falling behind their peers by an average of 0.4 SD/yr of therapy. Skeletal maturation was also significantly delayed. At puberty, growth remained slower than normal, but the pubertal period was prolonged, permitting some improvement in growth to occur and allowing a few children to reach the normal adult range for height. No clear associations between nutrition or medical treatment and growth were identified.

Another recent study of 15 children defined the protein and energy requirements for positive nitrogen balance on hemodialysis (56), but did not extend the observations over a long enough time to address the impact of optimal nutritional therapy on linear growth.

Since that time several series and reviews (57) have confirmed that growth on hemodialysis is generally poor as defined by subnormal growth velocities and declining SD scores. The most recent review of children's growth from the European Dialysis and Transplant Association (EDTA-ERA) registry indicated that among 61 prepubertal children on hemodialysis for at least one year, only 5 grew at rates at or above the mean height velocity for age and the vast majority were greater than 2 SD below the mean (58). But most children in that report did maintain weight for height ratios in the normal range.

In summary, although most children continue to grow, they grow poorly on hemodialysis. Older children who enter puberty while on hemodialysis do have a normal pubertal developmental sequence, but their progress is slowed. Importantly, puberty signals the impending completion of growth in these children and in fact, the Tanner stages correlate more closely with the patients' skeletal age than their chronological age (59). It should be remembered that despite delayed bone age and associated delay in epiphyseal fusion, the frequent blunting of the pubertal growth spurt results in a very diminished adult stature.

Continuous Peritoneal Dialysis

The pioneering work of Moncrief and Popovich (60) in the late 1970's established the usefulness of continuous peritoneal dialysis (PD) in uremic patients. This approach was rapidly adapted to children (61-63), even including small infants (64).

Most recently, the availability of peritoneal dialysis cycling equipment capable of warming, infusing, draining, and accurately measuring dialysate volumes has allowed children and infants to be treated at home with continuous cycling PD regimens (65-68).

The application of continuous cycling PD has dramatically altered the care of young children with CRF. Fluid intake and diet are now virtually unrestricted. Additionally, oral caloric intake maybe bolstered by supplemental nasogastric feedings which are widely available and accepted. Additional calories are available from the dextrose absorbed from the peritoneal cavity. Against this background, initial studies of growth in children on continuous PD were very optimistic (69, 70). Patients frequently seemed to grow at normal or near normal rates.

However, as the numbers of patients and the duration of follow up increased, two things became clearer. First, there were not substantial differences in growth between children treated with CAPD and those receiving CCPD (65, 71, 72). Second, while the growth documented in many continuous PD patients was comparable or even better than that seen on hemodialysis, growth was still suboptimal by comparison to normal children (65, 68, 73).

Current information suggests that supplemental tube-feeding providing more than 100% of the RDA for protein and calories (74) may be of benefit in at least some PD patients. At the same time significant overfeeding leads to frank obesity, without substantial improvements in the child's height (75).

Again another important variable may be the impact of patient age on both growth velocity (65) and SD score (68). But if age has an effect it may not yet be detectable since present studies do not stratify the patients by age.

Finally, although uremia in young children may be associated with a progressive encephalopathy, there are only fragmentary data available to assess brain growth, as well as the developmental and cognitive functioning of children on continuous PD (68, 74, 76, 77). Hopefully, future studies will address these important questions. Some of the variables which will need to be controlled include age, underlying disease, overall nutritional state, infections, duration and type of treatment, and center effects.

RENAL TRANSPLANTATION

Successful renal transplantation has generally been regarded as the ultimate goal of any therapeutic strategy for children with CRF. Theoretically, organ replacement should result in resolution of all the problems arising from CRF *per se* and might permit recovery of those potentially reversible lesions which developed as a consequence of chronic uremia (e.g. anemia, osteodystrophy, growth delay, and developmental delay).

Concern about growth was evident with the earliest studies of pediatric renal transplantation (78, 79) but the first results were mixed and transplantation could not be recommended for its positive impact on growth. However as the experience in individual centers expanded, the age and size of children undergoing transplantation decreased, at the same time however, the long term patient and allograft survivals improved. While these changes were occurring, reported growth results also improved and were better documented.

In 1987, Broyer and coworkers in Paris reported a consecutive series of 358 children who received renal allografts between 1973 and 1984 (80). Among 60 prepubertal children with data available up to seven years after transplantation, there was no improvement in the mean SD scores for height. However, the authors point out that individual growth patterns were quite variable, with 22 of these children experiencing actual "catch-up" growth. Adolescent growth spurts were documented in 18 of 56 pubertal patients in the same series. The remaining adolescents grew at stable or reduced rates, resulting in a reduction in their final adult height.

These authors pointed out that patient age, allograft function, as reflected by serum creatinine, and steroid dosage probably each affected individual growth velocity and final adult height. Although 25% of their transplant recipients experienced "catch-up" growth and most of the patients achieved improved growth with an allograft, they concluded that adequate growth still remained a major concern in all children receiving a renal transplant (80).

Another review of growth in 29 children with allograft function for more than ten years was even more discouraging, finding that the mean SD score actually decreased from -1.8 to -2.3 (81). In that series, only 38% of the patients were in the normal range of adult height at follow-up. Renal function in these patients was good, but it is likely that at least some patients were older at the time of their surgery, re-emphasizing that the loss of growth potential with increasing age is a major factor in reducing final adult height.

A recent Dutch study (82) presented more optimistic growth data on 68 patients, finding that among 35 patients who had reached their final adult height, 68% were within the normal range. Furthermore they demonstrated an increasing growth velocity in their patients after the first postoperative year as the steroid dosage was declining. However they were unable to detect a specific growth benefit from alternate day steroid therapy.

Recently, an editorial review (83) of pediatric renal transplantation reached similar conclusions. Citing growth as an important outcome variable in transplantation, these authors suggested that growth might be maximized if transplantation was performed at a relatively younger age, allograft function was excellent, and steroid dosage was maintained at a minimal level. These conclusions have been supported by a number of recent articles dealing with pediatric transplantation (20, 77, 84-87).

Age may also be an especially important determinant of growth rate in infants transplanted relatively early in the course of their CRF (20, 83, 84, 77). These young patients (20), at 1-7 years after transplantation, all had head circumferences in the normal range for age and height SD scores improved in all but three patients with primary oxalosis. In another series of children (86), a similar pattern was seen with height SD scores improving in 7 children transplanted at a mean age of 4.4 yrs versus a falling SD score for four older patients with an average age of 10 yrs at the time of transplantation. Another report indicated improved SD scores (mean increase = +1.4 SD) in eight of 18 children at 1 to 3 yrs after transplantation. Importantly the average age of these patients was 6 years and the daily dose of steroid averaged 0.2 mg/kg/day (88).

The impact of graft function was clear in the Paris report (80) and was noted again in a study of 59 of 82 children who received their renal transplant at the University of Florida between 1973 and 1982 (85). In this latter report (although height SD data were not given) it is clear that the best height velocities occurred in those patients with the lowest serum creatinine values and the best creatinine clearances. An earlier report (73) focusing only on those patients with relatively "good" renal function (creatinine < 2.5 mg/dl) demonstrated the same association. Similar results are found in pooled data from EDTA-ERA (89) where 138 boys demonstrated better growth if their serum creatinines at least one year following transplantation were below 150 μmol/l.

The impact of reduced steroid dosage or its correlate, reduced severity and frequency of rejection, on growth is most clear in a recent study of children from Hannover (87). Thirty three consecutive patients were transplanted from 1982-1985 and treated with cyclosporine and prednisone. Growth was markedly better at one year for these patients than a group of 34 children transplanted prior to 1982 in the same institution. Height SD scores and velocity data both indicated true "catch-up" growth in these cyclosporine treated children. This occurred despite a documented early and persistent reduction in inulin and PAH clearance. The authors indicate that these patients received only about one-half of the steroid dose used in the earlier non-cyclosporine treated patients and believe that is a major reason for the improved growth. Not all centers using cyclosporine have had documented improvement in growth (90), but the experience to date seems very encouraging (91).

Other factors including; age at onset of renal disease, duration of dialysis treatment before transplantation (89), the primary renal disease, recurrence of the primary disease in the allograft, alternate day steroid therapy (80, 89), donor kidney source (83), race, and blood pressure (85), have all been suggested as important variables. Studies reported to date have not been stratified for these factors nor have these factors been subjected to controlled, prospective study.

MISCELLANEOUS

Considerable attention has recently been focused on the use of growth hormone (GH) in children with CRF and a controlled trial of GH in these children is presently underway in the United States. Preliminary results reported in abstract (92), indicate an increase in growth velocity from 4.9 to 9.06 cm/yr in five boys with an average GFR of 18 ml/min. These investigators have also presented preliminary data suggesting that intraperitoneal administration of GH may be feasible in patients on chronic PD (93).

Carefully done studies (94) have indicated that recombinant GH effectively stimulates improved weight gain and linear growth in uremic rats. These same studies demonstrated more efficient conversion of ingested food to body mass. Since supraphysiologic amounts of GH are required for this effect, this observation supports the hypothesis that there may be circulating inhibitor(s) of growth hormone or its secondary messengers, the insulin-like growth factors in CRF. Recently, such an inhibitor, with an approximate molecular weight of 940 daltons, has been partially characterized (95).

At present there are a number of unresolved issues surrounding the rationale (96) and risks (97) involved in GH treatment in uremic children. What will be the long-term results of GH treatment? Will the final adult height be increased? What is the optimal dose and timing of GH administration? Will it be more effective if given before dialysis or transplantation, to maintain patients in the normal range? What is the role of GH therapy in the dialysis or post-transplant patient? Are there additive risks to GH therapy following transplantation in regard to rejection, malignancy, steroid-induced diabetes, epiphyseal injury? Some of these questions will likely be addressed by studies in the near future, but until the answers are available, GH treatment should be considered experimental except for children with demonstrated GH deficiency.

Recently another recombinant hormone, erythropoietin (EPO) has become available and the response in uremic children has been dramatic (98). As with GH, this may also be a situation in which uremic inhibitors (99) play important roles, since endogenous EPO levels are frequently not reduced in CRF (100). Also unknown at present is what effect either EPO or EPO plus GH supplementation might have on growth failure in uremic children.

RECOMMENDATIONS

Present recommendations for management must obviously be modified by the time and circumstances under which the child with CRF is seen. Initially, a precise diagnosis is the cornerstone of treatment. When dialysis is not clearly required, aggressive medical management with strict attention to appropriate caloric intake, dietary composition, vitamins, fluid and electrolyte balance should be instituted (38). As necessary, tube feedings should be used to achieve the dietary goals. With progressive deterioration of renal function, dialysis treatment should be anticipated and viewed as a "bridge" to early renal transplantation. Serious consideration should be given to transplantation before dialysis is actually required. If that is not practical, then once dialysis is initiated, prompt thought must be given to preparation, timing, and donor source in an effort to minimize delays prior to renal transplantation. Post-transplantation immunosuppression should be chosen with a conscious effort to minimize the daily and total dosage of steroid consistent with optimal graft survival and function. Since successful transplantation, occurring early in the patient's course is expected to optimize growth (80, 82, 83), the recognition of poor growth in the presence of adequate renal allograft function should trigger a renewed search for another cause of growth retardation.

CONCLUSION

We are no longer view all uremic children as sentenced to severe stunting and early death. While at present the optimal therapy for a uremic child remains empirical, the future especially for younger children with CRF is considerably more optimistic.

ACKNOWLEDGMENT

This work has been supported in part by NIH grants HD 17386 and AM 13083.

REFERENCES

1 Betts PR, and Magrath G: Growth pattern and dietary intake of children with chronic renal insufficiency. Br Med J, 2: 189-193, 1974.

2 Rotundo A, Nevins TE, Lipton M, Lockman LA, Mauer SM, Michael AF: Progressive encephalopathy in children with chronic renal insufficiency in infancy. Kidney Int, 21: 486-491, 1982.
3 McGraw ME and Haka-Ikse K: Neurologic-developmental sequelae of chronic renal failure in infancy. J Pediatr, 106: 574-583, 1985.
4 Bock GH, Conners CK, Ruley J, Samango-Sprouse CA, Conry JA, Weiss I, Eng G, Johnson EL, David CT: Disturbances of brain maturation and neurodevelopment during chronic renal failure in infancy. J Pediatr, 114: 231-238, 1989.
5 Tanner JM: Human Growth,(2nd ed.). Plenum, New York, 1986
6 Potter DE, Broyer M, Chantler C, Gruskin A, Holliday MA, Roche A, Scharer K, Thissen D: Measurement of growth in children with renal insufficiency. Kidney Int, 14: 378-382, 1978.
7 Barrett TM, Broyer M, Chantler C, Gilli G, Guest G, Marti-Henneberg C, Preece MA, Rigdon SPA: Assessment of growth. Am J Kidney Dis, 7: 340-346,1986.
8 Tanner JM: Growth at Adolescence, (2nd ed.). Appleton Century Crofts, New York, 1966.
9 Tanner JM, Whitehouse RH, Cameron N, Marshall WA, Healy MJR, Goldstein H: Assessment of Skeletal Maturity and Predictions of Adult Height (TW2 method), 2nd ed., Academic Press, London, 1983.
10 Tanner JM, Whitehouse RH, Hughes PCR, Vince FP: Effect of human growth hormone treatment for 1 to 7 years on growth of 100 children, with growth hormone deficiency, low birthweight, inherited smallness, Turner's syndrome, and other complaints. Arch Dis Child, 46: 745-782, 1971.
11 Hamill PVV, Drizd TA, Johnson CL, Reed RR, Roche AF: NCHS Growth Curves for Children. DHEW publication (PHS) 78-1650, US Govt. Printing Office, Washington, 1977.
12 Tanner JM and Davies PSW: Clinical longitudinal standards for height and height velocity for North American children. J Pediatr, 107: 317-329, 1985.
13 Tanner JM, Whitehouse RH, Takaishi M: Standards from birth to maturity for height velocity and weight velocity: British children. Arch Dis Child, 41: 454-471, 613-635, 1965.
14 Guo S, Roche AF, Moore WM: Reference data for head circumference and 1-month increments from 1 to 12 months of age. J Pediatr, 113: 490-494, 1988.
15 Tanner JM: Catch-up growth in man. Br Med Bull, 37: 234-238, 1981.
16 Forbes GB: A note on the mathematics of "catch-up" growth. Pediat Res, 8: 929-931, 1974.
17 Mahan JD, Mauer SM, Sibley RK, Vernier RL: Congenital nephrotic syndrome: evolution of medical management and the results of renal transplantation. J Pediatr, 105: 549-557, 1984.
18 Gahl WA, Reed GF, Thoene JG, Schulman JD, Rizzo WB, Jonas AJ, Denman DW, Schlesselman JJ, Corden BJ, Schneider JA: Cysteamine therapy for children with nephropathic cystinosis. N Engl J Med, 316: 971-977, 1987.
19 Clarren SK and Smith DW: The fetal alcohol syndrome; a review of the world literature. N Engl J Med 298:1063-1067, 1978.
20 So SKS, Chang P-N, Najarian JS, Mauer SM, Simmons RL, Nevins TE: Growth and development in infants after renal transplantation. J Pediatr, 110: 343-350, 1987.
21 Smith DW: Recognizable Patterns of Human Malformation, (3rd ed.), Saunders, Philadelphia, 1988.
22 Jeune M, Beraud C, Carron R: Dystrophie thoracique asphyxiante de caractère familial. Arch Franc Pediat, 12: 886, 1955.
23 Eddy AA and Mauer SM: Pseudohermaphroditism, glomerulopathy, and Wilms tumor (Drash syndrome): frequency in end-stage renal failure. J Pediatr, 106: 584-587, 1985.
24 Keller RJ and Wolfsdorf JI: Isolated growth hormone deficiency after cerebral edema complicating diabetic ketoacidosis. N Engl J Med 316:857-859, 1987.
25 Cornblath M and Schwartz R: Disorders of Carbohydrate Metabolism in Infancy,(2nd ed.). Saunders, Philadelphia, 1976, pp 379-381
26 Chesney RW: Growth retardation in childhood renal disease: a hormonal or nutritional problem? Am J Nephrol, 7: 253-256, 1987.
27 Rizzoni G, Broyer M, Guest G, Fine R, Holliday MA: Growth retardation in children with chronic renal disease: scope of the problem. Am J Kidney Dis, 7: 256-261, 1986.
28 Mehls O, Ritz E, Gilli G, Kreusser W: Growth in renal failure. Nephron, 21: 237-247, 1978.
29 French CB and Genel M: Pathophysiology of growth failure in chronic renal insufficiency. Kidney Int, (Suppl) 30: S59-S64, 1984.
30 Bischoff F: The influence of the diet on renal and blood vessel changes. J Nutr, 5: 431-450, 1932.
31 Giovannetti S and Maggiore Q: A low-nitrogen diet with proteins of high biological value for severe chronic uremia: Lancet, i: 1000-1003, 1964.

32 Brenner BM, Meyer TW, Hostetter TH: Dietary protein intake and the progressive nature of kidney disease. N Engl J Med, 307: 652-659, 1982.
33 Maschio G, Oldrizzi L, Rugiu C: The effects of dietary protein restriction on the course of early chronic renal failure, In "Contemporary Issues in Nephrology", vol.14, W Mitch, BM Brenner and JH Stein (Eds), Churchill Livingstone, New York, 1986.
34 Holliday M: Protein intake, renal function, and growth in chronic renal failure, In "Contemporary Issues in Nephrology", vol.14, W Mitch, BM Brenner and JH Stein (Eds), Churchill Livingstone, New York, 1986.
35 Holliday MA: Calories, protein, and other nutrients: requirements and recommendations, In: "Pediatric Nephrology" 2nd ed., MA Holliday, TM Barrett and RL Vernier (Eds), Williams and Wilkins, Baltimore, 1987.
36 Wassner SJ, Abitbol C, Alexander S, Conley S, Grupe WE, Holliday MA, Rigden S, Salusky IB: Nutritional requirements for infants with renal failure. Am J Kidney Dis, 7: 300-305, 1986.
37 Chantler C: Nutritional assessment and management of children with renal insufficiency, In: "End Stage Renal Disease in Children", RN Fine and AB Gruskin (Eds), Saunders, Philadelphia, 1984.
38 Hellerstein S, Holliday MA, Grupe WE, Fine RN, Fennell RS, Chesney RW, Chan JCM: Nutritional management of children with chronic renal failure. Pediatr Nephrol, 11: 195-211, 1987.
39 Arnold WC, Danford D, Holliday MA: Effects of caloric supplementation on growth in children with uremia. Kidney Int, 24: 205-209, 1983.
40 Kleinknecht C, Broyer M, Huot D, Marti-Henneberg C, Dartois A-M: Growth and development of nondialyzed children with chronic renal failure. Kidney Int, (Suppl), 24: S40-S47, 1983.
41 Barratt TM, Fay J, Rigden SPA: Prognosis of renal disease in infancy, In: "Chronic Renal Disease", NB Cummings and S Klahr (Eds), Plenum, New York, 1985.
42 Ray PE and Holliday MA: Growth rate in infants with impaired renal function. J Pediatr, 113: 594-600, 1988.
43 Schwartz GJ, Feld LG, Langford DJ: A simple estimate of glomerular filtration rate in full-term infants during the first year of life. J Pediatr, 104: 849-893, 1984
44 Rizzoni G, Basso T, Setari M: Growth in children with chronic renal failure on conservative management. Kidney Int, 26: 52-58, 1984.
45 Strife CF, Quinlan M, Mears K, Davey ML, Clardy C: Improved growth of three uremic children by nocturnal nasogastric feedings. Amer J Dis Child, 140: 438-443, 1986.
46 Chesney RW, Moorthy AV, Mazess RB, Jax DK, Eisman JA, DeLuca HF: Increased growth after long-term oral 1-25-dihydroxyvitamin D_3 in childhood renal osteodystrophy. N Engl J Med, 298: 238-242, 1978.
47 Dabbagh S and Chesney RW: Treatment of renal osteodystrophy during childhood, In: "End Stage Renal Disease in Children", RN Fine and AB Gruskin (Eds), Saunders, Philadelphia, 1984.
48 Fine RN, De Palma JR, Lieberman E, Donnell GN, Gordon A, Maxwell MH: Extended hemodialysis in children with chronic renal failure. J Pediatr, 73: 706-713, 1968.
49 Potter D, Larsen D, Leumann E, Perin D, Simmons J, Piel CF, Holliday MA: Treatment of chronic uremia in childhood. II. Hemodialysis. Pediatr, 46: 678-689, 1970.
50 Ahola T, Bjorkman H, Makela P, Pasila M, Vilska J, Hallman N: The low-weight groups and haemodialysis. Acta Paediat Scand, 61: 1-4, 1972.
51 Broyer M, Loirat C, Kleinknecht C: Technical aspects and results of regular hemodialysis in children. Acta Paediat Scand, 61: 677-684, 1972.
52 Simmons JM, Wilson CJ, Potter DE, Holliday MA: Relation of calorie deficiency to growth failure in children on hemodialysis and the growth response to calorie supplementation. N Engl J Med, 285: 653-656, 1971.
53 Broyer M, Kleinknecht C, Loirat C, Marti-Henneberg C: Growth in children treated with long-term hemodialysis. J Pediatr, 84: 642-649, 1974.
54 London Children's Home Dialysis Group: Home hemodialysis in children. Lancet, i: 242-246, 1977.
55 Kleinknecht C, Broyer M, Gagnadoux M-F, Dartois A-M, Kermanach C, Pouliquen M, Degoulet P, Usberti M, Roy M-P: Growth in children treated with long-term dialysis. A study of 76 patients. Adv Nephrol, 9: 133-163, 1980.
56 Grupe WE, Harmon WE, Spinozzi NS: Protein and energy requirements in children receiving chronic hemodialysis. Kidney Int, 24 (Suppl): S6-S10, 1983.
57 Scharer K and Gilli G: Growth in children with chronic renal insufficiency, In: "End Stage Renal Disease in Children" RN Fine and AB Gruskin (Eds), Saunders, Philadelphia, 1984.

58 Broyer M, Donckerwolcke RA, Brunner FP, Brynger H, Challah S, Gretz N, Jacobs C, Kramer P, Selwood NH, Wing AJ: Combined report on regular dialysis and transplantation of children in Europe, XII, 1982. Proc EDTA-ERA, 20: 101-104, 1983.
59 Ferraris J, Saenger P, Levine L, New M, Pang S, Saxena BB, Lewy JE: Delayed puberty in males with chronic renal failure. Kidney Int, 18: 344-350, 1980.
60 Popovich RP, Moncrief JW, Nolph KD, Ghods AJ, Twardowski ZJ, Pyle WK: Continuous ambulatory peritoneal dialysis. Ann Intern Med, 88: 449-456, 1978.
61 Balfe JW, Vigneux A, Willumsen J, Hardy BE: The use of CAPD in the treatment of children with end-stage renal disease. Perit Dial Bull, 1: 35-38, 1981.
62 Alexander SR and Tank ES: Surgical aspects of continuous ambulatory peritoneal dialysis in infants, children, and adolescents. J Urol, 127: 501-504, 1982.
63 Kohaut EC: Continuous ambulatory peritoneal dialysis: a preliminary pediatric experience. Am J Dis Child, 135: 270-271, 1981.
64 Alexander SR: CAPD in infants less than one year of age, In: "End Stage Renal Disease in Children", RN Fine and AB Gruskin (Eds), Saunders, Philadelphia, 1984.
65 Southwest Pediatric Nephrology Study Group: Continuous ambulatory and continuous cycling peritoneal dialysis in children. Kidney Int, 27: 558-564, 1985.
66 Alliapoulos JC, Salusky IB, Hall T, Nelson PA, Fine RN: Comparison of continuous cycling peritoneal dialysis with continuous ambulatory peritoneal dialysis in children. J Pediatr, 105: 721-725, 1984.
67 Brem AS and Toscano AM: Continuous cycling peritoneal dialysis for children: an alternative to hemodialysis treatment. Pediatrics, 74: 254-258, 1984.
68 Salusky IB, von Lilien T, Anchondo M, Nelson PA, Fine RN: Experience with continuous cycling peritoneal dialysis during the first year of life. Pediatr Nephrol, 1: 172-175, 1987.
69 Kohaut EC: Growth in children with end-stage renal disease treated with continuous ambulatory peritoneal dialysis for at least one year. Perit Dial Bull, 2: 159-161, 1982.
70 Stefanidis CJ, Hewitt IK, Balfe JW: Growth in children receiving continuous ambulatory peritoneal dialysis. J Pediatr, 102: 681-685, 1983.
71 Hogg RJ: Comparison of CAPD and CCPD in children, In "Chronic Ambulatory Peritoneal Dialysis (CAPD) and Chronic Cycling Peritoneal Dialysis (CCPD) in Children", RN Fine (Ed), Martinus Nijhoff, Boston, 1987.
72 Kohaut EC and Waldo FB: Growth in children on CAPD, In "Chronic Ambulatory Peritoneal Dialysis (CAPD) and Chronic Cycling Peritoneal Dialysis (CCPD) in Children", RN Fine (Ed), Martinus Nijhoff, Boston, 1987.
73 Fennell RS, Orak JK, Hudson T, Garin EH, Iravani A, Van Deusen WJ, Howard R, Pfaff WW, Walker DW, Richard GA: Growth in children with various therapies for end-stage renal disease. Am J Dis Child, 138: 28-31, 1984.
74 Conley SB: Supplemental (NG) feedings of infants undergoing continuous peritoneal dialysis. In "Chronic Ambulatory Peritoneal Dialysis (CAPD) and Chronic Cycling Peritoneal Dialysis (CCPD) in Children", RN Fine (Ed), Martinus Nijhoff, Boston, 1987.
75 Brewer ED, Holmes S, Tealey J: Initiation and maintenance of growth in infants with end stage renal disease managed with peritoneal dialysis and nasogastric tube feedings. Kidney Int, 29: 230, 1986 (Abstract).
76 Polinsky MS, Kaiser BA, Stover JB, Frankenfield M, Baluarte HJ: Neurologic development of children with severe chronic renal failure from infancy. Pediatr Nephrol, 1: 157-165, 1987.
77 Kohaut EC, Whelchel J, Waldo FB, Diethelm AG: Aggressive therapy of infants with renal failure. Pediatr Nephrol, 1: 150-153, 1987.
78 Lilly JR, Giles G, Hurwitz R, Schroter G, Takagi H, Gray S, Penn I, Halgrimson CG, Starzl TE: Renal homotransplantation in pediatric patients. Pediatrics, 47: 548-557, 1971.
79 DeShazo CV, Simmons RL, Bernstein DM, DeShazo MM, Willmert J, Kjellstrand CM, Najarian JS: Results of renal transplantation in 100 children. Surgery, 76: 461-468, 1974.
80 Broyer M, Gagnadoux M-F, Guest G, Beurton D, Niaudet P, Habib R, Busson M: Kidney transplantation in children: Results of 383 grafts performed at Enfants Malades Hospital from 1973 to 1984. Adv Nephrol, 16: 307-334, 1987.
81 Potter D, Feduska N, Melzer J, Garvoy M, Hopper S, Duca R, Salvatierra O: Twenty years of renal transplantation in children. Pediatrics, 77: 465-470, 1986.
82 van Diemen-Steenvoorde R, Donckerwolcke RA, Brackel H, Wolff ED, de Jong MCJW: Growth and sexual maturation in children after kidney transplantation. J Pediatr, 110: 351-356, 1987.
83 Fine RN and Tejani A: Renal transplantation in children. Nephron, 47: 81-86, 1987.

84 Kohaut EC, Whelchel JR, Waldo FB, Diethelm AG: Living-related donor renal transplantation in children presenting with end-stage renal disease in the first month of life. Transplantation, 40: 725, 1985.
85 Fennell RS, Love JT, Carter RL, Hudson TM, Pfaff WW, Howard RJ, Van Deusen W, Garin EH, Iravani A, Walker RD, Richard GA: Statistical analysis of statural growth following kidney transplantation. Eur J Pediatr, 145: 86-89, 1986.
86 Tagge EP, Campbell DA, Dafoe DC, Merion RM, Sedman AB, Kelsch RC, Mollen E, Rocher LL, Turcotte JG: Pediatric renal transplantation with an emphasis on the prognosis of patients with chronic renal insufficiency since infancy. Surgery, 102: 692-698, 1987.
87 Brodehl J, Offner G, Hoyer PF: Cyclosporine in pediatric kidney transplantation. Adv Nephrol, 16: 335-350, 1987.
88 Ettenger RB, Blifeld C, Prince H, Ben-Ezer Gradus D, Cho S, Sekiya N, Salusky IB, Fine RN: The pediatric nephrologist's dilemma: growth after renal transplantation and its interaction with age as a possible immunologic variable. J Pediatr, 111: 1022-1025, 1987.
89 Rizzoni G, Broyer M, Brunner FP, Brynger H, Challah S, Kramer P, Oulès R, Selwood NH, Wing AJ, Balás ÉA: Combined report on regular dialysis and transplantation of children in Europe, XIII, 1983. Proc EDTA-ERA, 21: 69-95, 1984.
90 Ellis D, Avner ED, Rosenthal JT, Taylor RJ, Young LW, Palumbi MA, Hakala TR: Renal function and somatic growth in pediatric cadaveric renal transplantation with cyclosporine-prednisone immunosuppression. Am J Dis Child, 139: 1161-1167, 1985.
91 Offner G, Hoyer PF, Jüppner H, Krohn HP, Brodehl J: Somatic growth after kidney transplantation. Am J Dis Child, 141: 541-546, 1987.
92 Koch VH, Lippe BM, Sherman BM, Fine RN: Accelerated growth following recombinant human growth hormone (rhGH) therapy (Rx) in children with chronic renal failure (CRF). Ped Res, 23: 541A, 1988.
93 Fine RN, Fine SE, Sherman BM: Absorption of recombinant human growth hormone (rgGH) following intraperitoneal (IP) instillation. Kidney Int, 35: 269, 1989 (Abstract).
94 Mehls O, Ritz E, Hunziker EB, Eggli P, Heinrich U, Zapf J: Improvement of growth and food utilization by recombinant growth hormone in uremia. Kidney Int, 33: 45-52, 1988.
95 Phillips LS, Fusco AC, Unterman TG, del Greco F: Somatomedin inhibitor in uremia. J Clin Endocr Metab, 59: 764-772, 1984.
96 Lantos J, Siegler M, Cuttler L: Ethical issues in growth hormone therapy. J Amer Med Assoc 261: 1020-1024, 1989.
97 Rosenfeld RG, Hintz RL, Johanson AJ, Sherman B, and the Genentech Collaborative Group: Results from the first 2 years of a clinical trial with recombinant DNA-derived human growth hormone (Somatrem) in Turner's Syndrome. Acta Paediatr Scand (Suppl.), 331: 59-66, 1987.
98 Sinai-Trieman L, Salusky IB, Fine RN: Use of subcutaneous recombinant human erythropoietin in children undergoing continuous cycling peritoneal dialysis. J Pediatr, 114: 550-554, 1989.
99 McGonigle RJ, Boineau FG, Beckman B, Ohene-Frempong K, Lewy JE, Shadduck RK, Fisher JW: Erythropoietin and inhibitors of in vitro erythropoiesis in the development of anemia in children with renal disease. J Lab Clin Med, 105: 449-458, 1985.
100 Beckman BS, Brookins JW, Garcia MM, Fisher JW: Measurement of erythropoietin in anephric children. Pediatr Nephrol, 3: 75-79, 1989.

ACUTE RENAL FAILURE

10

RECENT ADVANCES IN THE TREATMENT OF RENAL DYSFUNCTION IN LIVER DISEASE (HEPATORENAL SYNDROME)

CARLOS A. VAAMONDE

Nephrology Section, Veterans Administration Medical Center and Department of Medicine, University of Miami School of Medicine, Miami, Florida 33125, U.S.A.

INTRODUCTION

A large body of information is available concerning the effects on the kidney of a diseased liver. The most grave expression of this interrelationship is the hepatorenal syndrome (HRS) (1, 2). The HRS is a form of unexplained acute renal failure occurring in patients with parenchymal end-stage or acute liver disease of diverse etiology in the absence of clinical, laboratory, or anatomic evidence of other known causes of renal failure. The relative frequency of different types of liver disease causing HRS, depends on geographic and other unknown factors. In the U.S.A. the most common cause of HRS is alcoholic liver disease (Laennec's cirrhosis), whereas in other countries in addition to an alcoholic etiology, postnecrotic, cryptogenic cirrhosis or fulminant acute hepatic failure are also frequently reported. The occurrence of the HRS is distinctly rare in children (3). Terms such as "renal failure of cirrhosis", "functional renal failure", "cirrhotic nephropathy", and others, have been used from time to time to identify this specific renal dysfunction of liver disease. Not having any desire to add to the controversy related to terminology, I will use in this review the more appealing and common term HRS. A comprehensive review of the clinical aspects and pathogenesis of the HRS can be found elsewhere (1, 2, 4). In this review, the emphasis will be on the treatment of this serious condition.

DIAGNOSIS

There are numerous conditions that can be confused with the HRS (Table 1). Some overlapping is apparent in this list. The term HRS may be used in a restrictive fashion, exclusively for patients with end-stage liver disease secondary to alcoholic, postnecrotic or cryptogenic cirrhosis; more frequently, its meaning will be expanded by the addition of acute fulminant liver disease [hepatitis or toxic injury (paracetamol)].

Table 1 Conditions with both liver and kidney involvement.

1.	Simultaneous hepatic and renal injury ("Pseudohepatorenal" syndrome) *
2.	Immune complex glomerulonephritis secondary to hepatitis B disease.
3.	Renal injury secondary to intravascular coagulation in patients with severe liver injury.
4.	Acute tubular necrosis in patients with obstructive jaundice.
5.	Prerenal azotemia in patients with liver disease.
6.	Hepatorenal syndrome.

* These include (a) generalized disorders: sepsis, hepatitis B, leptospirosis, Reye's syndrome, shock, heart failure, polycystic disease, SLE, polyarteritis, hyperthermia; (b) toxins: Carbon tetrachloride, acetaminophen (paracetamol), *Amanita phalloides* poisoning, methoxyflurane, etc; (c) Neoplasms: metastatic, renal cell carcinoma.

The clinical characteristics of HRS are well known: oliguric acute renal failure, which may develop rapidly with or without precipitating causes [mild gastrointestinal (GI) bleeding, abdominal paracentesis, induced diuresis], occurring in a decompensated cirrhotic patient with ascites, and usually becoming apparent during hospitalization. Other etiologies will somewhat alter the presentation (1, 2). Patients are usually hyponatremic, mildly hypotensive, with an initial concentrated urine and low urinary Na (< 10 mmol/l) and fractional excretion of Na (FE_{Na}) (< 1%). Transient improvement in renal function may occur with volume expansion. Reversal, however, occurs with a change in the hepatic environment: the kidney from patients with HRS may be used successfully as a donor for transplantation in a uremic patient with a normal liver (5). Conversely, a successful liver transplant in a cirrhotic patient with HRS results in improvement of renal function (6). A few patients may evolve into typical acute tubular necrosis (ATN) (7), but the vast majority do not exhibit overt morphologic changes of ATN.

Table 2 outlines the clinical and laboratory features that may help to differentiate the HRS from other conditions.

Note that there are no specific tests for the HRS, and that the diagnosis is essentially by exclusion, which includes negative criteria that are always difficult to assess. Note also, that the early urinary indexes of the HRS are indistinguishable from those of prerenal azotemia. Of crucial importance, in the HRS there is not a sustained response (diuresis, improved renal function) to acute expansion of the vascular volume. The latter, however, may correct prerenal azotemia confirming its diagnosis. Finally, in evaluating these patients it should be remembered that, because of poor nutrition, severe muscular wasting, and hepatic disease many cirrhotic patients have more severe renal dysfunction than indicated by the level of their serum creatinine (8). Thus, a serum creatinine concentration "within the range of normal" in these patients may actually be concomitant with important renal dysfunction.

Table 2 Clinical and laboratory features of the HRS.

1. Presence of liver disease (end-stage or fulminant)
2. Absence of pre-existing renal disease or known causes of renal failure.
3. Acute or subacute onset of renal functional impairment that is usually progressive in days or few weeks.
4. No sustained improvement with cautious expansion of the intravascular volume with colloid solutions.
5. Urinary indexes:

	Urine Na (mmol/l)	FE_{Na} (%)	U_{Osm}/P_{Osm}
Early HRS *	<10-20	<1	>1 (concentrated urine)
Late HRS	<10-20	<1	>1 to 1
Progression to ATN (rare)	>30-40	>2	1 (isosmotic urine)

* Cannot be distinguished from prerenal azotemia. In the HRS, the response to volume expansion is nil, minimal or not sustained.

PROGNOSIS - RECOVERY

The development of renal failure in the course of severe hepatic disease is of grave prognostic significance. The HRS, particularly in the alcoholic cirrhotic patient, is almost always a fatal complication. Although an uncommon event, spontaneous recovery from the HRS has been described in a few patients (9-11). We might have seen such a case in one out of 100 patients (1). In some of these published cases, however, as no doubt in many unpublished ones, it is difficult to differentiate true HRS from prerenal azotemia (10), drug-induced nephrotoxicity, or the follow-up was short and the patient's long-range outcome unknown. Recovery is somewhat better established after improvement of hepatic function with liver transplantation, portal decompression with portocaval shunts, or after insertion of peritoneovenous shunts, or dialytic procedures. Renal failure in most of these patients, however, complicated the course of fulminant rather than chronic liver disease. This will be discussed subsequently.

PREVENTION

The best treatment of the HRS is its prevention. Although in the absence of a completely defined pathogenesis it may be difficult to know with certainty how to prevent its development, two points, however, stand-out: (A) Avoidance of further reduction in effective circulating volume, and (B) Avoidance of nephrotoxic agents.

(A) Avoidance of further reduction in effective circulating volume

Since we cannot predict with any accuracy when a decompensated cirrhotic patient will develop HRS (1, 11), volume contraction secondary to diuretic therapy (often loop diuretics plus metolazone) should be avoided. Abdominal paracentesis beyond diagnostic, and strict therapeutic needs (tense ascites with respiratory distress) should be used carefully. More recent data, however, supports the use of large volume paracentesis together with intravenous administration of albumin in these patients (11a). Any other obvious volume loss, such as GI bleeding, vomiting, diarrhea [use of osmotic cathartics (lactulose) for treatment of encephalopathy (11)] should be promptly corrected.

(B) Avoidance of nephrotoxic agents

In recent years, we have become keenly aware of the role that many commonly used drugs have in causing renal dysfunction or disease. Patients with severe liver disease are no exception, and indeed, they may be more susceptible to the nephrotoxic effect of certain drugs.

It is now clearly established that nonsteroidal antiinflammatory agents, through their inhibitory action on prostaglandin synthetase activity, often have an adverse effect on renal function in decompensated cirrhosis (12), and should be used with extreme caution or not prescribed in these patients. Of the antibiotics, two should be considered with special concern. Demeclocycline, a broad spectrum antibiotic, can induce acute renal failure (4, 13), and the aminoglycosides have been reported as having an increased risk of inducing nephrotoxicity in patients with liver disease (14, 15). Of note, because of the suggested role of endotoxemia in the pathogenesis of the HRS (16), is the recent report of an association between Gram-negative sepsis and enhanced gentamicin nephrotoxicity (17). The authors attributed the effect to endotoxin and the enhanced renal cortical uptake of the aminoglycoside (17). Lactulose may produce volume loss by inducing diarrhea resulting in hypovolemia, hypernatremia, and azotemia when given to decompensated cirrhotics for the control of encephalopathy (11). Although suspected as potentially capable of causing renal dysfunction, it appears that ß-blockers (propranolol) do not reduce renal perfusion in patients with cirrhosis without overt ascites (18).

MANAGEMENT OF ESTABLISHED HRS

It is realistic to accept the fact that the management of the HRS is extremely frustrating. This is, after all, a complication of severe liver disease that is almost invariably fatal. Many approaches have been employed through the years with very limited success in an attempt to alter the dismal outcome of the HRS. These include: (a) attempts to increase effective circulating volume, (b) renal pharmacologic modulation, (c) dialytic techniques, and (d) liver transplantation.

(a) Attempts to increase effective circulating volume

Because of the prominent role that decreased effective circulating volume may have in the pathogenesis of the HRS (1, 2, 4), it is mandatory first to assess, and then to correct any volume deficiency that may exist. Even if no risk factors for precipitating the HRS are present (see Prevention) in all suspected patients, a volume challenge should be undertaken (Table 2). This, in itself, may be diagnostic and therapeutic at the same time.

Attempts at volume expansion beyond repair of deficits can be acute (single or intermittent) or continuous. A number of elaborated invasive maneuvers have been designed to sustain volume expansion. These are: paracentesis with ultrafiltration and reinfusion of ascites, creation of portocaval anastomosis and insertion of peritoneovenous shunts.

Acute volume expansion

Single or few repeated attempts at volume expansion with blood, plasma, albumin, dextran, and saline infusions have been almost uniformly disappointing in established HRS (1, 2). In few patients, a modest increase in urine volume and sodium excretion may occur, but with little impact on renal failure. Patients become rapidly refractory to repeated attempts.

Of great interest, because it was carried out in 11 patients with the HRS, is the recent work of Cade et al (19). The authors infused one liter of fresh frozen plasma (containing renin substrate) daily for 7 to 18 days to expand the blood volume to supranormal values. These repeated infusions resulted in increases in blood volume, renal plasma flow, creatinine clearance, urine volume, and sodium excretion with a decrease in plasma aldosterone levels. These renal changes were associated with improvement in the clinical status and clearing of encephalopathy in all patients. The changes were temporary, however, since as ascites continued to form reducing vascular volume, the improved variables slowly reverted. Although the practicality, complications, and cost of this treatment were not discussed, this contribution reemphasized the importance of a decreased effective circulating volume in the pathogenesis of the HRS, and the potential benefits obtained from its correction.

Head-out water immersion

In recent years, Epstein has extensively studied the effects of head-out water immersion as a mean of increasing by redistribution, central blood volume, in normal and cirrhotic patients (4). Bichet et al (20) immersed a patient with HRS for five hours to assess the role of blood redistribution on the HRS. As predicted from previous studies (4), immersion increased effective blood volume, and cardiac index with concomitant decreases in ADH, aldosterone and plasma renin activity. There were little changes, however, in renal plasma flow or GFR. These results are, however, not surprising in view of the very limited nature of the volume expansion stimuli. They should be contrasted with those of Cade et al (19) referred to above. Because of its transient nature, of the time commitment of attendant personnel, cost, and other unknowns, it appears that water immersion is not a practical mode of therapy for decompensated cirrhosis or the HRS.

Paracentesis with ultrafiltration and reinfusion of ascites

Historically, these intermittent techniques were devised and used for the treatment of intractable ascites, particularly in Europe and Japan. These include direct reinfusion of ascites or its infusion after prior concentration with various devices [Rhodiascit apparatus (21), or ultrafiltration (22)]. Details of the procedures can be found elsewhere (22). The early experience with these techniques in the HRS was very limited and the results disappointing. The procedures, because the potential for serious complications (bacterial peritonitis, intravascular volume depletion with aggravation [or induction] of HRS, hepatic encephalopathy, protein depletion) fell out of favor. More recent efforts, however, have shown promising results. Landini et al (23) reported on the weekly ambulatory treatment of five decompensated cirrhotic patients with ascitic ultrafiltration and reinfusion. None of these patients, however, had the HRS at the onset nor did they develop renal failure during a follow-up period up to 10 months. Others (24) reported similar experience. Thus, although the newer results are encouraging, these techniques have not been tested in patients with the HRS.

Portasystemic anastomosis

Few isolated reports of recovery from the HRS following decompression of portal hypertension with end-to-end portocaval shunts have been published. The mechanism(s) responsible for its effect on renal function remains unclear. Schroeder and coworkers (25) carefully studied five such patients. Three died within one to eight weeks after surgery, whereas two patients were well two and 10 years later. Others found that surgery actually precipitated renal failure or was of no therapeutic value (4). Because of the limited experience, the substantial morbidity and mortality of the procedure, it cannot be recommended as a standard treatment of the HRS.

Peritoneovenous shunt

Since the introduction of the peritoneovenous shunt (PVS), in 1974 by LeVeen et al (26), for the management of refractory ascites, numerous PVS have been placed for the original indication or for treatment of the HRS. A comprehensive recent review of the subject can be found elsewhere (4), and procedural details will not be given here. It has been estimated that over 30,000 (and more as of this writing) PVS have been placed worldwide since 1974 (4). Table 3 summarizes some of the information available regarding the use of PVS in the HRS. Analysis of the accumulated data is difficult because of uncertainty about the presence of HRS in some patients, incomplete information, and unknown follow-up. There are over 100 patients with alleged HRS reported. Long-term survival (defined as more than two months) is about 40%. When selected series are considered, average survival is also about 40% (18 out of 45), but there is considerable individual variation (Table 3) (19, 25, 27-29). In the prospective study of Linas et al (28), 20 patients with the HRS were randomized to PVS or conventional medical therapy. The results showed that while the PVS stabilized renal function, it did not prolong life. The study of Stanley et al (VA Cooperative study) in its preliminary report indicated that although there were seven long-term survivors in a group of 14 HRS patients treated with PVS, the results were not statistically different from those of 19 HRS patients randomized to medical therapy (29). It is clear, that a number of patients with HRS exhibit improvement of renal function following PVS implantation, but the benefits need to be balanced with the high occurrence of major adverse reactions, and mortality (4). Further controlled prospective randomized studies are necessary to assess the effects of PVS on liver and kidney function, complications, long-term survival, and quality of life obtained.

Table 3 Long-term survival with peritoneovenous shunt in the HRS.[(a)] Selected studies.[(b)]

	Nº Patients/Survival	Longest Survival
Schroeder et al, 1970 (25)	5/4	2 years
Smith et al, 1984 (27)	10/0	mean, 28±5 days
Stanley et al, 1985 (29) [(c)]	14/7	-
Linas et al, 1986 (28) [(c)]	10/1	7 months
Cade et al, 1987 (19) [(d)]	6/6	up to 2 years

[(a)] Long-term survival defined as more than 2 months; [(b)] Only studies with rigorous criteria for diagnosis of HRS are included; [(c)] Prospective randomized studies, compared PVS with medical therapy; [(d)] These patients were treated also with intermittent plasma infusions prior to PVS.

(b) Renal pharmacologic modulation of the HRS

Table 4 lists the numerous and varied pharmacologic agents that have been used to attempt to control renal cortical vasoconstriction and/or decrease vascular capacitance in patients with HRS.

Table 4 Renal pharmacologic modulation of the HRS.

Sympathomimetics (metaraminol, isoproterenol)
Parasympathomimetics (acetylcholine derivatives)
Dopaminergic (dopamine, levodopa)
Alpha adrenergic blockers (phenoxybenzamine, phentolamine)
Beta adrenergic blockers (propranolol)
Angiotensin II
Angiotensin blockers (captopril, saralasin)
Prostaglandins (PGE_1, PGA_1, PGI_2)
Thromboxane synthesis blockers (Daxoziben)
Antibiotics (anti-endotoxin)
Others (papaverine, glucocorticoids, furosemide)
Atrial natriuretic factor?
Calcium channel blockers?
Renin substrate?
Lumbar sympathectomy?

It is fair to say that none of these agents has shown effects that resulted in any sustained improvement of renal function or patients' outcome.

I would like to suggest that controlled trials of powerful intraarterial vasodilator agents should be attempted in the HRS. It is known, for example, that the atrial natriuretic factor can reverse early ischemic acute renal failure in the rat when given into the renal artery (30). Calcium channel blockers also ameliorate acute renal failure in animals, and have been suggested as ideally suited to reverse the episodic renal vasospasm of HRS (31). Administration of renin (renin-substrate rich-plasma), which usually is markedly depressed in the HRS, might be also of some benefit (19, 32). Amelioration of renal sympathetic nerve activity associated with lumbar sympathectomy has been reported as producing some benefit in patients with the HRS (33).

(c) Dialysis and ultrafiltration

The indication of dialytic procedures in the management of the HRS remains a controversial issue. Although most experts believe that dialysis has no role, there may be special circumstances when dialytic support is justified. (Table 5).

The potential benefits to be obtained from dialytic procedures in the HRS include:(a) correction of fluid, electrolyte and acid-base disturbances, facilitating prevention or treatment of pulmonary edema in patients in need of large volume replacement because of shock, bleeding, or coagulopathy; (b) supporting nutrition by permitting the sustained administration of parenteral nutrients; (c) improvement of the platelet dysfunction associated with uremia; (d) removal of metabolites that may contribute to uremic or hepatic toxicity (ammonia, mercaptans, amino acids, octopamine, etc), or of endotoxin fragments (that may play a role in the pathogenesis of the HRS). For example, in a recent study, Coratelli et al (16) utilized dialysis membranes with large pores (polyacrylonitrile) and demonstrated removal of endotoxin fragments from the circulation. Unfortunately, there were no survivors in the seven cirrhotic patients with HRS that were dialyzed.

The major problem encountered when employing dialytic techniques in cirrhotic patients is severe hypotension. This results, undoubtedly, from the known cardiovascular instability of these patients (contracted plasma volume, ascites-induced hemodynamic changes, bleeding, septic shock). Hypotension is difficult to control and frequently limits the usefulness of the dialysis. Other problems are increased risk of infection, worsening of coagulopathy, and changes in drug-protein binding associated with correction of uremia.

Peritoneal dialysis, hemodialysis and ultrafiltration techniques have been employed in the HRS with limited or varied success.

Peritoneal dialysis

The published experience is limited, although one must assume that most workers in the field have used these techniques at some time. The overall results with peritoneal dialysis are dismal. In HRS secondary to fulminant hepatic failure, only 4 of 47 patients survived in three studies, the largest being that of Wilkinson et al (34). A recent study (35) utilizing rapid exchange-peritoneal dialysis, however, reported encouraging results in five patients with fulminant hepatic liver failure (four of them had also renal failure). Three of these patients did recover. In chronic cirrhosis with encephalopathy the outcome is very poor. Only one of 35 reported patients survived (36) despite the correction in all of marked electrolyte abnormalities. Those considering the use of peritoneal dialysis in patients with severe liver disease with or without renal failure should remember that because of the bleeding tendency of these patients, the placement of the peritoneal catheter is best done by surgeons, that ascites decreases the efficiency of the procedure and increases protein losses, and that intraperitoneal sepsis may be a serious complication.

Hemodialysis

As with peritoneal dialysis, hemodialysis was considered to be ineffective in the treatment of the HRS by early investigators (34).

Table 5 Indications for dialytic therapy (Peritoneal dialysis, hemodialysis, CAVH) in patients with liver and kidney failure *

1. Acute fulminant liver disease when recovery from liver failure is expected.
2. While awaiting or undergoing consideration for liver transplantation.
3. When known or strongly suspected nephrotoxins (aminoglycosides, nonsteroidal antiinflamatory agents, radiocontrast, cyclosporine) are a major factor in the appearance of renal failure.
4. When etiology of the renal failure in a patient suspected of having the HRS is not clear, particularly if evidence of prerenal factors (diuretic therapy, blood loss due to GI bleeding) is prominent, or untreated rampant infection is present, and lessening the intensity and duration of uremia (hypercatabolic renal failure) is thought to be beneficial.
5. When obstructive jaundice is complicated by renal failure.
6. When a diagnostic or surgical procedure is necessary.

* It is possible that CAVH or one of its variants may be the dialytic modality of choice for these patients (see text).

Most of the patients on whom hemodialysis was employed had chronic rather than acute liver disease. Current experience suggests that a more selective approach should be used, and that hemodialysis should not be denied beforehand to patients with liver and renal failure. Table 5 outlines the specific clinical situations when dialytic procedures should be considered in these patients. In addition, Wilkinson et al (34) noted a favorable outcome (78% recovery) in patients with obstructive jaundice and renal failure (1). It should be particularly noted that the "typical" chronic alcoholic cirrhotic patient who has developed renal failure in the absence of the clinical situations outlined in Table 5 and failed to respond to volume expansion is not a candidate for dialytic therapy, and almost invariably will not benefit from the procedure.

Newer dialytic techniques (CAVH, CAVHD)

These combine ultrafiltration with hemodialysis and are administered in a continuous rather than in an intermittent fashion (37). Their major advantage is that they combine enhanced fluid and solute removal with hemodynamic stability. Thus, they appear *a priori* to be suited ideally for the severely decompensated cirrhotic patient with or without renal failure. These procedures are: slow continuous ultrafiltration (SCUF) for removal of fluid, at a slow rate; continuous arteriovenous hemofiltration (CAVH) for removal of water, and electrolyte, acid-base, and azotemia control using a higher rate of fluid removal tailored to the patient's needs; and continuous arteriovenous hemodialysis (CAVHD), a combination of CAVH and dialysis for patients with high urea generation. Of these, CAVH is the most popular because of its simplicity. Electrolytes and small-sized molecules are removed continuously from the patient by convective transport across highly permeable membranes. Because of their low internal resistance the filters use the arteriovenous pressure difference to maintain blood flow through them, making the use of pumps unnecessary. Usually, a filtrate flow of 20 to 30 ml/min can be maintained for hours or days. The volume ultrafiltrated is replaced by a modified Ringer's lactate solution, minus the amount necessary for the patient to achieve a negative fluid balance. The method is much simpler than other dialytic procedures and can be used in most intensive care units. Major indications of CAVH are: rapid removal of fluid in acute or chronic renal failure, congestive heart failure, and postoperative heart surgery; treatment of "intractable" edema (diuretic-resistant); severe hyponatremia, fluid overload complicated by hypotension, and provision of hyperalimentation (37).

CAVH has been used in patients with liver disease for the treatment of symptomatic ascites and in few patients with renal failure. Epstein and coworkers (38) and Kaplan (39) have recently reported on the successful use of CAVH in four cirrhotic patients with renal failure. Furthermore, Davenport et al (40) reported excellent results with CAVH in a patient with fulminant hepatic and renal failure, secondary to paracetamol intoxication. From this limited experience it appears that CAVH or one of its variants may be the preferable alternative when dialysis is indicated in combined liver and kidney failure. In the next few years, we will have hopefully, sufficient information to judge its true usefulness.

(d) Liver transplantation

Liver transplantation constitutes the definitive treatment of the HRS, since a major improvement in liver function after transplantation is associated with recovery from the HRS (3, 6, 41, 42). In the recent Pittsburgh study (41), the normalization of renal function occurred independently of whether there was a transient post-operative episode of early renal impairment (within six days of surgery), and it appeared, as originally described (6), over a period of several weeks.

Most reviewers of the HRS, however, discount this therapeutic modality, because at present, it is not considered a cost-effective procedure due to its complicated course, high expense, and limited availability to only few centers around the world. I believe that the age of the patient (children vs adults) and the type of liver disease may be additional factors to consider. The majority of the adult patients in two recent large series [77% (43) and 80% (44)] had liver disease secondary to chronic active hepatitis, primary sclerosing cholangitis or primary biliary disease, whereas as expected, biliary hypoplasia or atresia and metabolic disorders were dominant in children. No mention was made regarding these 200 liver transplantations to the specific presence of renal failure or the HRS (43, 44), although elevated pre-operative serum creatinine values were present in some patients (44). On the other hand, the HRS was present in 7 of 133 children (5.3%) who underwent liver transplantation at Children's Hospital in Pittsburgh (3). Four of these 7 patients recovered renal function 2 to 4 weeks after transplantation.

Earlier reports suggested that patient survival in liver transplantation appears to correlate unfavorably with elevated preoperative serum creatinine concentration, frank renal failure, the need of dialysis or with postoperative renal dysfunction or dialytic support (3, 36, 37). The former findings may tend to exclude patients with HRS from consideration for liver transplantation. Recent data from London and Cambridge, however, found no correlation between pre-operative elevated serum creatinine levels and outcome in 33 patients with acute hepatic failure (45). Furthermore, Gonwa et al

(42) have recently reported that patients with HRS and acute liver failure can safely and effectively undergo liver transplantation with results similar to those of patients without HRS (Table 6). Indeed, it appears that graft rejection was lower in the HRS patients.

Table 6 Effect of orthotopic liver transplantation on patients with acute liver disease and HRS [(a)]

	Non-HRS	p value	HRS
Number of patients	81		19
Age (yr)	44±8 [(b)]	NS	41±1
Serum creatinine (mg/dl)			
Pre-operative	1.0±0.04	<0.001	3.4±0.5
Post-operative (1 mo)	1.3±0.06	<0.02	1.7±0.3
Post-operative (1 yr)	1.4±0.4	NS	1.7±0.3
GFR (ml/min) [(c)]			
Pre-operative	98±5	<0.001	26±8
Post-operative (1 mo)	55±4 [(d)]	<0.02	31±4
Post-operative (1 yr)	55±4 [(d)]	NS	42±12
Hemodialysis (%)			
Pre-operative	0	<0.001	21
Post-operative	11	<0.001	58
3-month patient survival (%)	86	NS	79 [(e)]
Patients with rejection (%)	60	<0.02	32

[(a)] Adapted from Gonwa et al (42); [(b)] Mean ±SEM; [(c)] ^{135}Iothalamate technique; [(d)] The decreased GFR in the patients without HRS was attributed in part to their higher levels of cyclosporine; [(e)] 4 of 19 patients with HRS died.

In the U.S.A. and other countries, alcoholic liver disease remains the most common form of end-stage hepatic disease, contributing a large share to the etiology of the HRS. Notwithstanding the controversy about the wisdom of treating end-stage liver disease due to alcoholism with liver transplantation [because of moralistic, medical, rehabilitation, or economic considerations (46)], recent data on the subject is of interest. Starzl and coworkers (47) found no difference between the survival of 41 patients who received liver transplants for Laennec's cirrhosis and 625 adults transplanted for other causes in a recent study where all patients received cyclosporin treatment. Thus, at present, the vast majority of alcoholic cirrhotic patients with HRS are simply not considered for liver transplantation except under very unusual circumstances, whereas children and patients with acute liver disease, or other forms of chronic hepatic disease, as noted, fared better. A report of the long-term survival and renal outcome of patients with the HRS who received liver transplants should be extremely useful. This will permit the prescription of liver transplantation in these patients on a more rational basis.

OVERVIEW OF MANAGEMENT OF PATIENTS WITH THE HRS

The best treatment for the HRS remains its prevention, which is based on avoidance of circulating volume contraction and the use of drugs with potential for kidney damage. Treatment for established HRS remains a frustrating experience, with recovery being an uncommon event. More recent experience, however, indicates that every possible effort to alter the dismal outcome should be undertaken in patients with HRS associated with acute or subacute forms of hepatic failure who may have potential for recovery of liver function. The outcome for patients with chronic end-stage liver disease, particularly of the alcoholic variety, remains disheartening. Increasing the effective circulating blood volume in a sustained manner has been attempted with insertion of the peritoneovenous shunt, and dialytic procedures (preferably CAVH or one of its variants) have been used to control renal failure and volume perturbations, with varied, sometimes promising results. Most of these invasive procedures, however, need further assessment of their true clinical value by means of larger, controlled, randomized, prospective studies. The use of pharmacologic modulation of renal vasoconstriction in the HRS has been so far uniformly disappointing. Liver transplantation has been performed with increasing frequency and encouraging results, almost exclusively in non-alcoholic liver disease. The current management of the HRS remains a formidable challenge to the ingenuity and perseverance of physicians.

REFERENCES

1. Vaamonde CA, Papper S: The kidney in liver disease, In: "Diseases of the Kidney", Third edition, LE Earley and CW Gottschalk (Eds), Little, Brown & Co., Boston, 1979, pp 1289-1317.
2. Papper S: Hepatorenal syndrome, In: "Acute Renal Failure", VE Andreucci (Ed), Martinus Nijhoff Publishing, Boston, 1984, pp 233-250.
3. Wood RP, Ellis D, Starzl TE: The reversal of the hepatorenal syndrome in four pediatric patients following successful orthotopic liver transplantation. Ann Surg, 205: 415-419, 1987.
4. Epstein M: The Kidney in Liver Disease. Third edition, Williams & Wilkins, Baltimore, 1988.
5. Koppel MH, Coburn JW, Mims MM, Goldstein H, Boyle JD, Rubini ME: Transplantation of cadaveric kidneys from patients with hepatorenal syndrome. Evidence for the functional nature of renal failure in advanced liver disease. N Eng J Med, 280: 1367-1371, 1969.
6. Iwatsuki S, Popovtzer MM, Corman JL, Ishikawa MM, Putnam CW, Katz F, Starzl T: Recovery from "hepatorenal syndrome" after orthotopic liver transplantation. N Eng J Med, 280: 1155-1159, 1973.

7. Solez K, Racusen LC, Jewell LD: Pathology of acute renal failure occurring in liver disease. In: "The Kidney in Liver Disease", Third edition, M Epstein (Ed), Williams & Wilkins, Baltimore, 1988, pp 182-206.
8. Papadakis MA, Arieff AI: Unpredictability of clinical evaluation of renal function in cirrhosis. Am J Med, 82: 945-952, 1987.
9. Galambos JT, Wilkinson HA III: Reversible hyponatremia and azotemia in a patient with cirrhosis and ascites. Amer J Dig Dis, 7: 642-647, 1962.
10. Goldstein H, Boyle JD: Spontaneous recovery from the hepato-renal syndrome. Report of four cases. N Eng J Med, 272: 895-897, 1965.
11. Vaamonde CA: Renal water handling in liver disease. In "The Kidney in Liver Disease", Third edition, M Epstein (Ed), Williams & Wilkins, Baltimore, 1988, pp 31-72.
11a. Arroyo V, Ginés P, Planas R, Panés J, Rodés J: Paracentesis in the management of cirrhotics with ascites. In: "The Kidney in Liver Disease", Third edition, M Epstein (Ed), Williams & Wilkins, Baltimore, 1988, pp 578-592.
12. Boyer TD, Zia P, Reynolds TB: Effect of indomethacin and prostaglandin A_1 on renal function and plasma renin activity in alcoholic liver disease. Gastroenterology, 77: 215-222, 1979.
13. Carrilho F, Bosch J, Arroyo V, Mas A, Viver J, Rodes J: Renal failure associated with demeclocycline in cirrhosis. Ann Intern Med, 87: 195-197, 1977.
14. Cabrera J, Arroyo V, Ballesta AM, Rimola A, Gual J, Elena M, Rodes J: Aminoglycoside nephrotoxicity in cirrhosis. Value of urinary ß-microglobulin to discriminate functional renal failure from acute tubular damage. Gastroenterology, 82: 97-105, 1982.
15. Lietman PS: Liver disease, aminoglycoside antibiotics and renal dysfunction. Hepatology, 8: 966-968, 1988.
16. Coratelli P, Passavanti G, Munno I, Fumarola D, Amerio A: New trends in hepatorenal syndrome. Kidney Int, 17: S143-S147, 1985.
17. Zager RA, Prior RB: Gentamicin and gram-negative bacteremia. A synergism for the development of experimental nephrotoxic acute renal failure. J Clin Invest, 78: 196-204, 1986.
18. Bataille C, Bercoff E, Pariente EA, Valla D, Lebrec D: Effects of propranolol on renal blood flow and renal function in patients with cirrhosis. Gastroenterology, 86: 129-133, 1984.
19. Cade R, Wagemaker H, Vogel S, Mars D, Hood-Lewis D, Privette M, Peterson J, Schlein E, Hawkins R, Raulerson D, Campbell K: Hepato-renal syndrome. Studies of the effect of vascular volume and intra-peritoneal pressure on renal and hepatic function. Am J Med, 82: 427-438, 1987.
20. Bichet DG, Groves BG, Schrier RW: Effect of head-out water immersion on hepatorenal syndrome. Am J Kidney Dis, 3: 258-263, 1984.
21. Wilkinson SP, Davidson AR, Henderson J, Williams R: Ascites re-infusion using the Rhodiascit apparatus - clinical experience and coagulation abnormalities. Postgrad Med J, 51: 583-587, 1975.
22. Perez GO, Epstein M, Oster JR: Role of dialysis and ultrafiltration in the treatment of the renal complications of liver disease. In:"The Kidney in Liver Disease", Third edition, M Epstein (Ed), Williams & Wilkins, Baltimore, 1988, pp 613-624.
23. Landini S, Coli U, Fracasso A, Morachiello P, Righetto F, Scanferia F, Gallenda F, Bazzato O: Spontaneous ascites filtration and reinfusion (SAFR) as ambulatory chronic treatment for hepato-renal syndrome. Trans Am Soc Artif Intern Organs, 31: 439-443, 1985.
24. Lai KN, Leung JWC, Vallance-Owen J: Dialytic ultrafiltration by hemofilter in treatment of patients with refractory ascites and renal insufficiency. Am J Gastroenterol, 82: 665-668, 1987.
25. Schroeder ET, Anderson GH Jr, Smulyan H: Effects of portacaval or peritoneovenous shunt on renin in the hepatorenal syndrome. Kidney Int, 15: 54-61, 1979.
26. LeVeen HH, Christoudias G, Moon JP, Luft R, Falk G, Grossberg S: Peritoneovenous shunting for ascites. Ann Surg, 180: 580-591,1974.
27. Smith RE, Nostrant TT, Eckhauser FE, Wilson JP, Knol JA, Strodel WE: Patient selection and survival after peritoneovenous shunting for nonmalignant ascites. Am J Gastroenterol, 79: 659-662, 1984.
28. Linas SL, Schaefer JW, Moore EE, Good JT Jr, Giansiracusa R: Peritoneovenous shunt in the management of the hepatorenal syndrome. Kidney Int, 30: 736-740, 1986.
29. Stanley MM, and members of the VA Cooperative Study Group 142: Peritoneovenous shunting vs medical treatment of alcoholic cirrhotic ascites. Hepatology, 5: 980, 1985.
30. Nakamoto M, Shapiro JI, Shanley PF, Chan L, Schrier RW: *In vitro* and *in vivo* protective effect of atriopeptin III on ischemic acute renal failure. J Clin Invest, 80: 698-705, 1987.

31. Edelson JT: Calcium-channel blockers and the hepatorenal syndrome. Med Hypothesis, 22: 335-340, 1987.
32. Berkowitz HD, Miller LD, Rosato EF: Letter: Renin substrate depletion in hepatorenal syndrome. N Eng J Med, 290: 461, 1974.
33. Solis-Herruza JA, Duran A, Favela V, Castellano G, Madrid JL, Muñoz-Yagüe MT, Morillas JD, Estenoz J: Effects of lumbar sympathetic block on kidney function in cirrhotic patients with hepatorenal syndrome. J Hepatology, 5: 167-173, 1987.
34. Wilkinson SP, Weston MJ, Parsons V, Williams R: Dialysis in the treatment of renal failure in patients with liver disease. Clin Nephrol, 8: 287-292, 1977.
35. Mactier RA, Dobbie JW, Khanna R: Peritoneal dialysis in fulminant hepatic failure. Perit Dial Bull, 6: 199-202, 1986.
36. Ring-Larsen H, Clausen E, Ranek L: Peritoneal dialysis in hyponatremia due to liver failure. Scand J Gastroenterol, 8: 33-40, 1973.
37. Quellhorst EA: Hemofiltration. In: "Textbook of Nephrology", Second edition, SG Massry and RJ Glassock (Eds), Williams & Wilkins, Baltimore, 1989, pp 1426-1433.
38. Epstein M, Perez GO, Bedoya LA, Molina R: Continuous arterio-venous ultrafiltration in cirrhotic patients with ascites or renal failure. Int J Artif Organs, 9: 253-256, 1986.
39. Kaplan AA: Clinical trials with predilution and vacuum suction: enhancing the efficiency of the CAVH treatment. Trans Am Soc Artif Intern Organs, 32: 49-51, 1986.
40. Davenport A, Will EJ, Losowsky MS, Swindells S: Continuous arteriovenous haemofiltration in patients with hepatic encephalopathy and renal failure. Br Med J, 295: 1028, 1987.
41. Rimola A, Gavaler JS, Schade RR, El-Lankany S, Starzl TE, Van Thiel DH: Effects of renal impairment on liver transplantation. Gastroenterology, 93: 148-156, 1987.
42. Gonwa TA, Poplawski S, Paulsen W, Brajtbord D, Goldstein R, Husberg B, Klintmalm GB: Pathogenesis and outcome of hepatorenal syndrome in patients undergoing orthotopic liver transplant. Transplantation, 47: 395-397, 1989.
43. Busuttil RW, Colonna JO II, Hiatt JR, Brems JJ, El Khoury G, Goldstein LI, Quiñones-Baldrich WJ, Abdul-Rasool IH, Ramming KI: The first 100 liver transplants at UCLA. Ann Surg, 206: 387-399, 1987.
44. Krom RA, Wiesner RH, Rettke SR, Ludwig J, Southorn PA, Hermans PE, Taswell HF. The first 100 liver transplantations at the Mayo Clinic. Mayo Clin Proc, 64: 84-94, 1989.
45. O'Grady JG, Alexander GJM, Thick M, Potter D, Calne RY, Williams R: Outcome of orthotopic liver transplantation in the aetiological and clinical variants of acute liver failure. Q J Med, 69: 817-824, 1988.
46. Flavin DK, Niven RG, Kelsey JE: Alcoholism and orthotopic liver transplantation. JAMA, 259: 1546-1547, 1988.
47. Starzl TE, Van Thiel D, Tzakis AG, Iwatsuki S, Todo S, Marsh JW, Koneru B, Staschak S, Stieber A, Gordon RD: Orthotopic liver transplantation for alcoholic cirrhosis. JAMA, 260: 2542-2544, 1988

CHRONIC RENAL FAILURE

11

RECENT ADVANCES IN THE TREATMENT OF RENAL OSTEODYSTROPHY

ALBERT FOURNIER, PHILIPPE MORINIERE, BERNARD BOUDAILLIEZ, MARTINE ESTHER COHEN-SOLAL, RAIFAH MAKDASSI, PIERRE FRANÇOIS WESTEEL, JEAN LUC SEBERT AND JOHN B. EASTWOOD

Departments of Nephrology, Rheumatology and Pediatrics, CHU Amiens, France
Department of Biochemical Medicine, St George's Hospital Medical School, London, England

TREATMENT OF CLINICALLY SIGNIFICANT RENAL OSTEODYSTROPHY

Renal osteodystrophy becomes clinically significant when the following features are present: clinical symptoms (pain, muscle weakness, pruritus), radiological signs (subperiosteal erosions, osteopenia, fractures or pseudofractures, slipped epiphysis with *coxa vara* or *genu valgum* in children, metastatic calcification) and marked plasma abnormalities, particularly uncontrollable hyperphosphatemia. Clinically significant bone disease is not usually seen in adults until they have been on dialysis for several years but may be seen earlier (even before dialysis has been started) in children. Such bone disease may be due either to hyperparathyroidism or to aluminum (Al) bone disease. In favor of hyperparathyroidism are the following features (1, 2): rarity of pain and fractures, greater elevation of alkaline phosphatase, greater elevation of parathyroid hormone (PTH) plasma concentration and lower basal plasma concentration of Al (<300 μg/l) with smaller increase of plasma Al after i.v. administration of desferoxamine (increase <175 μg/l). It is only by bone biopsy, however, that it is possible to differentiate with certainty osteitis fibrosa, the bone expression of hyperparathyroidism, from osteomalacia or adynamic bone disease, both of which have been linked to Al intoxication (1, 2).

Whereas osteitis fibrosa is a consequence of hyperparathyroidism secondary to the disturbances in divalent ion metabolism induced by uremia (see below), aluminum bone disease appears to be an iatrogenic and therefore entirely avoidable form of bone disease. Since the discovery by Kerr's group (3) that the "epidemic" osteomalacia often associated with dialysis encephalopathy is related to the Al concentration of the dialysate, it has been possible to avoid the problem by adequate treatment of the water used to prepare the dialysate. However, it has become apparent that Al overload in uremic patients can also arise from Al-containing phosphate binders since sporadic aluminum bone disease is sometimes observed in patients who have either never been dialysed or have always been dialysed with Al-free dialysate. A bone histomorphometric study performed by Llach and Coburn (2) showed that, in 142 asymptomatic patients dialysed against a dialysate containing little or no Al for 56 ± 37 months, the prevalence of aluminum bone disease was high (27% of patients had osteomalacia and 7% adynamic bone disease), some of the patients subsequently becoming symptomatic.

The treatment of these forms of aluminum bone disease is now generally agreed (1, 2). The patients should be treated with desferoxamine in a dose of 20-30 mg/kg once a week during the last hour of a dialysis and such treatment should continue for several months. Treatment of osteomalacia with $24{,}25(OH)_2\ D_3$ has been less successful, the main effect being a decrease of plasma phosphate and plasma calcium (Ca) which allows a larger dose of calcitriol (1,25 dihydroxyvitamine D_3, the biologically active form of vitamin D) to be given (2). The results with desferoxamine have generally been satisfactory in osteomalacia though hyperparathyroid bone disease may sometimes develop during treatment; in such cases 1α hydroxylated D metabolites may be useful but, if not, parathyroidectomy may become necessary. In contrast, adynamic bone disease does not respond as well to desferoxamine and some authors have advocated transient stimulation of PTH secretion by a low dialysate Ca. Severe hyperparathyroidism, where the plasma Ca is still low or normal, should be treated by providing more efficient dialysis, increasing doses of PO_4-binders including Ca carbonate ($CaCO_3$), greater dietary restriction in PO_4 and 1α OH vitamin D derivatives. A controversy exists as regards the superiority of i.v. versus oral administration of these vitamin D derivatives. An advantage of the i.v. route is the certainty of treatment, at least in hospital, since it can be administered by a nurse at the end of each dialysis. There is also the possibility that the metabolites when given i.v. might, by inducing higher plasma calcitriol levels than by the oral route, cause a greater stimulation of the calcitriol receptors in the parathyroid glands. Indeed, PTH levels often fall before there has been a rise in ionized Ca as a result of the stimulated Ca absorption by the gut (4). This might result in more effective suppression of PTH than by using the oral route. However, according to Quarles et al (5), equally good suppression of hyperparathyroidism (as assessed by measuring intact plasma PTH but without histological data) can be achieved with oral calcitriol + $CaCO_3$ + $Al(OH)_3$. If the plasma Ca is normal at the start of treatment, there is usually a rapid rise above 11.0 mg/dl and the dose of $CaCO_3$ and calcitriol have to be decreased even when a low dialysate Ca is used. Because this hypercalcemia often occurs before the alkaline phosphatase has returned to normal, parathyroidectomy may have to be considered. Before surgery, Al overload must, however, first be excluded. This must be done not only by bone biopsy with Al staining, but also using a desferoxamine test since parathyroidectomy can precipitate low bone turn over disease with relocation of the Al buried in the bone at the calcified/osteoid interface, even if the pre-parathyroidectomy biopsy showed predominant osteitis fibrosa with little positive Al staining (2). One should be careful therefore to perform parathyroidectomy only when post-desferoxamine plasma Al values are known to be below 150 µg/l. When using desferoxamine one should be aware of its potential hazards, namely hypotension, allergic skin rashes, iron depletion, retinal abnormalities, early cataract formation, ototoxicity, precipitation of dialysis dementia, yersiniosis and fungal infections with the *rhizopus* responsible for the usually fatal mucormycosis (2). The frequency of these severe complications has been reduced by lowering the dose to 20-30 mg/kg per week, but one must be aware that a single challenge test may induce an irreversible complication such as ocular toxicity (6).

The present treatment of severe renal osteodystrophy is unsatisfactory because of the iatrogenic vicious cycle induced by the use of Al PO_4-binders: these binders lead to Al overload with consequences not only on bone but also on the brain (dementia), bone marrow (anemia), soft tissues (calcinosis) (7) and on the joints (Al overload has been recently incriminated in the pathogenesis of erosive arthropathies with β2 microglobulin amyloidosis) (8). Treatment of this Al overload necessitates desferoxamine administration which brings its own hazards. In spite of a large literature on the pathophysiology of aluminum bone disease, no treatment other than desferoxamine has been evaluated on a long term basis. Removal of Al by biocompatible hemoperfusion on Al/Fe Clark® specific cartridges prevents side-effects of systemic use of desferoxamine, but this treatment needs long term evaluation and is expensive. Therefore, the major challenge in the treatment of renal osteodystrophy is how to prevent hyperparathyroidism without exposing the patients to the risk of iatrogenic Al intoxication. In 1982 we proposed (9) that oral Ca supplement should be used not only to correct the negative Ca balance, but also more importantly as a PO_4-binder by giving it with meals at doses proportional to their PO_4 content. Before discussing the clinical efficacy and safety of this approach we shall consider the rationale of the use of oral Ca supplements.

ORAL CALCIUM SUPPLEMENTATION AND ITS EFFECTS ON THE PATHOGENESIS OF HYPERPARATHYROIDISM, OSTEOMALACIA AND ADYNAMIC BONE DISEASE

Metabolic effects of calcium supplements as $CaCO_3$

First, oral Ca supplements can be used to increase the passive absorption of Ca, a process that remains normal in uremia (10-12), in contrast to the calcitriol dependent absorption which is usually impaired. The negative Ca balance in uremic individuals can be prevented if the total intake of elemental Ca is greater than 1.5 g/day, especially if the supplemental Ca is taken fasting or between meals (11). It should be pointed out that, when the supplement is taken with meals, Ca can become bound to PO_4, which decreases the absorption and increases the fecal elimination of both Ca and PO_4 (10, 12, 13). The importance of this schedule for administration of oral Ca as a PO_4-binder (9) has received support recently from the data of Schiller et al (13) in their study of net absorption of Ca and PO_4 by the technique of intestinal lavage. Although the decrease of plasma PO_4 with oral Ca may be explained by gut PO_4 being complexed by Ca in the gut, it should be remembered that the early balance data of Clarkson et al (10) showed that, during high intake of $CaCO_3$, not only the Ca balance but also the PO_4 balance became positive (because the decrease of the intestinal absorption of PO_4 was compensated for by a greater reduction of phosphaturia consequent upon a fall in plasma PTH). Therefore it is possible that the decrease of plasma PO_4 seen by Clarkson et al (10) was explicable partly on the basis of Ca phosphate deposition within the body, though which tissue was involved (bone or soft tissues) was not clear in this short term study. It must be kept therefore in mind that soft tissue calcification may increase without being preceded by increase in the plasma concentrations of Ca and PO_4 and that innocuity of high doses of $CaCO_3$ will be proven only by long term observation. We will see below that it is fortunately the case with a follow up of 2-4 years. Finally the study of Clarkson et al (10) showed also an increase in plasma bicarbonate with a decrease of urinary excretion of H^+ suggesting a gastrointestinal mechanism for the alkalinizing effect of $CaCO_3$ administration. This alkalinizing effect results from the fact that in the stomach HCl reacts with $CaCO_3$ to give $CaCl_2$ and CO_2 + H_2O. Some of the $CaCl_2$ is absorbed by the gut while the remainder is converted back to $CaCO_3$ or to Ca PO_4H. It is clear that the amount of Ca absorbed with Cl^- and therefore not combined with CO_3H^- to form $CaCO_3$ (according to the equation $CaCl_2 + 2NaHCO_3 = CaCO_3 + 2NaCl + H_2O + CO_2$), corresponds to the amount of net H^+ secretion into the gut and therefore to the alkalinizing effect.

Pathogenesis of hyperparathyroidism in uremia

Figure 1 gives our current view of the pathogenesis of hyperparathyroidism in uremia. It differs only slightly from that proposed in 1985 (14). The main difference concerns the role of PO_4 retention in early renal failure and the mechanisms involved in the resetting upwards of Ca-regulated PTH secretion. In early renal failure there is a trend towards hypophosphatemia, not hyperphosphatemia. Therefore, the trade-off theory of Bricker and Slatopolsky, by which stimulation of PTH secretion is explained solely by the physico-chemically mediated decrease of ionised Ca when plasma PO_4 transiently increases because of the decrease in GFR, can no longer be regarded as entirely valid. The following explanation has been proposed by Llach et al (2) and Bonjour (15). Reduction of nephron mass leads to a rise in the intracellular concentration of PO_4 in the proximal tubule by an unprecised mechanism, which, however, probably depends on an increased filtered load of PO_4 per nephron mainly explained by an increase of single nephron GFR and not necessarily by a transient hyperphosphatemia. This induces, with the acidosis, a depression of 1α hydroxylase activity. The resulting deficiency in calcitriol contributes to: 1/ the negative intestinal Ca balance (because of lack of active Ca absorption in conjunction with a low dietary intake of Ca, which may be spontaneous as a result of anorexia or secondary to the dietary restriction in protein and PO_4) (11); 2/ the blunted hypercalcemic effect of PTH; 3/ the upper resetting of Ca-regulated PTH secretion. It has been shown that calcitriol depresses the synthesis of the mRNA of prepro PTH by its action on the parathyroid receptors and that the expression of calcitriol receptors in parathyroid glands is reduced in renal failure (16). Thus, even in the absence of continued hyperphosphatemia, PTH secretion is hyperstimulated, an observation that explains why patients with early renal failure (40-80 ml/min) have relatively low fasting plasma PO_4 levels and are able to excrete a PO_4 load more rapidly than a normal individual. When renal failure progresses (GFR <25 ml/min) plasma PO_4 increases and contributes to the hypocalcemia by

Figure 1 : PATHOGENESIS OF OSTEITIS FIBROSA AND HYPERPARATHYROIDISM IN UREMIA

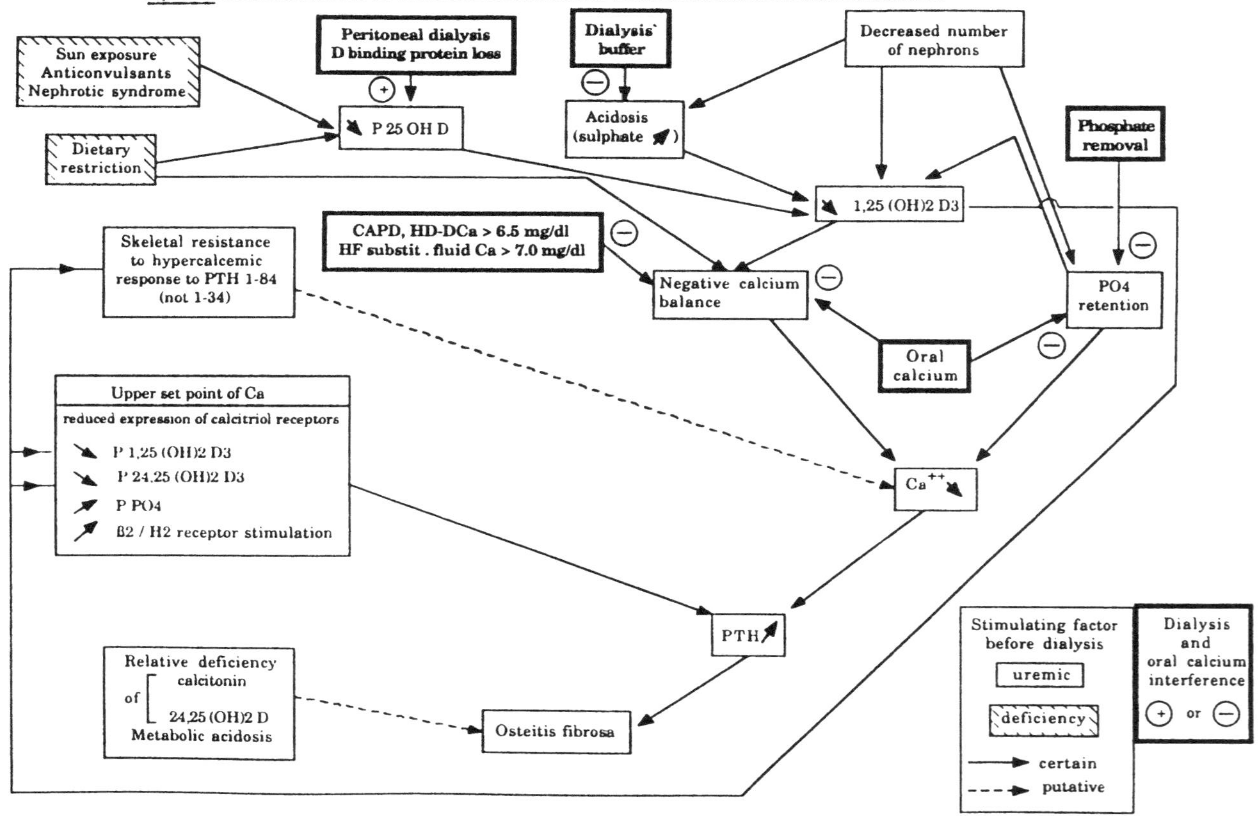

physico-chemical mechanisms. Furthermore, increased plasma PO_4 may independently contribute to the upper resetting of Ca-regulated PTH secretion (17).

When a patient is on chronic dialysis, Ca balance may be influenced by the intradialytic Ca balance depending on dialysate Ca. Assuming a normal ultrafiltrable Ca of 6.0 mg/dl and a body weight loss of about 3 kg, there will be a Ca loss of 180 mg by ultrafiltration per procedure. Under these circumstances a dialysate Ca of 6.5 mg/dl will probably maintain Ca balance in equilibrium over the course of a dialysis. A recent study has shown that during a 4 hour dialysis there was a Ca loss of 98 mg with a dialysate Ca of 6.0 mg/dl and a gain of Ca of 110 mg using a dialysate Ca of 7.0 mg/dl (18). For patients being treated by hemofiltration the recommended ultrafiltration is approximately 30 liters per treatment. Therefore, the Ca concentration in the substitution fluid should be higher than in hemodialysis fluid so that there is no net loss of Ca during the hemofiltration session. To give an example: if body weight loss is 3 kg and 1 liter of fluid is used to prime the circuit, the Ca loss during a hemofiltration session will be given by: 30 liters x 6 mg/dl = 1800 mg of Ca. Since the amount of substitution fluid in the same session should be: 30 - (3+1) = 26 liters, to maintain a null balance, Ca concentration in substitution fluid should be: 6.9 mg/dl (in fact, 26 liters x 6.9 mg/dl = about 1800 mg of Ca).

In addition to the above mentioned factors directly related to uremia and its treatment, hyperparathyroidism may be aggravated by vitamin D depletion as detected by a low plasma 25 OH vitamin D. Uremia is unique in that there is a direct correlation between the plasma concentrations of 25 OH D and calcitriol; hence a low plasma 25 OH D can have an adverse effect on hyperparathyroidism by inducing a low plasma concentration of calcitriol (19).

Interference of oral Ca supplements with the pathogenesis of hyperparathyroidism

If given between meals in a dose sufficient to overcome the negative intestinal Ca balance, oral Ca will restore plasma Ca to normal but will not prevent PO_4 retention. Since calcitriol deficiency is not corrected by oral Ca, the blunted calcemic response to PTH and upward shift of the set point of Ca-regulated PTH secretion, which are dependent upon normal plasma concentrations of calcitriol, will remain. If the supplement of Ca is given with meals rich in PO_4 so that intestinal PO_4 is complexed, oral Ca will tend to prevent PO_4 retention and increase calcitriol synthesis, thereby tending to correct the disturbances linked to calcitriol deficiency. That it is possible to correct the pathophysiological events of hyperparathyroidism in early renal failure by dietary PO_4 restriction alone has been demonstrated by Llach and Coburn in 4 patients (2). We shall see below that such effects are also possible with $CaCO_3$, which has been found by Turner et al (20) to decrease plasma PO_4 and increase plasma calcitriol in early renal failure as effectively as $Al(OH)_3$, when combined with similar moderate restriction of dietary PO_4.

Interference of oral Ca supplements with the pathogenesis of osteomalacia and adynamic bone disease (Figure 2)

Al PO_4-binders appear to be the major cause of osteomalacia and adynamic bone disease both in uremic patients not yet on dialysis and in those dialyzed using dialysate known to contain little or no Al. Clearly in these individuals, substitution of $CaCO_3$ for $Al(OH)_3$ should avoid such complications. Furthermore, since in patients not yet on dialysis administration of $CaCO_3$ causes a positive Ca balance, an increase in calcitriol synthesis in vitamin D replete patients and overcomes the acidosis and hypocalcemia, there should be a beneficial effect on the osteomalacia in such patients (14). In anephric hemodialysis patients who had normal plasma Ca and mild hyperphoshatemia we reported, with Bordier and de Wardener (21), the absence of histological evidence of osteomalacia. This evidence suggests that, provided the Ca x PO_4 product is high enough and the individuals are vitamin D replete, normal levels of calcitriol are not necessary for the maintenance of normal bone mineralization (21). Abolition of the negative Ca balance by dialysis and/or $CaCO_3$, however, will not benefit a vitamin D deplete state which may be associated with deficient synthesis of potentially useful vitamin D metabolites at the bone or cartilage levels. In other words it is important to keep vitamin D depletion in mind in individuals with osteomalacia; similarly the toxic effect of barbiturates on bone will not be affected by improvements in the balance or plasma levels of Ca and PO_4.

If Ca supplements are given as PO_4-binder it will be possible to avoid completely the use of magnesium (Mg) antacids as a PO_4-binder in uremic individuals not yet on dialysis. It will also be possible to reduce the dose of Mg salts given to dialysis patients who are being dialysed using a low Mg dialysate. The risk of Mg-induced osteomalacia (reported only in experimental animals) will therefore be decreased by Ca supplements. In fact, after 18 months of mild hypermagnesemia (1.5 mmol/l) induced by low doses of $Mg(OH)_2$ in association with oral Ca, no adverse effect on bone mineralization was observed in our dialysed patients (22).

Figure 2 : PATHOGENESIS OF OSTEOMALACIA IN UREMIA

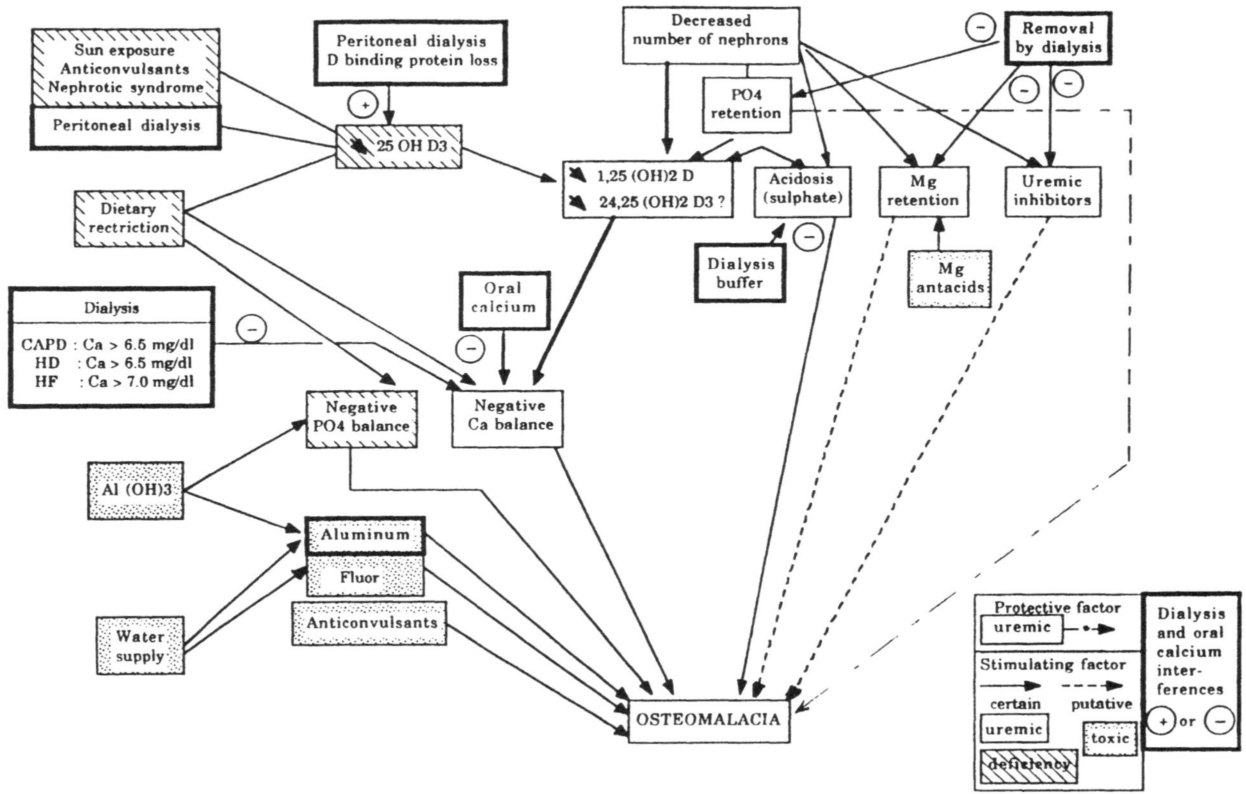

Adynamic bone disease has up to now (in the absence of iron overload, parathyroidectomy, corticosteroid, diabetes) been causally related only to Al intoxication. Such a cause and effect relationship has been suggested even when no stainable Al was present in a bone biopsy because the patients were taking Al hydroxide [$Al(OH)_3$] and had moderately increased plasma Al (4 times normal) (23). The occurrence of adynamic bone disease in patients taking Ca supplements alone should be exceptional unless marked PTH suppression is induced.

PREVENTION OF RENAL OSTEODYSTROPHY BEFORE DIALYSIS: $CaCO_3$ OR SMALL DOSES OF CALCITRIOL?

Before discussing the respective roles of $CaCO_3$ and calcitriol, it is important to stress that all possible measures should be instituted with a view to slowing down any decline in renal function. These measures include: 1/ diagnosis and treatment of urinary tract obstruction, dehydration and drug intoxication; 2/ good control of blood pressure; 3/ dietary restriction of protein and PO_4. As regards the last mentioned, we recommend, in adults, moderate reduction of dairy products and a protein intake of 1 g/kg/day when the GFR is 60 ml/min. We recommend a protein intake of 0.7 g/kg/day when the GFR has reached 40 ml/min and 0.4 g/kg/day with the addition of essential aminoacids or ketoanalogs when the GFR is between 15 and 5 ml/min.

PREVENTION OF HYPERPARATHYROIDISM

This is based on measures which can be grouped according to their major aims: 1/ prevention of PO_4 retention and Ca deficiency without inducing Al intoxication; 2/ prevention of vitamin D deficiency; 3/ prevention of metabolic acidosis. To what extent these goals can be achieved by appropriate oral supplements of alkaline salts of Ca will be discussed below.

1/ Prevention of phosphate retention and Ca deficiency without Al intoxication.

The PO_4 intake of an adult in industrialized countries is between 1.0 and 1.8 g/day. By exclusion of dairy products and reduction of protein intake to 0.7 g/kg/day (i.e. to 40 g/day for a 60 kg patient) the PO_4 intake can be reduced to 600 - 900 mg/day, i.e. 60% of the normal intake. This reduction of PO_4 intake will be proportional to the reduction of GFR (as recommended by Slatopolsky) only for a reduction of GFR to 60%, i.e. 72 ml/min, if one assumes a normal GFR of 120 ml/min/1.73 m^2. Therefore, at a GFR of as high as 60 ml/min the above mentioned restrictions will already be insufficient. Furthermore, since patients with a GFR of 60 ml/min have a normal or even low plasma PO_4 and a normal plasma Ca, we believe that protein restriction is not yet appropriate and would delay such restriction till the GFR is below 40 ml/min. Therefore, in patients with a GFR of 60 ml/min eating 1g/kg/day of protein, prevention of PO_4 retention will have to be achieved using PO_4-binders. In order to avoid Al, it would seem appropriate to use an oral supplement of an alkaline salt of Ca, for example $CaCO_3$ for which there is the widest clinical experience.

In what dose and how should Ca carbonate be given to uremic patients before dialysis?

A positive Ca balance can be achieved in patients with renal failure by increasing elemental Ca intake to 1500 mg/day. Assuming a Ca intake in the food of 400 mg, most uremic patients will need a supplement of around 1200 mg of elemental Ca, i.e. 3 g of $CaCO_3$, 40% of which is elemental Ca. As discussed above, it is important that the daily dose should be taken with meals in order to better complex the PO_4 and decrease the amount of Ca absorbed, since hypercalcemia can be a limiting factor of the use of $CaCO_3$ as a PO_4-binder (13).

This therapy with $CaCO_3$ should be monitored by periodic measurements of Ca and PO_4 not only in the plasma but also in the urine. Plasma values of Ca and PO_4 are usually in the normal range as long as GFR has not decreased <25 ml/min. However, the urinary excretion of Ca and PO_4 is in the main a reflection of intestinal absorption of these substances, provided there is no excessive release of Ca and PO_4 from bone as happens when there is severe hyperparathyroidism. Therefore determination of urine Ca and urine PO_4 gives indirect information on the effectiveness of dietary restriction and chelation of PO_4 and on Ca absorption. From the data of ourselves (24), Baker et al (25) and Tessitore et al (26) it appears that the urine Ca of patients with a GFR of 40 ml/min should be increased but no more than up to 120 mg/24 hr since above this level there is a risk of hypercalcemia with possible deterioration of renal function. Ideally, urine PO_4 should be around 500 mg/24 hr and urine urea around 13 g/24 hr reflecting a daily dietary intake of 800 mg of PO_4 and 40 g of protein. $CaCO_3$ is usually well tolerated and only occasionally causes diarrhea or constipation. With doses of less than 6 g/day taken with meals, hypercalcemia is exceptional.

Though some non commercial preparations of $CaCO_3$ are moderately palatable, $CaCO_3$ palatability has undoubtedly been improved in certain commercial preparations (in France Calcidia®, Lefranc - Calcium Forte®, Sandoz).

Can other salts of calcium be used?

Although $CaCl_2$ binds well with PO_4 it should not be used because it causes acidosis. Alkaline salts of Ca other than $CaCO_3$ may be used, but since these salts are lower than $CaCO_3$ as regards Ca content the doses are bulkier. They have no intrinsic superiority except, perhaps, Ca acetate which, because of solubility in both acid and alkaline solutions, has a greater effect as regards PO_4 chelation and a lesser Ca absorption (27). Ca citrate is claimed to be more palatable than $CaCO_3$ but, if it is used, $Al(OH)_3$ should not be given at the same time since Bakir et al (28) have shown that the citrate ion promotes Al absorption. The development of Ca alginate (or polyuronate) described by Schneider et al (29) has been hampered by technical problems; unfortunately also it has been unpopular with patients because it is taken in the form of a large number of big capsules.

Since the report of Mitch et al (30) pointing out the hypophosphatemic and hypercalcemic effects of the Ca salts of aminoacid-ketoanalogs (Ca KA of Fresenius laboratory), there have been several reports which have also shown that these analogs have an important, although ill understood, suppressive effect on hyperparathyroidism (31). It is possible that the supplementation of biologically important aminoacid-ketoanalogs induces incorporation of PO_4 into intracellular structures or alternatively ketoanalogs may have a direct effect on the parathyroid glands. Recent work by Schaeffer et al (32) suggests that the most likely explanation for the suppressive effect on the parathyroid glands is by virtue of their action as PO_4-binders as a result of their Ca content (the 18 tablets of mixed ketoanalogs or of pure ketovalin taken daily contain respectively 900 and 1680 mg of elemental Ca). Ketoanalogs may, however, undergo a more favorable pH dependent dissociation in the gut than $CaCO_3$ so that the complexing capacity for PO_4 may be greater. Trials are at present under way in which ketovalin is being compared with $CaCO_3$ in order to evaluate its potential superiority over $CaCO_3$ as regards its efficacy and tolerance. It is very likely that the hypophosphatemic effect of Ca free ketoanalogs (*Synthelabo*) is due just to the decreased intake of PO_4 associated with the decreased intake of protein that they allow and not to a PO_4 binding effect.

Can magnesium hydroxide or carbonate be used in uremic patients not yet on dialysis?

Mg hydroxide and Mg carbonate should never be used as PO_4-binders in uremic patients not yet on dialysis, since they will aggravate the mild hypermagnesemia which is usually already present. Furthermore, by increasing the volume of the stools they may stimulate Ca secretion by the gut and induce a negative Ca balance.

2/ Prevention of vitamin D deficiency

The term "vitamin D deficiency" when used in the context of uremia can lead to confusion since it has two different meanings: 1/ it may mean low plasma 25 OH D, and this state would be better called "vitamin D depletion", 2/ it may also mean low plasma calcitriol.

The prevalence of vitamin D depletion in uremic patients is different in different countries and depends on the extent of solar exposure and nutritional habits of the inhabitants. Thus, it is rare in countries such as the USA, where it is common for foods to be fortified with vitamin D_2, but relatively frequent in Northern European industrial countries like Britain or France where there are low levels of solar irradiation and little or no fortification of food. A tendency to vitamin D depletion may further be aggravated by a nephrotic syndrome since heavy proteinuria is associated with loss of 25 OH vitamin D binding protein into the urine; another adverse factor is treatment with barbiturates, phenytoin and gluthetimide, all of which induce hypercatabolism of 25 OH vitamin D. Restriction of protein and dairy products and the use of fiber-rich bread (since ligninine chelates not only Ca but also vitamin D metabolites interrupting the enterohepatic cycle of vitamin D) also lead to vitamin D depletion. Prevention of vitamin D depletion by giving either parent vitamin D or 25 OH vitamin D_3 in adequate doses (400 IU of vitamin D_2 or 10 μg of 25 OH D_3 are physiological daily doses in the normal adult) is crucial since in uremia plasma calcitriol critically depends on plasma 25 OH D (19). Also we have found that the incidence of subperiosteal resorption is higher in those uremic patients with the lower levels of plasma 25 OH D (14). It is therefore advisable to monitor plasma 25 OH D in uremic patients and to keep it in the upper range of normal by using appropriate supplements of vitamin D or 25 OH D_3.

However, even in vitamin D replete uremic patients, plasma calcitriol falls with the decrease of GFR (2). Can this calcitriol deficiency be prevented simply by ensuring that PO_4 retention is avoided? Portale et al (33) were the first to demonstrate that plasma calcitriol in children with early renal failure could be increased by lowering the plasma PO_4 with $Al(OH)_3$. Turner et al (20) have confirmed these findings, recently, also in children with early renal failure, but showed in addition that the increase of plasma calcitriol could be obtained as easily with $CaCO_3$. These findings are particularly interesting since in patients with more advanced renal failure (GFR 5-20 ml/min) to whom much higher doses of $Al(OH)_3$ where given than the patients of Portale et al (33), Takamoto et al (34) have shown that the decrease of plasma PO_4 with $Al(OH)_3$ administration was associated with a decrease in plasma calcitriol. This decrease is probably attributable to suppression of PTH induced not only by the lower plasma PO_4 but also by a direct toxic effect of Al on the parathyroid glands as well as to a direct toxic effect of Al on the renal 1α hydroxylase system. In contrast we have shown (24) in 12 patients with moderate uremia [plasma creatinine (Cr) = 3.3 ± 0.6 mg/dl] that it is possible to maintain plasma calcitriol in the normal range for 1 year by the following measures: prevention of PO_4 retention by moderate dietary restriction of protein (0.8 g/kg/day) and PO_4 (17 mg/kg/day), use of 3 g of $CaCO_3$ as a PO_4-binder, and supplementation with 10-20 μg of 25 OH D_3 in order to raise plasma 25 OH D to the upper limit of normal (30 ng/ml). Using this regimen plasma Ca remained at 9.4 mg/dl and urine Ca increased from 40 to 80 mg/24 hr though the plasma PO_4 did increase slightly (3.5→4.4 mg/dl) because of the decrease of GFR (plasma Cr increased to 4.2 mg/dl but with a decrease in the slope of 1/plasma Cr suggesting that the rate of decline of GFR decreased). These observations are in agreement with those of Tessitore et al (26).

The practice of maintaining normal and sometimes high plasma calcitriol values without Al PO_4-binders has the advantage of interrupting the vicious cycle between calcitriol administration and intestinal absorption of Al and Ca by the gut. In this context we have recently published (35) indirect clinical evidence that 1α OH vitamin D_3 increases intestinal absorption of Al by showing that 1α OH D_3 increases plasma Al only in patients taking simultaneously a constant dose of $Al(OH)_3$ but not in those not taking $Al(OH)_3$. On the other hand, Merke et al (36) have shown that Al intoxication leads to a post receptor resistance of enterocytes to calcitriol with the result that active Ca absorption is impeded.

Is there a need for 1α hydroxylated vitamin D derivatives when Ca carbonate is given and vitamin D depletion prevented?

Theoretically yes since, by ensuring high plasma calcitriol levels, it should be possible to compensate for the reduced expression of calcitriol receptors in the parathyroid glands and adjust downwards the set point of Ca-regulated PTH secretion. Furthermore, in practice it may not be possible to achieve normal-high plasma calcitriol levels in more advanced uremia, because of reduced nephron mass, even if hyperphosphatemia is avoided. However, in adults given $CaCO_3$, who have no radiographic signs of renal osteodystrophy and normal plasma alkaline phosphatase, 1α OH vitamin D derivatives tend to cause hypercalcemia. In general therefore 1α derivatives, if given, should be given on their own. Occasionally, however, especially in children, $CaCO_3$ overcomes hyperphosphatemia without correcting the hypocalcemia; in these individuals it should be safe to give 1α OH D derivatives, and their administration is then recommanded.

Is treatment with small doses of 1α hydroxylated vitamin D metabolites alone safer and more efficacious than administration of an oral Ca supplement?

It is impossible to answer this question with any degree of certainty although three studies have produced useful data: 1/ the study of Coen et al (37) who compared 15 patients treated with 0.25 μg/day of calcitriol with 23 controls, their initial mean plasma Cr being 4.9 mg/dl and their diet restricted in protein (0.8 g/kg/day), PO_4 (12 mg/kg/day) and Ca (500 mg/day); 2/ the study of Massry (38), in which 17 patients, with milder renal insufficiency (15-50 ml/min of GFR), received 0.5 μg/day of calcitriol; 3/ the recent study by Baker et al (25), in which 8 patients with early renal failure (plasma Cr = 2.4±1.2 mg/dl) received small doses of calcitriol (0.25 μg/day). The biochemical changes, reported by Coen et al (37) and Baker et al (25), with 0.25 μg/day of calcitriol, are similar to those that we observed in 12 uremic patients with a plasma Cr of 3.5 mg/dl, i.e.with a renal function between that of the above studies. The bone histological changes also were similar, since we found a significant decrease of osteoid volume and osteoblastic surface (in keeping with a decrease in alkaline phosphatase). There was also a non significant decrease in osteoclasts and no increase of C terminal PTH in spite of the decrease of GFR (which decreases C terminal fragment catabolism) suggesting a real decrease in PTH secretion. Mineral apposition which was normal initially was unchanged at 1 year. Furthermore, we observed adynamic bone disease in two patients in association with plasma PTH levels which were equal to those of patients with normal bone but with higher plasma Cr, suggesting that adynamic bone disease may be due to an insufficient hyperparathyroidism, i.e. a relative hypoparathyroidism in relation to the degree of renal failure. This adynamic bone disease was probably due, in the absence of hypercalcemia or hypophosphatemia, to the high levels of plasma calcitriol secondary to the high levels of 25 OH D induced by 25 OH D_3 administration. These observations are in agreement with the decrease in bone formation rate observed by Baker et al (25) in their patients treated with calcitriol.

3/ Prevention of metabolic acidosis

Metabolic acidosis is associated with deleterious effects on bone. There is a negative Ca balance, a rise in plasma PO_4 and a fall in 1α hydroxylase activity (2, 14).

$CaCO_3$ may have a role in raising plasma bicarbonate (10), although in some individuals with chronic interstitial nephritis or polycystic disease an adequate rise of plasma bicarbonate is difficult to achieve. In such cases, therapy with other alkali, such as sodium, bicarbonate or citrate, may be the only way of ensuring that the plasma bicarbonate returns to or remains within the normal range. Combined Ca and alkali therapy can be achieved by using *Calcium Forte Sandoz* ® each tablet of which contains 500 mg of elemental Ca and 12 mEq of Na bicarbonate. In France "Vichy" alkaline waters, which are still very popular for the control of acidosis in uremia, should be abandoned since they are rich in fluoride and known to cause fluorosis in patients with renal failure. Shohl's solution, which contains citric acid, can be used with $CaCO_3$ but should never be given in association with $Al(OH)_3$ since citrate ions promote Al absorption, which may lead to fatal Al encephalopathy within months (28).

PREVENTION OF OSTEOMALACIA AND ADYNAMIC BONE DISEASE

In keeping with our current knowledge of pathophysiology, osteomalacia did not develop in our patients treated with $CaCO_3$ + 25 OH D nor in those of Baker et al (25) treated with 0.25 µg/day of calcitriol alone. The efficacy of calcitriol in curing osteomalacia is not well demonstrated, on the other hand, by the study of Coen et al (37), since he found no difference between control group and group treated with 0.25 µg of calcitriol as regards osteoid parameters. When $Al(OH)_3$ is used in the treatment of uremic patients not yet on dialysis, a deleterious effect on bone mineralisation is usually observed. Thus, Turner et al (20), who gave $Al(OH)_3$ for 6 months after 6 months of $CaCO_3$, found on the second biopsy both positive Al staining and decreased mineral apposition rate. Also, Nordal and Dahl (39) found a significant decrease of the mineral apposition rate to the lower limit of normal in their group of 15 patients treated with a mean dose of 0.36 µg of calcitriol for 8 months, whereas this parameter remained stable and normal in the placebo group. Eight patients of each group had received $Al(OH)_3$ in order to control their plasma $PO_4 < 5.1$ mg/dl while their mean plasma Cr was 4.0 ± 1.0 mg/dl. It is noteworthy that the dose of $Al(OH)_3$ had to be increased only in the calcitriol group. New Al staining occurred in two patients in the calcitriol group, whereas in the control group Al staining developed *de novo* in only one, and in one other patient (a diabetic one) there was a decrease of the widespread Al staining present initially thanks to a decrease in the dose of $Al(OH)_3$. From the experiences of Baker et al (25) and ourselves (40) it is clear that adynamic bone disease is a possible consequence of over enthusiastic attention to suppression of hyperparathyroidism. It is to be hoped that the long term prognosis of this adynamic bone disease is very different from that of aluminum adynamic bone disease.

PRACTICAL CONCLUSIONS FOR THE PREVENTION OF RENAL OSTEODYSTROPHY IN EARLY AND MODERATE RENAL FAILURE

The *primum non nocere* principle should always be respected and therefore the only patients one should treat are those in whom plasma and urinary Ca, PO_4, urea and creatinine can be adequately monitored in order to maintain plasma Ca between 10.0 and 10.5 mg/dl, plasma PO_4 between 3.5-4.5 mg/dl, urine Ca between 80-120 mg/24 hr and urine PO_4 around 500 mg/24 hr. Clearly one should first correct any possible vitamin D depletion so yet it is not clear from the literature which of the two therapeutic measures, $CaCO_3$ or calcitriol administration is preferable. We would favor giving $CaCO_3$, not only because it is less expensive, but because it is capable on its own of preventing PO_4 retention, increasing plasma calcitriol and improving the acidosis. Furthermore, since $CaCO_3$ alone is capable of preventing clinically significant hyperparathyroidim in dialysis patients (see below), it is a treatment that can be continued throughout the life of a uremic individual. In contrast administration of calcitriol promotes PO_4 retention, since it causes an increase in intestinal absorption of PO_4 (11). This increase in PO_4 absorption may not at first be apparent since the plasma PO_4 may remain normal or even fall as a result of suppression of hyperparathyroidism with the consequent reduction in bone resorption. It has been shown that it is possible to prevent calcitriol-induced hyperphosphatemia in early (25) and even moderate renal failure but then by imposing a diet very restricted in PO_4 (37). Such good control of plasma PO_4 is difficult to achieve in patients with more advanced renal failure, especially if they do not adhere to the low PO_4 diet. This means that 1α OH D_3 derivatives may be dangerous in patient with advanced renal failure (GFR $<$ 15 ml/min) as has been shown by Christiansen et al (41) and Toogard et al (42), who found that renal function deteriorates with calcitriol or 1α as a result of the increase in PO_4 and plasma Ca. Furthermore, it should be remembered that there is experimental evidence that calcitriol may increase the Ca content of the aorta and of the kidneys even if plasma Ca and PO_4 are kept within the normal range (43). In contrast, our experience with $CaCO_3$ in dialysis patients is reassuring in this regard (see below).

Until further studies are performed in which 1α OH vitamin D derivatives are compared with $CaCO_3$, the role of 1α OH vitamin D derivatives in the preventive treatment of renal osteodystrophy is uncertain. As will be discussed below in relation to patients on dialysis, vitamin D derivatives without hypercalcemic effects [for example 24,25 $(OH)_2$ D_3 and 22-oxa-calcitriol] may prove, in combination with $CaCO_3$, to be the ideal preventive treatment of renal osteodystrophy.

PREVENTION OF RENAL OSTEODYSTROPHY DURING MAINTENANCE DIALYSIS

Classical treatment with $Al(OH)_3$ + low doses of oral Ca with or without 1α OH vitamin D derivatives and a dialysate Ca of 7.0 mg/dl

Since the early 1970's prevention of hyperparathyroidism in dialysis patients has been based on the notion that one could compensate for the negative intestinal Ca balance by ensuring a positive intradialytic Ca balance using a dialysate Ca of 7.0 mg/dl and secondly control predialysis hyperphosphatemia by oral Al PO_4-binders (44). In addition, small amounts of oral Ca and 1α hydroxylated D derivatives have been given with the intention of better suppressing the parathyroid glands. Two double blind trials of oral calcitriol versus placebo in asymptomatic dialysis patients (45, 46) have clearly shown on radiological and biochemical grounds that calcitriol in low doses (0.25-0.5 μg/day) is effective in preventing osteitis fibrosa. Unfortunatcly, worsening hyperphosphatemia often led to increased use of Al PO_4-binders. Bone histology in the study of Baker et al (46) suggested that the price of curing osteitis fibrosa might be induction of osteomalacia. In the 10 control patients, 5 of the 8 with initially normal bone developed osteitis fibrosa, whereas in the 10 treated patients only 1 of the 5 with initially normal bone developed osteitis fibrosa, but 3 of them developed osteomalacia and 3 who started osteomalacic remained osteomalacic. In most cases, the osteomalacia was associated with positive Al staining even when the dialysate Al levels were low. Since exposure to Al was comparable in the two groups, the higher prevalence of osteomalacia in the treated group suggests that calcitriol in these patients may have unmasked Al toxicity by decreasing hyperparathyroidism. These observations are in agreement with those of Delmez et al (47), who showed that adequate control of hyperparathyroidism by maintaining the plasma PO_4 in the normal range using Al PO_4-binders was associated with the development of histological osteomalacia.

New treatment with oral Ca supplements as phosphate binders

In 1980 we became aware of the hazards of $Al(OH)_3$ for two reasons. First, two of our patients, who were known to be taking $Al(OH)_3$ regularly, died from an encephalopathy and secondly the treatment of our water by reverse osmosis in 1978 had not been followed by a decrease in plasma Al which continued to be correlated with the intake of Al PO_4-binder (48). It was decided, therefore, at that time to discontinue $Al(OH)_3$ completely in all our dialysis patients and to replace it by a higher dose of $CaCO_3$ in order to complex PO_4. In 1982 we reported our experience of 6 months in 23 patients in whom we showed that an increase of $CaCO_3$ dose from 3 to 9 g/day was as effective as 4 g of $Al(OH)_3$ with or without 1α OH D_3 in maintaining plasma PO_4 < 6.0 mg/dl without hypercalcemia. In the majority there was no increase in plasma PTH or alkaline phosphatase suggesting reasonable control of hyperparathyroidism in spite of the decrease in plasma Al (9). These data have since been confirmed by others (see review 49). Furthermore, in a second study we compared in a randomized 6 months' trial the control of hyperparathyroidism obtained with either 9 g of $CaCO_3$/day alone or $CaCO_3$ 3g/day together with 1α OH D_3 and $Al(OH)_3$; the plasma PTH remained stable and comparable in the two groups in spite of lower plasma Al in the $CaCO_3$ group (50). When high doses of $CaCO_3$ are used as PO_4-binder, 1α OH vitamin D derivatives should not be given routinely because of potential hypercalcemia. However, when as little as 3 g of $CaCO_3$ is sufficient to prevent hyperphosphatemia (as is the experience of an Italian group), small doses of calcitriol can be given without producing hypercalcemia in the majority of patients (51). In all cases vitamin D depletion should be avoided by adequate supplement of vitamin D_2 or 25 OH D_3 in order to bring plasma 25 OH in the upper limit of normal. As a matter of fact we have observed an osteomalacia in a dialysed women given $CaCO_3$ alone which was due to vitamin D depletion, since it was cured by physiological doses of 25 OH D_3 (50).

Limits of oral Ca supplements as phosphate binder. Complementary measures

Reviewing our experience and that of others it appears that, in about half the patients given high doses of $CaCO_3$ with meals, it is not possible to prevent hyperphosphatemia either because of non compliance or because of hypercalcemia. If hypercalcemia occurs before a satisfactory fall in plasma PO_4 has been achieved, it is important to look for other causes of hypercalcemia than oral Ca. Besides the most frequent causes which are not directly related to chronic dialysis (cancer, myeloma, sarcoidosis) one should exclude the causes more specific of this condition: vitamin D intoxication, severe hyperparathyroidism, granulomatous disease induced by silicone and incipient aluminum bone disease. This latter possibility justify a desferoxamine test and a long term treatment with desferoxamine until post-desferoxamine plasma Al becomes < 150 μg/l (52). When these causes have been excluded and that hypercalcemia appears to be related exclusively to a too big amount of Ca being absorbed, precluding the use of the appropriate dose of oral Ca to control hyperphosphatemia, there are three possible therapeutic options: 1/ decrease in dialysate Ca; 2/ use of phosphate-binders other than Al hydroxide or alkaline salts of Ca; 3/ use of 24,25 dihydroxyvitamin D_3 or 22 oxa-calcitriol.

1/ Decrease in dialysate Ca

How much should dialysate Ca be decreased when $CaCO_3$ is used as phosphate binder? Doses of $CaCO_3$ sufficient to produce adequate PO_4 binding also overcome the negative Ca balance. If $CaCO_3$ is given, therefore, it is not necessary to ensure a positive intradialytic Ca balance and a dialysate Ca of 6.5 mg/dl is appropriate. In the event of hypercalcemia in hemodialysis or peritoneal dialysis patients one can reduce dialysate Ca progressively to 5.0 or even 4.0 mg/dl as suggested by Mactier et al (53). Slatopolsky et al (17) have suggested that a dialysate Ca of 5.0 mg/dl is adequate for all patients. This remains unresolved at present since Malberti et al (18) have found that, even with a dialysate Ca of 6.0 mg/dl, oral $CaCO_3$ (3 g/day) and 0.13 μg/day of calcitriol, there was an increase in the alkaline phosphatase. When using a dialysate Ca of 5.0 mg/dl, therefore, one should always use high doses of oral $CaCO_3$ and probably 1α OH vitamin D_3 derivatives as well. Thus Oettinger et al (54) were unable to correct hypocalcemia and suppress PTH and alkaline phosphatase when using a dialysate Ca of 5.0 mg/dl and oral Ca to control hyperphosphatemia. Suppression of hyperparathyroidism was only possible in their hands when calcitriol was given by the i.v. route (54). However, Slatopolsky et al (55) have recently reported their experience of using a dialysate Ca of 5.0 mg/dl for their patients. The mean daily dose of $CaCO_3$ required for the prevention of hyperphosphatemia was 10 g; with this regimen and without calcitriol it was possible to maintain plasma alkaline phosphatase and PTH levels more or less unchanged over the 7 months period of the study.

Kaye et al (56) have recently suggested another method of maintaining Ca balance in equilibrium during a dialysis treatment, namely using a Ca-free dialysate and replacing the Ca loss by i.v. administration of $CaCl_2$. This approach is particularly appropriate when bicarbonate is used as the buffer, since an ordinary dialysis machine with a single proportioning dilution system can be used. The problem, however, is how to predict the optimal Ca balance for each patient at each treatment. Kaye et al (56) found that in a 4 hour dialysis using Ca free dialysate (blood flow: 200 ml/min, dialysate flow: 500 ml/min) there was a mean Ca loss of approximately 40 mmol (1600 mg). These authors therefore recommend 40 mmol of Ca should be infused over the 4 hours of each dialysis. If oral $CaCO_3$ is being used to prevent hyperphosphatemia, this strategy, devised by Kaye et al, enables one, should there be hypercalcemia, to reduce the amount of $CaCl_2$ infused during dialysis.

With hemofiltration, a negative Ca balance can easily be produced by decreasing the Ca concentration in the substitution fluid below 7.0 mg/dl.

It is important to stress again that all these measures, aiming at producing a negative Ca balance during a dialysis or hemofiltration treatment, have the inherent hazard of inducing a chronic negative Ca balance in patients non compliant with these high doses of $CaCO_3$, and that this phenomenon will be overlooked for many months or years until significant radiological bone disease appears, because it is not necessarily accompanied by a decrease in plasma Ca (44). As a matter of fact this negative Ca balance will stimulate PTH secretion which will maintain normocalcemia. Therefore a more scrupulous monitoring of the plasma alkaline phosphatase and PTH concentrations is mandatory in these patients. Because of this risk we prefer to use this strategy, based on intradialytic negative Ca balance, only when hypercalcemia is present and proved to be related exclusively to increased Ca absorption because of the oral Ca supplements.

2/ Use of phosphate-binders other than Al hydroxide or alkaline salts of Ca

In dialysis patients, O'Donnovan et al (57) have suggested using Mg-carbonate in a dose of 7.5±2.5 g/day with a Mg free dialysate in order to prevent hypermagnesemia. This treatment which is said not to induce diarrhea or hyperkalemia, has the advantage of keeping 1α OH vitamin D derivatives in reserve should there be a rise in the alkaline phosphatase as happened in their study. The problem of, in effect, replacing the dialysate Mg by oral Mg salts is that the maintenance of a normal plasma Mg will depend on the uninterrupted regular ingestion of Mg salts. If the Mg salts were to be stopped by mistake or simply not taken by the patient without informing the doctor, there is the distinct danger of developing symptoms of hypomagnesemia including cramps and arrythmias.

Because of this possible hazard we have chosen a middle course in which Mg administration is divided between the dialysate and oral route. In this way a smaller oral dose of Mg [2.5 g/day of $Mg(OH)_2$] was given in combination with $CaCO_3$ and a dialysate Mg of 0.375 mmol/l was used. By this regimen it was hoped to avoid hypomagnesemia in those patients who failed to take their oral Mg salts. This approach resulted in a small increase of plasma Mg from 1 to 1.5 mmol/l. There was also the expected rise in plasma potassium necessitating increased use of a potassium chelator. For this purpose we gave Ca polystyrene sulfonate and reduced the dose of $CaCO_3$; sodium polystyrene sulfonate was not used since, when given with $CaCO_3$ or $Mg(OH)_2$, it is known to induce an alkalosis by complexing Ca and Mg and liberating OH^-. This approach of using moderate oral doses of Ca and Mg without 1α OH D_3 in the prevention of osteodystrophy was compared with our former therapeutic regimen of using $Al(OH)_3$ + small doses of $CaCO_3$ with or without 1α OH D_3 in 2 groups of 30 patients for 2-4 years. It appeared that the Ca + Mg treatment was as efficacious as the Al + Ca + 1α OH D treatment in the prevention of hyperparathyroidism and did not induce aluminum bone disease nor non aluminic osteomalacia. The Ca + Mg treatment, however, was accompanied by the emergence in 4 patients of adynamic bone disease not otherwise explained by iron overload, diabetes, previous parathyroidectomy or corticosteroid therapy (58). Compared with the osteitis fibrosa patients those with idiopathic adynamic bone disease had a shorter duration on dialysis, a slightly higher age and lower plasma PTH. Their relative hypoparathyroidism was not explained by higher doses of oral Ca or Mg, by higher plasma Ca and plasma Mg nor by lower plasma PO_4 or plasma bicarbonate. The long term prognosis of this histological disease is unknown but it may be hoped that it has not the disastrous prognosis of aluminum adynamic bone disease since the patients were asymptomatic, had no fracture and a normal trabecular bone volume. Since this histological pattern was mainly seen in the patients with shorter duration on dialysis, it is likely that with longer duration on dialysis secondary hyperparathyroidism will eventually stimulate again their bone turn over.

The use of oral Ca alone or in combination with oral Mg was not associated with any greater risk of soft tissue calcification (vascular and periarticular calcification as assessed on X rays) than the treatment with $Al(OH)_3$ + small doses of Ca with or without 1α OH vitamin D derivatives (59). Furthermore, it has been shown that the increase in vascular calcifications was related mainly to age, male sex, blood pressure level, blood concentration of triglycerides and glucose and, only at a borderline level, with plasma concentrations of Ca and PO_4 (60). The increase in vascular calcification was, however, not related to the dose of $CaCO_3$. Therefore, the fear that soft tissue calcification may develop incipiently, in spite of no increase in the plasma Ca x PO_4 product, because of the simultaneous deposition of Ca and PO_4, does not seem to be justified, since in that case a relation of vascular extension with the $CaCO_3$ dose should have been found. It can, therefore, be reasonably concluded that oral $CaCO_3$ per se is not toxic as long as it does not induce hypercalcemia without decreasing plasma PO_4.

Ca salts of ketoanalogs may have a place in the management of hyperphosphatemia in hemodialysis patients, since even without protein restriction, Ca salts of ketoanalogs can exert a hypophosphatemic effect and produce a fall in plasma PTH (32). Clearly these substances are exciting prospects for the future management of hyperparathyroidism.

3/ Use of 24,25 dihydroxyvitamin D_3 or 22 oxa-calcitriol

The 24,25 dihydroxyvitamin D_3 [24,25 $(OH)_2$ D_3] is known to have hypophosphatemic and hypocalcemic effects and a direct suppressive effect on parathyroid secretion as a result of binding to specific receptor. This latter effect is much weaker than that of calcitriol and does not result (61) in adequate prevention of hyperparathyroidism when the substance is given alone. However, we feel that the use of 24,25 $(OH)_2$ D_3 should be re-evaluated as an agent for lowering plasma PO_4 in uremic patients when hypocalcemia has been corrected by high doses of $CaCO_3$. Very recently, Slatopolsky et al (55) have suggested that 22-oxa-calcitriol, a new vitamin D derivative, may have a place in combination with oral $CaCO_3$ in the prevention and treatment of renal osteodystrophy. The particular advantage of this substance is that, like 24,25 $(OH)_2$ D_3, it is devoid of a hypercalcemic effect in experimental animals, yet has a suppressive effect on PTH synthesis and release similar to that of calcitriol (62).

Practical conclusions

Thus the nephrologist responsible for patients on chronic hemodialysis now has several means of controlling hyperphosphatemia without Al PO_4-binders. Because of the problem of Al overload we now feel that Al PO_4-binders should be completely withdrawn from use in uremic patients. Al toxicity may only be relatively mild when, because of strict adherence to a PO_4 restricted diet and efficient removal of PO_4 by dialysis, only small doses are needed [< 3 g/day of $Al(OH)_3$] and when the suppression of hyperparathyroidism is not particularly good (63). However, since many of these patients may be on dialysis for more than 10 years, their Al stores will progressively increase [the bone aluminium content has been shown to be correlated with the cumulative dose of $Al(OH)_3$ (64)], and, if hyperparathyroidism is not adequately suppressed and parathyroidectomy becomes necessary, there will be a risk of inducing aluminum bone disease after surgery (2). Desferoxamine may prevent this complication but has its own hazards (6). Therefore, in order to prevent this vicious therapeutic circle, we strongly suggest that Al containing PO_4-binders are not used in uremic patients. As regards the choice between the alternative treatments, we will have to wait for adequate controlled comparative studies of their cost/safety- effectiveness ratios.

In practice, for the moment, we propose to start to dialyse the patients with a dialysate Ca of 6.5 mg/dl, a dialysate Mg of 0.9 mg/dl and to control their phosphatemia with $CaCO_3$ at increasing doses (3-12 g/day) taken with the meals. If their initial plasma PO_4 is higher than 6.0 mg/dl, transient administration of $Al(OH)_3$ is advised to bring it below 6.0 mg/dl, before giving doses of $CaCO_3$ greater than 3 g in order to prevent the risk of soft tissue calcification. Then $Al(OH)_3$ is definitively withdrawn. Weekly monitoring of predialysis plasma Ca and PO_4 is recommanded in order to maintain plasma Ca between 10.0-10.5 mg/dl and plasma PO_4 between 4.5-5.5 mg/dl (i.e. at a level higher than for patients not yet on dialysis, in order to compensate for the postdialytic hypophosphatemic phase). In addition adequate amount of vitamin D_2 or 25 OH D_3 will maintain plasma 25 OH D at the upper limit of normal to prevent vitamin D depletion-1α hydroxylated vitamin D derivatives will be added (orally or by the i.v. route) only if hypocalcemia persists in spite of a plasma PO_4 at 4.5 mg/dl or if plasma alkaline phosphatase increases whereas plasma Ca remains < 10.5 mg/dl and plasma $PO_4 < 5.5$ mg/dl. When plasma alkaline phosphatase increases above normal together with highly elevated PTH (levels of C terminal PTH above 5-10 times the upper limit of normal) while plasma Ca is > 10.5 mg/dl and plasma $PO_4 > 6.0$ mg/dl in spite of all the above preventive measures, failure of medical prevention of hyperparathyroidism must be admitted and parathyroidectomy considered.

TREATMENT OF RENAL OSTEODYSTROPHY IN CHILDREN

Children not yet on dialysis

In spite of the fact that renal osteodystrophy in children is often manifested clinically as classical "renal rickets", bone histology rarely shows a defect in bone mineralization but rather hyperparathyroidism (65). The increased uncalcified woven bone secondary to hyperparathyroidism is responsible for the radiolucent rickets-like appearances at the ends of long bones and for the slipped epiphyses. The latter can give rise to major skeletal deformity. In severe cases small size is explained by a combination of these deformities and stunted growth. In children with mild renal bone disease, however, it is not clear whether renal osteodystrophy per se is responsible for the stunted growth, since its treatment is often not followed by a catching up subsequently, in contrast to what is usually observed in children with vitamin D dependent rickets type 1 treated with 1α OH vitamin D_3. Skeletal growth in uremic children appears to be more dependent upon appropriate salt and water balance (sometimes requiring nocturnal tube feeding), correction of acidosis (plasma bicarbonate > 22 mmol/l using alkali supplements) and adequate protein and calorie intakes according to the Recommended Diet Allowance (66). These measures should be attended to when the GFR is < 80 ml/min/1.73 m^2.

Early PO_4 restriction is theoretically indicated as in the adult but is almost impossible in practice since it is important to adhere to the "recommended daily allowance" of protein. PO_4-binders, therefore, are very important. As for adults with renal failure, $Al(OH)_3$ should be avoided completely (especially when Shohl's solution is given for alkalinization) since children and particularly infants are highly susceptible to exogenous Al which has been reported to cause fatal aluminum encephalopathy with fracturing osteomalacia within a few months (67). Priority, therefore, should be given to $CaCO_3$ as a PO_4-binder. The successful experience of Alon et al (68) in 12 children with a plasma Cr of 3.7 to 5.1 mg/dl suggests that one should start with a dose of 0.1 g/kg/day and introduce 1α OH vitamin D_3 at a dose of 0.25 μg/day when plasma PO_4 has been lowered to below 5.5 mg/dl. The dose of $CaCO_3$ can then be increased to 0.3/kg/day in order to maintain a normal plasma Ca (10.3 mg/dl) and maintain plasma PO_4 at about 4.2 mg/dl. Urinary Ca should be measured regularly so that hypercalciuria can be avoided [Ca (mg/dl)/Cr (mg/dl) < 0.21]. When $CaCO_3$ is given, even low doses of $Al(OH)_3$ should not be added since their beneficial effect on hyperparathyroidism will be counterbalanced by the occurrence of aluminum bone disease (20).

Children on dialysis

When a child is on hemodialysis or CAPD the principles of treatment are much the same as for adults. In order to allow for the administration of adequate oral doses of Ca salts it is sometimes necessary to decrease dialysate Ca. Supplements of vitamin D or 25 OH D_3 should be given in order to prevent vitamin D depletion especially in children on CAPD. 1α OH vitamin D derivatives should be added once the predialysis plasma PO_4 is under good control (plasma PO_4 between 4.5 - 5.5 mg/dl for children over 2 years, and between 5.0 - 6.0 mg/dl for children under 2 years) provided plasma Ca is below 10.0 mg/dl. An acceptable level for plasma Ca in children on 1α OH D_3 is 10.5 mg/dl.

Parathyroidectomy is rarely required in children. There is no consensus in the literature as to which type of operation is preferable: total parathyroidectomy with autotransplantation of parathyroid tissue into the forearm or the classical 7/8 parathyroidectomy. Whatever procedure is chosen, it is crucial to cryopreserve parathyroid tissue in case significant hypoparathyroidism ensues. Gross deformities and slipped epiphyses should not be corrected surgically until the hyperparathyroidism is showing signs of healing. In general children on dialysis with crippling osteopathy should be considered for early renal transplantation since corrective osteotomy can be done more safely thereafter.

CONCLUSIONS

1/ Conventional Al containing PO_4-binder should no longer be used in the long term treatment of renal osteodystrophy since the price of their successful use in preventing hyperparathyroidism is the induction of an aluminum bone disease.

2/ Preventive treatment of renal osteodystrophy now has two therapeutic components (i) oral Ca salts used as a PO_4-binder and (ii) supplements of vitamin D or 25 OH D_3 to ensure adequacy of vitamin D.

3/ 1α (OH) vitamin D derivatives can also be used in addition either orally or intravenously provided plasma PO_4 is not high and the plasma Ca remains < 10.5 mg/dl. It is important to remember, however, that administration of 1α hydroxylated derivatives is probably less important than control of plasma PO_4 and correction (if present) of vitamin D depletion.

4/ Such an approach should greatly reduce the prevalence of both aluminum bone disease and osteitis fibrosa.

5/ It is important to look for the development of "relative hypoparathyroidism" for the degree of renal failure so that adynamic bone disease can be prevented. The safe range for biological bone markers is not known and will have to wait future studies.

6/ New PO_4-binders including insoluble forms of Al (boemite form of aluminum hydroxide) are now available. We would suggest that these should not be used generally until it is clear that they are less toxic than conventional Al salts. For the present, therefore, oral Ca salts should be regarded as the mainstay of the management of hyperphosphatemia and hyperparathyroidism.

ACKNOWLEDGMENTS

The authors thanks Professor Slatopolsky E. and Drueke T. for critically reviewing the manuscript and Mme Contart M. for excellent typing assistance.

REFERENCES

1. Sherrard DJ, Andress DL : Renal osteodystrophy. In: "Diseases of the kidney", Schrier RW and Gottschalk CW (Eds). Little, Brown and Company, Boston 1988, p 3035-3061.
2. Llach F, Coburn JW : Renal osteodystrophy and maintenance dialysis. In: "Replacement of renal function by dialysis". JF Maher(Ed), Kluwer Acad Publ, Dordrecht, p 911-952, 1989.
3. Ward MK, Feest TG, Parkinson IS, Ellis HM, Kerr DNS: Osteomalacic dialytic osteodystrophy: evidence for a water born aetiological agent, probably aluminum. Lancet, i: 841-845, 1978.
4. Slatopolsky E, Weert SC, Thielan J et al: Marked suppression of secondary hyperparathyroidism after IV administration of calcitriol in uremic patients. J Clin Invest, 74: 2136-2140, 1984.
5. Quarles LD, Davidai GA, Schwab SJ et al: Oral calcitriol and calcium: efficient therapy for uremic hyperparathyroidism. Kidney Int, 34: 840-844, 1988.
6. Bene C, Manzler A, Bene D, Krani AS: Irreversible occular toxicity from single challenge dose of deferoxamine. Clin Nephrol, 31: 45-48, 1989.
7. Zins B, Petitclerc T, Basile C et al: Tumoral calcinosis in hemodialysis patients: role of aluminum. Kidney Int, 35: 267, 1989 (Abstract).
8. Yver L, Blanchier D, Buiquang D et al: Does aluminum induce dialysis amyloidosis. Nephrol Dial Transpl, 2: 450-451, 1987.
9. Moriniere PH, Roussel A, Tahiri Y, Fournier A: Substitution of $Al(OH)_3$ by high doses of CaCO3 in patients on chronic hemodialysis, desappearances of hyperaluminemia and equal control of hyperparathyroidism. Proc EDTA, 19: 784-787, 1982.
10. Clarkson EM, Mc Donald SJ, de Wardener HE: The effects of high intake of calcium carbonate in normal subjects and patients with chronic renal failure. Clin Sci, 30: 425-438, 1966.
11. Coburn JW, Harten Bower DL, Brickman AS, et al: Intestinal absorption of calcium, magnesium and phosphorus in chronic renal insufficiency. In: "Calcium metabolism in Renal Failure and nephrolithiasis" David SD (Ed). Wiley Son NY, pp 77-99, 1977.
12. Clarkson EM, Eastwood JB, Koutsaimanis KG, de Wardener HE: Net intestinal absorption of calcium in patients with chronic renal failure. Kidney Int, 3: 258-263, 1973.
13. Schiller LR, Santa Ana C, Sheikk MS et al: Effect of the time of administration of calcium acetate on phosphorus binding. N Eng J Med, 320: 1110-3, 1989.
14. Fournier A, Moriniere Ph, Sebert JL, et al: Renal osteodystrophy: general concepts and current issues. In: Nephrology, Robinson R (Ed), Springer Verlag, New York 1985, Vol II, pp 1357-1373.
15. Bonjour JP: 1,25 $(OH)_2D_3$ and phosphate homeostasis in early chronic renal failure: "the trade-off hypothesis revisited". In: Nephrology, A. Davison (Ed), Baillère T and all. London, 1988, pp 1059-1065.
16. Feinfeld DA, Sherwood LM: Parathyroid hormone and 1,25 $(OH)_2$ D_3 in chronic renal failure. Kidney Int, 33: 1049-1058, 1988.
17. Slatopolsky E, Lopez-Milker S, Dusso A, et al: Parathyroid hormone secretion: Perturbations in chronic renal failure. In: "Bone and renal insufficiency" De Broe (Ed), Contr Nephrol, Karger, Basel, 64: 414-421, 1988.
18. Malberti F, Surian M, Mercantini F, et al: Effect of DCa changes on plasma calcium and PTH in dialysis patients treated with $CaCO_3$ as a phosphate binder. EDTA Abstracts,.Madrid, 1988, p 239.
19. Lucas PA, Woodhead JS, Brown RC: Vitamin D_3 metabolites in chronic renal failure and after renal transplantation. Nephrol Dial Transplant, 3: 70-76, 1988.

20. Turner C, Compston J, Mak RHK, et al: Bone turn over and 1,25 dihydroxycholecalciferol during treatment with phosphate binders. Kidney Int, 33: 989-995, 1988.
21. Bordier PJ, Tunchot S, Eastwood JB, Fournier A, de Wardener HE: Lack of histological evidence of vitamin D abnormality in the bones of anephric patients. Clin Sci, 44: 33-41, 1973.
22. Moriniere PH, Vinatier I, Abdulmassih Z, et al: Magnesium hydroxide as a complementary aluminum free phosphate-binder to high doses of oral calcium in uremic patients on chronic hemodialysis. Lack of deleterious effect on bone mineralization. Nephrol Dial Transplant, 3: 651-656, 1988.
23. Parisien M, Charhon SA, Arlot M, Chapuy MC, Meunier JP: Evidence for a toxic effect of aluminum on osteoblasts: a histomorphometric study in hemodialysis patients with aplastic bone disease. J Bone Min Res, 3: 259-267, 1988.
24. Fournier A, Idrissi A, Sebert JL, et al: Preventing renal bone disease in moderate renal failure by calcium carbonate and 25OH vitamin D. Kidney Int, 33, supl.24: S178-S179, 1988.
25. Baker LR, Abrams L, Roe C, et al: 1,25 $(OH)_2$ D_3 administration in moderate renal failure: a prospective double blind trial. Kidney Int, 35: 661-669, 1989.
26. Tessitore N, Venturi A, Adami S, Bonucci E, Maschio G: Relationship between serum vitamin D metabolites and dietary intake of phosphate in patients with early renal failure. Mineral Electrolyte Metab, 13: 38-44, 1987.
27. Sheikh MS, Maguire JA, Emmett M et al: Reduction of dietary phosphorus absorption by phosphate binders : a theoretical in vitro and in vivo study. J Clin Invest, 83: 66-73, 1989.
28. Bakir AA, Hryhorczuk DD, Berman E, Dunea G: Acute fatal hyperaluminemia encephalopathy in undialyzed and recently dialyzed uremic patients. Trans Am Soc Artif Intern Organs, 32: 171-176, 1986.
29. Schneider H, Kulbe KD, Weber H, Streicher E: *In vitro* and *in vivo* studies with a non-aluminum phosphate binding compound. Kidney Int, 28: S120-S122, 1986
30. Mitch WE, Gelman B, Walser M: Hypercalcemia and hypophosphatemia in uremic patients receiving essential aminoacids and N-free ketoanalogues. Kidney Int, 12: 530-535, 1988.
31. Fröhling PT, Kokot F, Schmicker R, Lindenau K, Vetter K: Influence of ketoacids on serum parathyroid hormone levels in patients with chronic renal failure. Clin Nephrol, 20: 212-217, 1989
32. Schaeffer K, von Herrath D, Asmus G, Umlauf L: The beneficial effect of ketoacid on serum phosphate and parathyroid hormone in patients with chronic uremia. Clin Nephrol, 30: 93-96, 1988.
33. Portale A, Booth B, Halloran B, Morris R: Effect of dietary phosphate on circulating concentration of 1,25 dihydroxy vitamin D and immunoreactive parathyroid hormone in children with moderate renal insufficiency. J Clin Invest, 73: 1580-1581, 1984.
34. Takamoto S, Onishi T, Morimoto S, Imanaka S, Kumahara Y: Serum phosphate, parathyroid hormone and vitamin D metabolites in patients with chronic renal failure: effect of aluminium hydroxide administration. Nephron, 40: 286-291, 1985.
35. Demontis R, Leflon A, Fournier A, et al: Indirect clinical evidence that 1α OH vitamin D3 increases the intestinal absorption of aluminum. Clin Nephrol, 31: 123-127, 1989.
36. Merke J, Lucas P, Drueke T, Ritz A: 1,25$(OH)_2$ D_3 receptors and end organ response in experimental aluminium intoxication. Kidney Int, 32: 204-211, 1987.
37. Coen G, Muzzaferro S, Bonucci E, Ballantini P, Massimetti C: Treatment of secondary hyperparathyroidism of predialysis chronic renal failure with low doses of 1,25 $(OH)_2D_3$: humoral and histomorphometric results. Mineral Electrolyte Metab, 12: 375-382, 1986.
38. Massry SG: Assessment of 1,25$(OH)_2D_3$ in the correction and prevention of renal osteodystrophy in patients with mild to moderate renal failure. In: "Vitamin D chemical, biochemical and clinical update " A Norman (Ed), de Gruyter, Berlin, pp 936-937, 1985.
39. Nordal KB, Dahl E: Low dose calcitriol versus placebo in patients with predialysis chronic renal failure. J Clin Endocrinol Metab, 67: 929-936, 1988.
40. Cohen Solal M, Westeel PF, Boudaillez Ph, Moriniere Ph, Marie A, Sebert JL, Gueris J, Garabedian M, Fournier A: Non aluminic adynamic bone disease in non dialyzed patients: a new type of osteopathy due to over-treatment? EDTA-ERA (Abstract), Göteborg, 1989.
41. Christiansen C, Rodbro P, Christensen MS, Hartnack B, Transbol I: Deterioration of renal function during treatment of chronic renal failure with 1,25 $(OH)_2D_3$. Lancet, i: 700-703, 1978.
42. Toogard L, Sorensen E, Brochner-Mortensen I, et al: Controlled trial of 1α hydroxycholecalciferol in chronic renal failure. Lancet, i: 1044-1047, 1976.

43. Tvedegaard E, Ladefoged O, Nielsen M, Kamstrup O: Effect of 1α hydroxyvitamin D_3 and dietary calcium and phosphate on the aorta mineral content in rabbits with mild uremia. Nephron, 34: 185-191, 1983.
44. Fournier AE, Arnaud C, Johnson WJ, Goldsmith RS: Etiology of hyperparathyroidism and bone disease during chronic hemodialysis. J Clin Invest, 30: 599-605, 1971.
45. Memmos DE, Eastwood J, Talner et al: Double blind trial of oral $1.25(OH)_2$ D_3 versus placebo in asymptomatic hyperparathyroidism in patients on maintenance haemodialysis. Brit Med J, 282: 1919-1924, 1981.
46. Baker LR, Muir JW, Sharman VL, Abrams SML, Greenwood RN, O'Riordan JLM: Controlled trial of calcitriol in hemodialysis patients. Clin Nephrol, 26: 185-191, 1986.
47. Delmez JA, Fallon MD, Harter HR, Hruska KA, Slatopolsky E, Teitelbaum SL: Does strict phosphorus control precipitate renal osteomalacia? J Clin Endoc Metab, 62: 747-752, 1986.
48. Tahiri Y, Moriniere P, Fournier A: Hyperaluminémie des hémodialysés chroniques. Evaluation du rôle respectif de l'aluminium du dialysat et de la prise orale d'$Al(OH)_3$. Nephrologie, 4: 129-133, 1983.
49. Moriniere PH, Fournier A, Idrissi A, Renaud H, et al: Calcium carbonate and magnesium hydroxide in the prevention of renal osteodystrophy or the demise of aluminum intoxicity in uremia. In "Bone and renal insufficiency", de Broe (Ed), Cont Nephr, Karger, Basel, 64: 58-73, 1988.
50. Fournier A, Moriniere Ph, Sebert JL, et al: Calcium carbonate, an aluminum free agent for control of hyperphosphatemia, hypocalcemia and hyperparathyroidism in uremia. Kidney Int, 29, 18: S114-S119, 1986.
51. Malberti F, Surian M, Poegio F et al: Efficacy and safety of long term treatment with $CaCO_3$ as a phosphate binder. Am J Kidney Dis, 12: 487-491, 1988.
52. Hercz G, Kraut J, Andress DA et al: Use of calcium carbonate as a phosphate binder in dialysis patients. Miner Electrolyte Metab, 12: 314-319, 1981.
53. Mactier RA, Vanstone M, Twaroowski Z: Calcium carbonate is an effective phosphate binder when dialysate calcium concentration is adjusted to control hypercalcemia. Clin Nephrol, 28: 222-226, 1987.
54. Oettinger CW, Macon EJ, Oliver JC: Effects of oral intravenous $1.25(OH)_2$ Vit D_3 in hemodialysis patients treated with $CaCO_3$ as sole PO_4 binder. A.S.N., (Abstract) 247 A, 1988.
55. Slatopolsky E, Weerts C, Norwood K et al: Long term effects of calcium carbonate and 2.5 mEq/l calcium dialysate on mineral metabolism in hemodialysis patients. Kidney Int, 1989 (in press).
56. Kaye M, Barber E, Vasilevsk Y, Langer K: Calcium free dialyzate: development and application. Clinical Nephrol, 31: 132-138, 1989.
57. O'Donnovan R, Monitz C, Baldwin D et al: Control of hyperphosphatemia by oral magnesium carbonate on zero manesium dialyzate without aluminium binders. Lancet, i: 880-881, 1986.
58. Moriniere Ph, Cohen Solal M, Belbrik S, Boudailliez B, Marie A, Sebert JL, Fournier A: Histological bone disease in a long term asymptomatic dialysis population restricting $Al(OH)_3$ intake : lack of aluminic osteomalacia, emergence of an idiopathic adynamic bone disease not related to aluminum. Nephron (in press) 1989.
59. Moriniere Ph, Hocine Ch, Boudailliez B, Fournier A: Long term efficacy and safety of oral calcium ± $Mg(OH)_2$ as phosphate binder as compared to $Al(OH)_3$ in dialysis patients. Kidney Int, 1989,- Suppl. with the Strasbourg workshop on nutrition in renal disease (in press)
60. Renaud H, Atik A, Herve M, Moriniere Ph, Hocine C, Belbrik S, Fournier A: Evaluation of vascular calcinosis risk factor in patients on chronic hemodialysis: lack of influence of calcium carbonate. Nephron, 48: 28-32, 1988.
61. Fournier A, Moriniere Ph, Boudailliez B, et al: $1.25(OH)_2$ vit D_3 deficiency and renal osteodystrophy: should its well-accepted pathogenetic role in secondary hyperparathyroidism lead to its systematic preventive therapeutic use? Nephrol Dial Transplant, 2: 498-503, 1987.
62. Brown A, Ritter C, Morrissey J et al: A novel non calcemic vitamin D analog .22 oxacalcitriol for the treatment of hyperparathyroidism. J Clin Invest, 1989 (in press).
63. Jenkins DAS, Gouldesbrough D, Smith GD, Cowie JF, Winney RJ: Can low dosage $Al(OH)_3$ control the plasma phosphate without bone toxicity? Nephrol Dial Transplant, 4: 51-56, 1989.
64. Sebert JL, Fournier A, Leflon P, et al: Comparative evaluation of bone aluminium content and bone histology in patients on chronic hemodialysis and hemofiltration. Nephron, 42: 34-40, 1986

65. Mehls O, Salusky B: Recent advances and controversies in childhood renal osteodystropy. Pediatr Nephrol, 1: 212-223, 1987.
66. Revised recommended dietary allowances. J Am Diet Ass, 75: 623-625, 1979.
67. Andreoli SP, Bergstein JM, Sherrard DJ: Aluminum intoxication from aluminum-containing phosphate binders in children with azotemia not undergoing dialysis. N Eng J Med, 310: 1079-1084, 1984.
68. Alon U, Davidai G, Bentur L, Berant M, Better O: Oral calcium carbonate as phosphate-binder in infants and children with chronic renal failure. Mineral Electrolyte Metab, 12: 320-325, 1986.

DIALYSIS

12

NEW DISEASES OF DIALYSIS PATIENTS: AMYLOIDOSIS

MICHEL JADOUL AND CHARLES VAN YPERSELE DE STRIHOU

Cliniques Universitaires St-Luc, Service de Néphrologie, 1200 Bruxelles, Belgium

Dialysis amyloidosis, a now well defined clinical entity, results from the accumulation of ß2-microglobulin (ß2m) fibrils mainly along synovial membranes. In long-term dialysis patients, it causes carpal tunnel syndrome, arthralgias and cystic bone lesions leading occasionally to pathological fractures (1-7).

THE EXTENT OF ß2-MICROGLOBULIN AMYLOID DEPOSITS IN DIALYSED PATIENTS.

ß2m amyloid deposits have been conclusively demonstrated in the carpal tunnel, in the synovial membranes and in peri-articular bone cysts of symptomatic patients (8-12). Occasionally, however, despite a careful search, they could not be identified in the material removed by surgery for a carpal tunnel syndrome (5, 13) or for a destructive arthropathy (2) or by puncture of peri-articular bone cysts (14). Although usually ascribed to inadequate sampling, this finding may alternatively point to the fact that both the carpal tunnel syndrome and the bone lesions sometimes result from another cause. Symptomatic amyloid deposits have also been described in popliteal synovial cysts (15, 16).

Synovial deposits may also be asymptomatic as illustrated by their presence in the sternoclavicular synovium of 9 out of 22 long-term dialysis patients biopsied systematically during parathyroidectomy (17).

The relationship between ß2m amyloidosis and destructive spondylarthropathy, a recently described complication of long-term dialysis (18), remains a moot point. Although amyloid deposits have been observed in the disks as well as in the vertebral ligaments of patients with this disease (19), this finding is not constant (20). Furthermore, destructive spondylarthropathy, ascribed to severe secondary hyperparathyroidism, has been recently reported before the onset of dialysis (21) at a time when no ß2m amyloidosis has been convincingly demonstrated. Even if destructive spondylarthropathy is not initiated by amyloidosis, the superimposition of ß2m amyloid deposits is not necessarily benign: massive extradural cervical deposits have resulted in tetraparesis in one patient (22) whereas amyloid infiltration of the yellow ligament has been associated in another with narrow lumbar canal syndrome, relieved after laminectomy (23).

ß2m amyloid deposits have also been identified outside the synovia and bone in over twenty patients (12, 24-35). These "systemic" deposits are usually minute and localized within the vessel walls of several organs. Rarely, they are large enough to invade the parenchyma (24, 33). Almost all organs, except the central and the peripheral nervous system have been implicated : rectum (11 cases), heart (8 cases), lungs and liver (6 cases each), colon (5 cases), kidneys and small intestine (4 cases each), stomach and prostate (3 cases each), spleen, adrenals and tongue (2 cases each), pancreas, testes, thyroid, bladder, uterus, large ligament, lymph nodes, vulva and skin (1 case each).

It is important to remember that all deposits with the morphologic characteristics of amyloid are not necessarily due to ß2m precipitation: both AA and AL amyloidosis have been occasionally observed in long-term dialysis patients (29). The amyloid substance identified by Suda et al. (36) in the pancreas of 6 out of 10 long-term dialysis patients may be related to peptides other than ß2m such as Diabetes-associated peptide (DAP) previously recognized in type II diabetes (37). Only specific immunostaining for ß2m provides a definitive answer. Strict histologic criteria should also be applied before retaining a diagnosis of amyloid. Thus Kachel et al.'s initial report (38) of frequent deposition of amyloid in the skin has not been confirmed, the deposits being eventually identified as altered collagen (39). In fact, neither Noël (29) nor Campistol (25) could recognize ß2m amyloid in the skin of 9 and 16 patients respectively.

The prevalence of systemic ß2m deposits remains unknown in the absence of a systematic study with well defined patient selection and pathological sampling criteria. For example, subcutaneous abdominal fat punctures yield ß2m amyloid deposits in 0 to 50% of patients (25, 29, 31, 32, 40). Similarly, rectal biopsy is positive in 10 (2 out of 21 samples in one study) (28) to 40% of patients (4 out of 11 samples in another study but no submucosa was available in the 7 negative samples) (25). It was hoped that the prevalence of cardiac amyloid deposits could be defined on the basis of the echocardiographic pattern: Campistol et al. reported evidence of amyloidosis in 7 out of 14 patients (25). However the size of the deposits, evaluated in autopsy series, is too small to account for such a high prevalence and suggests a high false positive rate in the reported results (29, 32).

Autopsy studies also yield conflicting results : Fenves (6) found no systemic deposits in 3 patients with synovial amyloidosis. Noël et al. (29) reported minute but widespread deposits in only one out of 8 long-term dialysis patients, 4 of whom with dialysis arthropathy. Sethi et al. identified systemic ß2m amyloid deposits in 2 out of 7 patients with synovial amyloidosis (32). More reports taking into account the duration of dialysis and the age of the patients will be needed to document the prevalence and the extent of visceral ß2m amyloidosis.

Whatever the results of such an investigation it is already evident that the clinical manifestations of visceral ß2m amyloidosis are minimal at least with the presently available follow-up. A single case of spontaneous rupture of the spleen (31), a known complication of AL amyloidosis (41) has been reported. Further jejunal hemorrhage and chronic diarrhea have been observed in a single patient each. In both cases, the only pathologic feature was the presence of intestinal amyloid ß2m deposits (35).

Clinical and X-ray signs of synovial amyloidosis

Dialysis arthropathy is not equal to ß2m amyloidosis. A variety of ill-defined joint symptoms and signs have been gathered under this heading. Thus, Brown et al. define dialysis arthropathy as all joint symptoms appearing in patients without hyperparathyroidism (42), including various conditions such as aluminic osteomalacia, microcristalline arthropathy etc. Charra et al. include in their "late dialysis periarticular syndrome" (43) such heterogeneous clinical manifestations as shoulder pain and stiffness, carpal tunnel syndrome, hemarthroses, spondylarthropathies, objective joint deformities, periarthritis, radiological bone cysts and a history of orthopedic surgery.

In order to better delineate the characteristics of ß2m amyloid arthropathy, we have evaluated 9 patients in whom we had histological and/or radiological evidence of amyloidosis (44). The clinical manifestations include the carpal tunnel syndrome (after an average of 9 years on dialysis), scapulohumeral (average 9 years) and/or hip pain (average 12 years) extending to both sides, with nocturnal and intra-dialytic exacerbation, leading occasionally to femoral neck pathological fractures. Other symptoms clearly related to ß2m amyloidosis, have also been reported such as chronic fluid effusion in the shoulders, knees, ankle and elbow (3) or, more rarely, flexor tenosynovitis of the fingers (44), bilateral temporomandibular aching (44), painful swelling of the sternoclavicular joint (45), popliteal synovial cysts (15, 16), tendon rupture of the biceps (23), swelling of a metacarpal bone (46), tetraparesis and narrow lumbar canal symptoms (23).

The radiological signs of documented amyloid osteoarthropathy have been recently reviewed (44). The soft periarticular tissue is swollen with frequent lateral displacement of the periarticular fat pad. Juxtaarticular bone lesions include erosions, marginal defects and expanding cysts. These alterations tend to become symetric, involving mainly the shoulders, the hips and the wrists.

The differential diagnosis between amyloid and hyperparathyroid cysts should take into account the concomitant signs of subperiosteal resorption, the evolution of the lesions after parathyroidectomy and, most important, by their presence or absence in the carpal bone, a target usually spared by hyperparathyroidism (47). Finally, it is of note that multiple brown tumors are most unusual in dialysis patients, only one case being reported up to 1986 (47).

Epidemiology

The association between ß2m amyloidosis and both the carpal tunnel syndrome and typical X-ray signs has provided the basis for a non invasive assessment of the epidemiology of this complication. The prevalence of carpal tunnel syndrome increases over time reaching virtually 100% after 18 to 20 years of hemodialysis (13, 43, 44), although Hirasawa (personal communication) observes a lower prevalence in Japan.

The prevalence of radiological signs of bone amyloidosis increases in parallel with that of the carpal tunnel syndrome. In a personal series of 58 cases, they increase from 10% between 7 and 10 years to 40% between 11 and 15 years and 100% beyond 15 years (44)

Neither the prevalence of the CTS nor that of bone lesions are 100% specific indicators of amyloid disease. Still, their association with amyloidosis is very strong so that their evolution over time provides a useful, non invasive tool to analyze the different factors responsible for ß2m deposition.

Factors influencing the prevalence of dialysis amyloidosis

Suggestive evidence that membranes play a significant role in the genesis of ß2m amyloidosis was provided by two studies. The first reported dialysis amyloidosis only in patients treated with cuprophane whereas patients treated for the same duration with AN69 (polyacrilonitrile) were spared (48). The second demonstrated that, among patients dialyzed with various membranes for the same overall duration, those who had a carpal tunnel syndrome had spent significantly more time on cuprophane and less on a synthetic membrane, AN69, than those who did not develop this complication (49).

More recently, a multicentre study of 165 patients dialyzed throughout either with cuprophane (n = 92) or with AN69 (n = 73) has recognized a significantly lower prevalence of carpal tunnel syndrome, bone lesions or any combination thereof within 8 years of dialysis in the AN69 treated subjects (50). The risk of developing significant lesions is three times lower with AN69 than with cuprophane.

It should be pointed out that membranes have at most a modulating effect as ß2m amyloidosis may develop in patients treated exclusively by peritoneal dialysis (51, 52). ß2m amyloidosis has also been reported in a patient treated only with hemofiltration (53). The prevalence of ß2m amyloidosis remains unknown in CAPD and hemofiltration: this will require the follow-up of large groups of long-term patients.

The multicentre study (50) also considered the effect of age independently of the dialysis membranes. It reported that the relative risk of developing amyloidosis within the first 8 years of dialysis rises strikingly with age: it is 9 fold higher in a patient aged 60 than in a patient aged 20 at the onset of dialysis.

ß2-MICROGLOBULIN CHEMISTRY IN DIALYZED PATIENTS

Several investigations have focused on the nature of the amyloid deposits. The early studies of Geyjo (10) and Gorevic (11) demonstrated that the amyloid fibrils were identical with ß2m. The presence of substance P was further recognized (54). Subsequent studies have tried to elucidate the structure of the circulating and of the precipitated ß2m.

Circulating serum β2-microglobulin

ß2m circulates in the serum as an intact monomer with an isoelectric point of 5.6 (54-56). Recently Ogawa et al. (56) have detected in the serum of dialysed patients alongside the normal ß2m, the presence of a small amount of lower molecular weight ß2m with an isoelectric point of 5.2. They suggest that the original moiety has undergone partial proteolysis to yield what they call "novel ß2m". The existence of such altered forms of serum ß2m has also been reported in various autoimmune and neoplastic diseases (57, 58). Nissen et al. have identified the presence, in the serum of patients with small cell lung carcinoma, of a ß2m molecule amputated of a single amino acid (58).

Structure of β2-microglobulin in amyloid deposits

Both Gorevic (54) and Linke (59) have demonstrated respectively by immunoblotting and by immunodiffusion together with western blotting, the presence of various ß2m polymers in the amyloid deposits. Polymerisation must occur locally as only the monomeric form is recognized both in serum (54) and in synovial fluid (60).

Whether ß2m also undergoes partial proteolysis in the deposition process remains debated. Gorevic (11, 54) failed to recognize "novel ß2m" in the deposits evaluated by immunoblotting. By contrast, Linke (59) utilizing a different purification procedure demonstrated the presence of intact ß2m together with a ß2m molecule amputated from its last 6 terminal aminoacids. Ogawa (56) recently confirmed this finding and reported that a high proportion of the deposited ß2m was "novel" ß2m. Interestingly, ß2m fragments are also the constituents of the amyloid kidney stones recognized in dialyzed patients (61).

If proteolysis is confirmed and proves to be the initial step of ß2m deposition, dialysis amyloidosis would be analogous to AA and AL amyloidosis where cleavage of a precursor molecule is a prerequisite for fibril formation (62). Furthermore, if proteolysis is achieved by synovial cells the preferential articular deposition of ß2m could be accounted for.

Argiles et al. further have described in the deposits the presence of globin chains in addition to ß2m and P substance (63). These as yet not confirmed data would be at variance with the other types of amyloidosis where only one serum precursor has been identified.

METABOLISM OF ß2-MICROGLOBULIN

ß2m is an 11.8 kilodalton, 100 aminoacids peptide. It is expressed within the HLA class I antigens at the cell surface (64) and contained within neutrophil specific granules (65). Its role is under scrutiny. Katoaka has provided evidence that ß2m inhibits bone mineralization *in vitro* (66), whereas Canalis suggested that ß2m is identical with the bone derived growth factor (BDGF) (67). More recently, Brinckerhoff et al. have isolated from fibroblast culture an autocrine 12 kilodalton protein able to induce collagenase synthesis. Interestingly, the amino-terminal sequence of this protein is 80% homologous with ß2m, a finding of potential interest in the elucidation of dialysis arthropathy (68). Further information is needed to evaluate the significance of these findings.

Daily endogenous ß2m production averages 150 mg irrespective of the level of renal function (69). No data, however, are available in patients treated by dialysis. Production is increased in states associated with lymphocyte stimulation such as lymphoproliferative, autoimmune and viral diseases. Cytokines are probably the mediators of this effect (70).

Several studies have documented, *in vitro*, that interferons a and g, tumor necrosis factor (TNF), and Interleukin-2 (IL_2) stimulate the synthesis and the expression of class I HLA antigens, as well as the release of ß2m. Ramadori et al. demonstrated in hepatoma cells that interferons a and g increase the synthesis of messenger RNA for HLA I antigens and, within 6 hours, the release of ß2m in the culture medium (70). Collins et al. provided evidence of TNF induced synthesis of HLA I antigens by endothelial and fibroblastic cells cultures (71). Nachbaur et al. analyzing the effect of several cytokines on ß2m release by lymphocytic and monocytic cell lines (72) observed that both interferon a and g as well as IL_2 were potent stimuli but that TNF was less active. The effect of Interleukin-1 (IL_1) remains debated. Lovett et al. reported that *in vitro*, IL_1 stimulates the expression of HLA I antigens on myeloid and lymphomatous cells (73). However, neither Pober et al. (74) nor Ramadori et al. (70) or Nachbaur et al. (72) working respectively with umbilical vein endothelial cells, hepatoma cells and lymphocytic or monocytic cells confirmed these findings. The latter two studies relied on recombinant cytokines (70, 72) whereas Lovett utilized natural IL_1, possibly contaminated by other cytokines (73) Finally, Interleukin-6 (IL_6) does not stimulate the synthesis of HLA I antigens by endothelial cells (75).

Results of *in vivo* studies agree with those obtained *in vitro* despite the difficulties inherent to the complex interactions existing *in vivo* between the various cytokines. Nachbaur et al. (76) and Aulitzky et al. (77) have demonstrated that therapeutic doses of recombinant interferons a and g and TNF raise ß2m serum level. Of course, *in vivo*, IL_1 might also stimulate ß2m production by inducing the release of other cytokines, like interferon (78).

ß2-microglobulin and renal failure

The kidney is the main catabolic site of ß2m (55). As a result, renal failure results in increased serum ß2m levels. In dialyzed patients without residual renal function, serum levels may reach up to sixty times the normal values (55). They are influenced by the patients' residual renal function (55) as well as by the technique of dialysis but remain stable over time as long as these factors are constant.

Provided that patients with the same residual renal function are compared, the serum levels tend to be approximately 30% lower in patients treated with AN69 than in those dialyzed with cuprophane membrane (79, 80). In the same patient group, an analogous lowering of ß2m is observed within 2 weeks after the replacement of cellulosic membrane by a synthetic, highly permeable membrane such as AN69 or polysulfone (81). Patients treated by peritoneal dialysis also have ß2m levels lower than subjects hemodialyzed with cuprophane matched for residual renal function (82). Switching patients from cuprophane hemodialysis to peritoneal dialysis similarly decreases ß2m serum levels (83) These observations suggest that the permeability characteristics of the dialysis membrane are important determinants of serum ß2m levels. The amount of ß2m, removed weekly varies from zero with cuprophane dialysis (79) to about 250 mg for peritoneal dialysis (84), 450 mg for AN69 dialysis (79) and 1000 to 1200 mg for hemofiltration (85), values to be compared with a weekly production around 1050 mg. During dialysis ß2m is removed not only by diffusion but also by adsorption to the membrane. This phenomenon is most striking for AN69 where up to 47 mg can be adsorbed on 1.1 m^2 (86). It is unaffected by reuse if sodium hypochlorite is utilized but markedly reduced if peracetic acid is utilized (86).

The changes of serum ß2m levels during dialysis are only partly accounted for by adsorption to or diffusion through the membrane. Changes in the distribution volume and alterations in the release of ß2m have also been considered. During dialysis, ß2m levels fall by 5 to 20% and 30 to 50% when either AN69 or polysulfone membranes are used (79, 81, 87, 88). By contrast, a 5 to 40% rise is observed in the presence of a cuprophane membrane (81, 87, 89). This increase has been initially ascribed to an augmented release of ß2m (89) but the timing of the rise, already evident within the first hour of dialysis (81, 87) is not compatible with an enhanced mRna mediated protein synthesis. Alternatively it has been suggested that the intra-dialytic increment results from hemoconcentration (90), a hypothesis contradicted by the fact that the percentage rise in ß2m exceeds the simultaneous changes in hematocrit or serum protein concentration in many studies (89, 91). More recently, however, it has been demonstrated that the changes in ß2m concentration during cuprophane dialysis are correlated ($r = 0.98$) with a parallel modification in the inulin distribution volume achieved with dialysates of varying Na content (92). Further support for the hypothesis that ß2m intra-dialytic kinetics are influenced by complex changes in the extracellular volume accrue from Flöge's observation that during cuprophane dialysis myoglobin (MW 17.2 KD) rises by 19.9%, a fractional change virtually identical with the 22.1% increment observed simultaneously for ß2m (91). The role played by changes in the distribution volume of ß2m in the intra-dialytic kinetics is supported by the observation that ß2m levels remain unchanged during cuprophane dialysis performed either *in vitro* with recirculating blood (93) or *in vivo* without dialysate flow (91).

Although the intra-dialytic changes in ß2m reflect mainly the balance between changes in distribution volume and the clearance of the polypeptide, it remains possible that the dialysis procedure itself affects ß2m production or deposition. No data concerning interdialytic ß2m synthesis are available. However, it has been demonstrated that the dialysis procedure itself influences the release of cytokines. As discussed earlier, these substances are able to stimulate ß2m production. Luger et al. have reported an augmented production of IL_1 and IL_2 during dialysis on cellulosic membranes (94). This could perhaps be ascribed to C3a and C5a generation, known inducer of cytokines release (95, 96). More recently, Lonnemann et al. (97) reported a greater production of IL_1 by mononuclear cells incubated on AN69 membranes than on cuprophane membranes. However, their study also demonstrated that AN69 membranes clear and adsorb IL_1 whereas cellulosic membranes don't. The integration in terms of clinical consequences of these contradictory properties of dialysis membranes will require further study. In this respect, we have recently observed that the TNF serum level rises significantly during cuprophane dialysis but remains unchanged during AN69 dialysis (98). Cytokines release during dialysis may also be affected by dialysate, if it contains endotoxin (99). It has also been suggested that acetate might enhance cytokine release (100).

The cytokines also influence various cell types such as macrophages and perhaps synoviocytes. If the latter play a critical role in the proteolysis of ß2m and if proteolysis or polymerisation is a prerequisite to ß2m amyloid fibril deposition, it is conceivable that the dialysis induced release of cytokines enhances local ß2m amyloid formation.

Factors responsible for β2-microglobulin deposition in dialysed patients

Obviously, the augmented pool of ß2m is a predisposing factor to ß2m precipitation. Even *in vitro*, ß2m may form fibrils with the characteristics of amyloidosis (101). However, additional factors must play a critical role as ß2m levels are not different in patients with or without amyloidosis (102). These additional factors must also account for the elective synovial precipitation of ß2m. The fact that ß2m concentration is virtually identical in the synovial fluid and in the serum makes the hypothesis of an enhanced articular ß2m production unlikely (103). A local stimulation of macrophages or synoviocytes capable of ß2m proteolysis or polymerisation has been considered above. Of note is the description of fibrillar material within the cytoplasm of macrophages adjacent to amyloid deposits (104, 105). Whether these inflammatory cells contribute to the local production of amyloid or are attracted secondarily by the deposit remains an open question. Still, it is of interest to remember that in AL amyloidosis the macrophages secrete the amyloid fibrils in close contact with the myeloma cells (106).

Alternatively, several other factors have been implicated in the synovial deposition of ß2m amyloid. The inflammatory effect of intraarticular aluminum (107) has raised the possibility that aluminum promotes dialysis amyloidosis. Aluminum accumulates in the synovia and cartilage of dialyzed patients, the highest concentration being reported in subjects with amyloidosis (107). Yver et al. (108) observed a larger desferrioxamine induced aluminum rise in patients with than in patient without carpal tunnel syndrome or dialysis arthropathy. A similar predisposing role has been proposed for iron by Cary (109). Foissac-Gegoux et al. also reported iron deposits within the synovia of 9 out of 14 dialysed patients, several of whom had coexistent amyloid deposits (110). In our own patients, however, we found no correlation between ferritin levels and the presence of amyloidosis (44). Furthermore the radiologic picture of iron overload arthropathy (111) is different from that of ß2m amyloid osteoarthropathy.

Finally, Bardin et al. have proposed that intraarticular apatite crystal may enhance amyloid precipitation. Munoz et al. (3), however, failed to observe crystals in the synovial fluid of ß2m amyloid arthropathy.

EARLY MARKERS OF ß2-MICROGLOBULIN AMYLOIDOSIS

Both the confirmation of the various factors incriminated in the genesis of dialysis amyloidosis and the evaluation of preventive or therapeutic strategies should rely on prospective controlled trials. Unfortunately such studies are difficult to implement as a result of the long delay of onset, 5 to 10 years, of the clinical manifestation of the disease. Several techniques aiming at an early diagnosis have thus been tested.

Bone scintigraphy with Technetium methylene diphosphonate has been investigated (112). The mechanism whereby this compound is fixed in the deposits has not been elucidated. Hawkins et al. have recently evaluated the fate of I^{123} labelled P substance, a component of all known amyloid deposits. In a preliminary communication on 13 patients with various types of amyloidosis including 2 with ß2m amyloidosis, the authors report that the substance is specifically bound by the amyloid deposits (113). Flöge et al. have utilized I^{131} labelled purified ß2m in an attempt to visualize by scintigraphy the amyloid deposits of 3 patients with demonstrated ß2m amyloidosis (114). The accumulation of the injected compound was demonstrated in an amyloid mass removed several days later. However, scintigraphy disclosed fixation of the labelled ß2m both in and outside deposits suspected on radiological or clinical grounds. The sensitivity and the specificity of these various methods remain to be documented.

Histologic studies of easily obtainable specimens are under way. It should be stressed again that the mere presence of ß2m demonstrated by immunofluorescence on a biopsy specimen is not sufficient to indicate the presence of amyloid deposits (115): the traditional tinctorial and electron microscopic criteria of amyloid should also be met.

TREATMENT OF ß2-MICROGLOBULIN AMYLOIDOSIS

The treatment of established dialysis amyloidosis remains disappointing. Hardouin et al. and Pengloan et al. have reported a subjective improvement of the clinical symptoms of dialysis arthropathy in uncontrolled studies of patients transferred from cuprophane to AN69 (116) or polysulfone (117) membrane dialysis. We failed to confirm this observation in 3 patients in whom cuprophane was replaced by high permeability membranes (AN69 or polysulfone). Laurent et al. have also reported a rapid improvement of the articular complaints of 5 patients transferred from cuprophane hemodialysis to peritoneal dialysis (118) We have observed the reverse sequence in a patient in whom peritoneal dialysis was initiated after 7 years of symptomless cuprophane hemodialysis. He developed within 6 years shoulder pain, bone cysts and a carpal tunnel syndrome (44).

Only a successful renal transplantation appears able to alter the relentless course of dialysis amyloidosis. Transplantation was followed within a few days by the disappearance of the osteoarticular complaints (119, 120). An objective assessment of the joints confirmed an improved mobility (120). Unfortunately, the bone cysts did not regress in five patients despite a follow-up extending up to 6 years after transplantation (119).

The disappearance of the joint symptoms is so rapid that it probably reflects the antiinflammatory effect of steroid treatment rather than any alteration of the ß2m deposits. Dialysis arthropathy has indeed an inflammatory component witnessed by a higher CRP concentration in the presence of dialysis arthropathy (121). It is encouraging, however, to note that the bone lesions do not progress and that the symptoms do not reappear when steroid therapy is tapered off.

CONCLUSION

Dialysis amyloidosis has been identified within the last 10 years. Within a few years its clinical symptoms, radiological signs and pathological extension have been delineated. At least two contributing factors have been identified: the age of the patient at the onset of dialysis and the characteristics of the dialysis membrane. The mechanisms of amyloid deposition have not yet been unraveled despite significant progresses. The only efficient therapy as yet is successful transplantation.

REFERENCES

1. Vandenbroucke JM, Huaux JP, Guillaume T, Noel H, Maldague B, van Ypersele de Strihou C: Capsular synovial and bone amyloidosis: complications of long-term haemodialysis. Proc EDTA-ERA, 22: 136-138, 1985.
2. Bardin T, Kuntz D, Zingraff J, Voisin MC, Zelmar A, Lansaman J: Synovial amyloidosis in patients undergoing long-term hemodialysis. Arthritis Rheum, 28: 1052-1058, 1985.
3. Munoz-Gomez J, Bergada-Barado E, Gomez-Perez R, Llopart-Buisan E, Subias-Sobrevia E, Rotés-Querol J, Solé-Arqués M: Amyloid arthropathy in patients undergoing periodical haemodialysis for chronic renal failure: a new complication. Ann Rheum Dis, 44: 729-733, 1985.
4. Huaux JP, Noel H, Bastien P, Malghem J, Maldague B, Devogelaer JP, Nagant de Deuxchaisnes C: Amylose articulaire, fracture du col fémoral et hémodialyse périodique chronique. Rev Rheumat, 52: 179-182, 1985.
5. Charra B, Calemard E, Uzan M, Terrat JC, Vanel T, Laurent G: Carpal tunnel syndrome, shoulder pain and amyloid deposits in long-term haemodialysis patients. Proc EDTA-ERA, 21: 291-295, 1984.
6. Fenves AZ, Emmett M, White MG, Greenway G, Michaels DB: Carpal tunnel syndrome with cystic bone lesions secondary to amyloidosis in chronic hemodialysis patients. Am J Kid Dis, 7: 130-134, 1986.
7. Huaux JP, Noel H, Malghem J, Maldague B, Devogelaer JP, Nagant de Deuxchaisnes C: Erosive azotemic osteoarthropathy: possible role of amyloidosis. Arthritis Rheum, 28: 1075-1076, 1985.
8. Bardin T, Zingraff J, Shirahama T, Noel LH, Droz D, Voisin MC, Drüeke T, Dryll A, Skinner M, Cohen AS, Kuntz D: Hemodialysis-associated amyloidosis and beta-2 microglobulin. Am J Med, 83: 419-424, 1987.
9. Casey TT, Stone WJ, Di Raimondo CR, Brantley BD, Di Raimondo CV, Gorevic PD, Page DL: Tumoral amyloidosis of bone of beta-2-microglobulin origin in association with long-term hemodialysis. Human Pathol, 17: 731-738, 1986.
10. Gejyo F, Yamada T, Odani S, Nakagawa Y, Arakawa M, Kunitomo T, Kataoka H, Suzuki M, Hirasawa Y, Shirahama T, Cohen AS, Schmid K: A new form of amyloid protein associated with chronic hemodialysis was identified as beta-2-microglobulin. Biochem Biophys Res Comm, 129: 701-706, 1985.
11. Gorevic PD, Casey TT, Stone WJ, Di Raimondo CR, Prelli FC, Frangione B: Beta-2-microglobulin is an amyloidogenic protein in man. J Clin Invest, 76: 2425-2429, 1985.
12. Shirahama T, Skinner M, Cohen AS, Gejyo F, Arakawa M, Suzuki M, Hirasawa Y: Histochemical and immunohistochemical characterization of amyloid associated with chronic hemodialysis as beta-2-microglobulin. Lab Invest, 53: 705-709, 1985.
13. Schwarz A, Keller F, Seyfert S, Pöll W, Molzahn M, Distler A: Carpal tunnel syndrome: a major complication in long-term hemodialysis patients. Clin Nephrol, 22: 133-137, 1984.
14. Di Raimondo CR, Casey TT, Gorevic PD, Di Raimondo CV, Stone WJ: Beta-2-microglobulin amyloidosis in chronic hemodialysis patients. Clin Res, 34: 82A, 1986.
15. Brancaccio D, Gallieni M, Padovese P, Anelli A, Coggi G, Uslenghi C: Dialysis amyloidosis with massive popliteal deposition of ß2-microglobulin amyloid. Lancet, ii: 802, 1988.
16. Reese W, Hopkovitz A, Lifschitz MD: ß2-Microglobulin and associated amyloidosis presenting as bilateral popliteal tumors. Am J Kidney Dis, 13: 323-325, 1988.

17. Zingraff J, Bardin T, Noel LH, Dubost C, Kuntz D, Drüeke: Occurrence of beta-2-microglobulin amyloid deposits in sternoclavicular synovium of chronic hemodialysis patients. Kidney Int, 33: 242, 1988.
18. Kuntz D, Naveau B, Bardin T, Drüeke T, Treves R, Dryll A: Destructive spondylarthropathy in hemodialyzed patients. Arthritis Rheum, 27: 369-375, 1984.
19. Lambrey G, Sebert JL, Bardin T, Shirahama T, Marie A, Gheerbrand JD, Moriniere P, Kuntz D, Zingraff J, Fournier A: Destructive spondylarthropathies of haemodialysis patients is associated with amyloidosis reacting with anti-beta-2-microglobulin antiserum. Nephrol Dial Transpl, 1: 106-107, 1986.
20. Kaplan P, Resnick D, Murphey M, Heck L, Phalen H, Egan D, Rutsky E: Destructive noninfectious spondylarthropathy in hemodialysis patients: a report of four cases. Radiology, 162: 241-244, 1987.
21. Alcalay M, Goupy MC, Azais I, Bontoux D: Hemodialysis is not essential for the development of destructive spondylarthropathy in patients with chronic renal failure. Arthr Rheum, 30: 1182-1186, 1987.
22. Allain TJ, Stevens PE, Bridges LR, Phillips ME: Dialysis myelopathy: quadriparesis due to extradural amyloid of ß2 microglobulin origin. Br Med J, 296: 752-753, 1988.
23. Bouteiller G, Ton That H, Goudable C, Goffinet F, Heche JP, Orfila C, Suc JM: Amyloidosis in chronic hemodialysis: rheumatological aspects. Contr Nephrol, 62: 67-74, 1988.
24. Campistol JM, Cases A, Torras A, Soler M, Munoz-Gomez J, Monoliu J, Lopez-Pedret J, Revert L: Visceral involvement of dialysis amyloidosis. Am J Nephrol, 7: 390-393, 1987.
25. Campistol JM, Torras A, Lopez-Pedret J: Systemic character and visceral involvement of dialysis amyloidosis. Clin Nephrol, 28: 261, 1987.
26. Fuchs A, Jagirdar J, Schwartz IS: Beta 2-microglobulin amyloidosis in patients undergoing long-term hemodialysis. Am J Clin Pathol, 88: 302-307, 1987.
27. Arakawa M, Gejyo F, Ohara K, Honma N: Systemic type of hemodialysis-associated amyloidosis. Kidney Int, 31: 227, 1987.
28. Hardouin P, Flipo RM, Lecomte-Houcke M, Foissac-Gegoux Ph, Delcambre B: Amylose des hémodialysés. Recherche d'une diffusion générale par biopsie rectale. Presse Méd, 16: 445-446, 1987.
29. Noël LH, Zingraff J, Bardin T, Atienza C, Kuntz D, Drüeke T : Tissue distribution of dialysis amyloidosis. Clin Nephrol, 27: 175-178, 1987.
30. Ogawa H, Saito A, Hirabayashi N, Hara K: Amyloid deposition in systemic organs in long-term hemodialysis patients. Clin Nephrol, 28: 199-204, 1987.
31. Orfila C, Goffinet F, Durroux R, Bouteiller G, Goudable C, Ton That Y, Manuel Y, Suc JM: Haemodialysis-associated amyloidosis and beta2 microglobulin deposits in long-term haemodialysis patients. Nephrol Dial Transplant, 2: 448, 1987.
32. Sethi D, Woodrow DF, Brown A, Cary NRB, Gower PE: Dialysis amyloid: systemic or local? Nephrol Dial Transplant, 3: 552, 1988.
33. Takahashi S, Morita T, Koda Y, Murayama H, Hirasawa Y: Gastrointestinal involvement of dialysis-related amyloidosis. Clin Nephrol, 30: 168-171, 1988.
34. Theaker JM, Raine AEG, Rainey AJ, Heryet A, Clark A, Oliver DO: Systemic amyloidosis of ß2-microglobulin type: a complication of long term haemodialysis. J Clin Pathol, 40: 1247-1251, 1987.
35. Maher ER, Hamilton Dutoit S, Baillod RA, Sweny P, Moorhead JF: Gastrointestinal complications of dialysis related amyloidosis. Br Med J, 297: 265-266, 1988.
36. Suda K, Ariwa R.: The islets of Langerhans in uremic patients receiving chronic hemodialysis. Nephron, 46: 134-136, 1987.
37. Clark A, Cooper GJS, Lewis CE, Morris JF, Willis AC, Reid KBM, Turner RC: Islet amyloid formed from diabetes-associated peptide may be pathogenic in type-2 diabetes. Lancet, ii: 231-238, 1987.
38. Kachel HG, Altmeyer P, Baldamus CA, Koch KM: Deposition of an amyloid-like substance as a possible complication of regular dialysis treatment. Contr Nephrol, 36: 127-132, 1983.
39. Kachel HG, Altmeyer P, Kühn KW, Koch KM, Baldamus CA: Deposition of nonamyloid material in connective tissue in uraemia. Blood Purification, 2: 142-148, 1984.
40. Varga J, Idelson BA, Felson D, Skinner M, Cohen AS: Lack of amyloid in abdominal fat aspirates from patients undergoing long-term hemodialysis. Arch Intern Med, 147: 1455-1457, 1987.
41. Polliack A, Hershko C: Spontaneous rupture of the spleen in amyloidosis. Israel J Med Sci, 8: 57-60, 1972.

42. Brown EA, Arnold IR, Gower PE: Dialysis arthropathy: complication of long term treatment with haemodialysis. Br Med J, 292: 163-166, 1986.
43. Charra B, Calemard E, Laurent G: Chronic renal failure treatment duration and mode: their relevance to the late dialysis periarticular syndrome. Blood Purification, 6: 117-124, 1988.
44. van Ypersele de Strihou C, Honhon B, Vandenbroucke JM, Huaux JP, Noel H, Maldague B: Dialysis amyloidosis. In "Advances in Nephrology" Grünfeld JP, Bach JF, Funck-Brentano JL, Maxwell Eds, Year Book Medical Publishers, Inc, 17: 1988, pp 401-422.
45. Sethi D, Maher ER, Cary NRB: Dialysis amyloid presenting as acute arthritis. Nephron, 50: 73-74, 1988.
46. Hadjipavlou A, Lander P, Begin L, Bercovitch D, Davidman M, Jakab E: Skeletal amyloidosis due to beta microglobulinemia in a patient on hemodialysis. J Bone Joint Surg, 70-A: 119-121, 1988.
47. Bohlman ME, Kim YC, Eagan J, Spees EK: Brown tumor in secondary hyperparathyroidism causing acute paraplegia. Am J Med, 81: 545-547, 1986.
48. Vandenbroucke JM, Jadoul M, Maldague B, Huaux JP, Noel H, van Ypersele de Strihou C: Possible role of dialysis membrane characteristics in amyloid osteoarthropathy. Lancet, i: 1210-1211, 1986.
49. Chanard J, Lavaud S, Toupance O, Roujouleh H, Melin JP: Carpal tunnel syndrome and type of dialysis membrane used in patients undergoing long-term hemodialysis. Arthritis Rheum, 29: 1170-1171, 1986.
50. van Ypersele de Strihou C, Maldague B and the Working Party on Dialysis Amyloidosis: Relation between membrane type and signs of dialysis-related amyloidosis. Nephrol Dial Transplant, 3: 552-553, 1988.
51. Gagnon RF, Lough JO, Bourgouin PA: Carpal tunnel syndrome and amyloidosis associated with continuous ambulatory peritoneal dialysis. Can Med Assoc J, 139: 753-755, 1988.
52. Benhamou CL, Bardin T, Noel LH, Cornelis F, Tourliere D, Maitre F, Pierre D: Beta-2-microglobulin amyloidosis as a complication of peritoneal dialysis treatment. Clin Nephrol, 30: 346, 1988.
53. Renaud H, Fournier A, Morinière Ph, Westeel PF, El Esper N, Belbrik S, Marie A, Cohen-Solal HE, Sebert JL: Erosive osteoarthropathy associated with ß2-microglobulin amyloidosis in a uraemic patient treated exclusively by long-term haemofiltration with biocompatible membranes. Nephrol Dial Transplant, 3: 820-822, 1988.
54. Gorevic PD, Munoz PC, Casey TT, Di Raimondo CR, Stone WJ, Prelli FC, Rodrigues MM, Poulik MD, Frangione B: Polymerization of intact ß2-microglobulin in tissue causes amyloidosis in patients on chronic hemodialysis. Proc Natl Acad Sci, 83: 7908-7912, 1986.
55. Vincent C, Revillard JP, Galland M, Traeger J: Serum ß2-microglobulin in hemodialyzed patients. Nephron 21: 260-268, 1978.
56. Ogawa H, Saito A, Oda O, Nakajima M, Chung TG: Detection of novel ß2-microglobulin in the serum of hemodialysis patients and its amyloidogenic predisposition. Clin Nephrol, 32: 158-163, 1988.
57. Plesner T, Wiik A: Demonstration of electrophoretic heterogeneity of serum ß2-microglobulin in systemic lupus erythematosus and rheumatoid arthritis: evidence against autoantibodies to ß2-microglobulin. Scand J Immunol, 9: 247-254, 1979.
58. Nissen MH, Thim L, Christensen M: Purification and biochemical characterization of the complete structure of a proteolytically modified ß-2-microglobulin with biological activity. Eur J Biochem, 163: 21-28, 1987.
59. Linke RP, Hampl H, Bartel-Schwarze S, Eulitz M: ß2-microglobulin, different fragments and polymers thereof in synovial amyloid in long-term hemodialysis. Biol Chem Hoppe Seyler, 368: 137-144, 1987.
60. Sethi D, Gower PE: Is ß2-microglobulin polymerised in the synovial fluid of patients with dialysis amyloid? Nephrol Dial Transplant, 3: 552, 1988.
61. Linke RP, Bommer J, Ritz E, Waldherr R, Eulitz M: Amyloid kidney stones of uremic patients consist of beta2-microglobulin fragments. Biochem Biophys Res Comm, 136: 665-671, 1986.
62. Cohen AS, Connors LH: The pathogenesis and biochemistry of amyloidosis. J Pathol, 151: 1-10, 1987.
63. Argiles A, Mourad G, Axelrud-Cavadore C, Derancourt J, Jauregui Adell J, Mion C, Cavadore JC: Haemodialysis-associated amyloidosis: ß2-microglobulin alone or associated with globin chains? Clin Sci, 73: 515-518, 1987.

64. Cresswell P, Springer T, Strominger JL, Turner MJ, Grey HM, Kubo RT: Immunological identity of the small subunit of HL-A antigens and β2-microglobulin and its turnover on the cell membrane. Proc Nat Acad Sci, 71: 2123-2127, 1974.
65. Bjerrum OW, Bjerrum OJ, Borregaard N: β2-Microglobulin in neutrophils: an intragranular protein. J Immunol, 138: 3913-3917, 1987.
66. Kataoka H, Gejyo F, Yamada S, Kunitomo, Arakawa M: Inhibitory effects of β2-microglobulin on *in vitro* calcification of osteoblastic cells. Biochem Biophys Res Comm, 141: 360-366, 1986.
67. Canalis E, McCarthy T, Centrella M: A bone-derived growth factor isolated from rat calvariae is beta2 microglobulin. Endocrinol, 121: 1198-1200, 1987.
68. Brinckerhoff CE, Mitchell TI, Karmilowicz MJ, Kluve-Beckerman B, Benson MD: Autocrine induction of collagenase by serum amyloid A-like and β2-microglobulin-like proteins. Science, 243: 655-657, 1989.
69. Karlsson FA, Groth T, Sege K, Wibell L, Peterson PA: Turnover in humans of beta-2-microglobulin: the constant chain of HLA-antigens. Eur J Clin Invest, 10: 293-300, 1980.
70. Ramadori G, Mitsch A, Rieder H, Meyer zum Büschenfelde KH: Alpha- and gamma-interferon (IFNa, IFNg) but not interleukin-1 (IL_1) modulate synthesis and secretion of β2-microglobulin by hepatocytes. Eur J Clin Invest, 18: 343-351, 1988.
71. Collins T, Lapierre LA, Fiers W, Strominger JL, Pober JS: Recombinant human tumor necrosis factor increases mRNA levels and surface expression of HLA-A,B antigens in vascular endothelial cells and dermal fibroblasts *in vitro*. Proc Natl Acad Sci, 83: 446-450, 1986.
72. Nachbaur K, Troppmair J, Bieling P, Kotlan B, König P, Huber C: Cytokines in the control of beta-2 microglobulin release. I. *In vitro* studies on various haemopoietic cells. Immunobiol, 177: 55-65, 1988.
73. Lovett D, Kozan B, Hadam M, Resch K, Gemsa D: Macrophage cytotoxicity: interleukin 1 as a mediator of tumor cytostasis. J Immunol, 136: 340-347, 1986.
74. Pober JS, Bevilacqua MP, Mendrick DL, Lapierre LA, Fiers W, Gimbrone MA Jr: Two distinct monokines, interleukin 1 and tumor necrosis factor, each independently induce biosynthesis and transient expression of the same antigen on the surface of cultured human vascular endothelial cells. J Immunol, 136: 1680-1687, 1986.
75. Lapierre LA, Fiers W, Pober JS: Three distinct classes of regulatory cytokines control endothelial cell MHC antigen expression. J Exp Med, 167: 794-804, 1988.
76. Nachbaur K, Troppmair J, Kotlan B, König P, Aulitzky W, Bieling P, Huber C: Cytokines in the control of beta-2-microglobulin release. II. *In vivo* studies with recombinant interferons and antigens. Immunobiol, 77: 66-75, 1988.
77. Aulitzky WE, Tilg H, Herold M, Berger M, Vogel W, Judmaier G, Gastl G, Mull B, Flener R, Wiegele J, Pichler E, Denz H, Böheim E, Aulitzky WK, Huber C: Enhanced serum levels of β-2-microglobulin, neopterin and interferon-g in patients treated with recombinant tumor necrosis factor-a. J Interferon Res, 8: 655-664, 1988.
78. Dinarello CA, Mier JW: Lymphokines. N Engl J Med, 317: 940-945, 1987.
79. Zingraff J, Beyne P, Urena P, Uzan M, Khoa Man N, Descamps-Latscha B, Drüeke T: Influence of haemodialysis membranes on β2-microglobulin kinetics: *in vivo* and *in vitro* studies. Nephrol Dial Transplant, 3: 284-290, 1988.
80. Caverle Y, Simon P, Ang KS, Cam G, Catheline M: Serum β2 microglobin levels in hemodialysed uremics depend on permeability of dialysis membranes. Kidney Int, 31: 229, 1987.
81. Bommer J, Seelig P, Seelig R, Geerlings W, Bommer G, Ritz E: Determinants of plasma β2-microglobulin concentration: possible relation to membrane biocompatibility. Nephrol Dial Transplant, 2: 22-25, 1987.
82. Tielemans C, Dratwa M, Bergmann P, Goldmann M, Flamion B, Collart F, Wens R: Continuous ambulatory peritoneal dialysis vs haemodialysis: a lesser risk of amyloidosis? Nephrol Dial Transplant, 3: 291-294, 1988.
83. Sethi D, Brown EA, Gower PE: CAPD, protective against developing dialysis-associated amyloid? Nephron, 50: 85-86, 1988.
84. Blumberg A, Bürgi W: Behavior of β2-microglobulin in patients with chronic renal failure undergoing hemodialysis, hemodiafiltration and continuous ambulatory peritoneal dialysis (CAPD). Clin Nephrol, 27: 245-249, 1987.
85. Flöge J, Wilks M, Shaldon S, Koch KM, Smeby LC: β2-Microglobulin kinetics during haemofiltration. Nephrol Dial Transplant, 3: 784-789, 1988.
86. Goldman M, Dhaene M, Amraoui Z, Thayse C, Vanherweghem JL: Adsorption of β2-microglobulin on new and reused dialysis membranes. Nephrol Dial Transplant, 3: 551, 1988.

87. Vandenbroucke JM, van Ypersele de Strihou C: Relationship between membrane characteristics and dialysis-induced changes in beta-2-microglobulin levels. Nephrol Dial Transpl, 1: 105, 1986.
88. Flöge J, Granolleras C, Bingel M, Deschodt G, Branger B, Oules R, Koch KM, Shaldon S: ß2-Microglobulin kinetics during haemodialysis and haemofiltration. Nephrol Dial Transplant, 1: 223-228, 1987.
89. Hauglustaine D, Waer M, Michielsen P, Goebels J, Vandeputte M: Haemodialysis membranes, serum beta-2-microglobulin and dialysis amyloidosis. Lancet, i: 1211-1212, 1986.
90. Bergström J, Wehle B: No change in corrected ß2-microglobulin concentration after cuprophane haemodialysis. Lancet, i: 628-629, 1987.
91. Flöge J, Granolleras C, Merscher S, Eisenbach GM, Deschodt G, Colton CK, Shaldon S, Koch KM: Is the rise in plasma beta-2-microglobulin seen during hemodialysis meaningful? Nephron, 51: 6-12, 1989.
92. Hönig R, Marsen T, Schad S, Barth C, Pollok M, Baldamus CA: Correlation of beta-2-microglobulin concentration changes to changes of distribution volume. Int J Art Organs, 11: 459-464, 1988.
93. Dratwa M, Galand L, Tielemans C, Bergmann P, Colle P: Absence of *in vitro* generation of ß2-microglobulin by cuprophane dialyser. Nephrol Dial Transplant, 2: 447, 1987.
94. Luger A, Kovarik J, Stummvoll HK, Urbanska A, Luger TA: Blood-membrane interaction in hemodialysis leads to increased cytokine production. Kidney Int, 32: 84-88, 1987.
95. Haeffner-Cavaillon N, Cavaillon JM, Laude M, Kazatchkine MD: C3a(C3adesArg) induces production and release of interleukin 1 by cultured human monocytes. J Immunol, 139: 794-799, 1987.
96. Okusawa S, Yancey KB, van der Meer JWM, Endres S, Lonnemann G, Hefter K, Frank MM, Burke JF, Dinarello CA, Gelfand JA: C5a stimulates secretion of tumor necrosis factor from human mononuclear cells *in vitro*. J Exp Med, 168: 443-448, 1988.
97. Lonnemann G, Koch KM, Shaldon S, Dinarello CA: Studies on the ability of hemodialysis membranes to induce, bind, and clear human interleukin-1. J Lab Clin Med, 112: 76-86, 1988.
98. Ghysen J, De Plaen JF, van Ypersele de Strihou C: Effect of membrane characteristics on TNFa kinetics during hemodialysis. Nephrol Dial Transplant (in press)
99. Bingel M, Lonnemann G, Shaldon S, Koch KM, Dinarello CA: Human interleukin-1 production during hemodialysis. Nephron 43: 161-163, 1986.
100. Bingel M, Lonnemann G, Koch KM, Dinarello CA, Shaldon S: Enhancement of *in vitro* human interleukin-1 production by sodium acetate. Lancet, i: 14-16, 1987.
101. Connors LH, Shirahama T, Skinnner M, Fenves A, Cohen AS: *In vitro* formation of amyloid fibrils from intact ß2-microglobulin. Biochem Biophys Res Comm, 131: 1063-1068, 1985.
102. Gejyo F, Homma N, Suzuki Y, Arakawa M: Serum levels of beta-2-microglobulin as a new form of amyloid protein in patients undergoing long-term hemodialysis. N Engl J Med, 314: 585-586, 1986.
103. Sethi D, Gower PE: Synovial-fluid beta-2-microglobulin levels in dialysis arthropathy. New Engl J Med, 315: 1419-1420, 1986.
104. Depierreux M, Goldman M, Fayt I, Richard C, Quintin J, Dhaene M, Vanherweghem JL: Osteoarticular amyloidosis associated with haemodialysis: an immunoultrastructural study. J Clin Pathol, 41: 158-162, 1988.
105. Morita T, Suzuki M, Kamimura A, Hirasawa Y: Amyloidosis of a possible new type in patients receiving long-term hemodialysis. Arch Pathol Lab Med, 109: 1029-1032, 1985.
106. Durie BG, Persky B, Soehnlen BJ, Grogan TM, Salmon SE: Amyloid production in human myeloma stem-cell culture, with morphologic evidence of amyloid secretion by associated macrophages. N Engl J Med, 307: 1689-1692, 1982.
107. Netter P, Kessler M, Gaucher A, Gillet P, Delons S, Burnel D, Benoit J, Got C: Aluminium and dialysis arthropathy. Lancet, i: 886-887, 1988.
108. Yver L, Blanchier D, Buiquang D, Cabanne JF, Charmes JP, Meftahi H: Does aluminium induce dialysis amyloidosis? Nephrol Dial Transplant, 2: 450-451, 1987.
109. Cary NRB, Sethi D, Brown EA, Erhardt CC, Woodrow DF, Gower PE: Dialysis arthropathy : amyloid or iron? Br Med J, 293: 1392-1394, 1986.
110. Foissac-Gegoux P, Flipo RM, Hardouin P, Dumont A, Duquesnoy B, Lecomte-Houcke M, Delcambre B: Aspects actuels de la pathologie ostéo-articulaire des hémodialysés. Néphrologie, 4: 157-163, 1986.
111. Huaux JP, Geubel A, Koch MC, Malghem J, Madague B, Devogelaer JP, Nagant de Deuxchaisnes C: The arthritis of hemochromatosis. A review of 25 cases with special reference to

chondrocalcinosis, and a comparison with patients with primary hyperparathyroidism and controls. Clin Rheumatol, 5: 317-324, 1986.
112. Grateau G, Zingraff J, Fauchet M, Mundler O, Raymond P, Berthelot JM, Bardin T, Kuntz D, DrüekeT: Radionuclide exploration of dialysis amyloidosis: preliminary experience. Am J Kidney Dis, 11: 231-237, 1988.
113. Hawkins PN, Myers MJ, Lavender JP, Pepys MB: Diagnostic radionuclide imaging of amyloid: biological targeting by circulating human serum amyloid P component. Lancet, i: 1413-1418, 1988.
114. Flöge J, Nonnast-Daniel B, Gielow P, Brandis A, Spindler E, Hundeshagen H, Koch KM, Shaldon S: Specific imaging of dialysis-related amyloid deposits using ^{131}I-beta-2-microglobulin. Nephron, 51: 444-447, 1989.
115. Assounga AGH, Bascoul S, Canaud B, Banya PA, Vendrell JP, Sciolla JP, Mourad G, Baldet P, Serre A, Mion C: Beta 2 microglobulin deposits in uremic patients: skin study. Kidney Int, 35: 238, 1989.
116. Hardouin P, Flipo RM, Foissac-Gegoux P, Dumont A, Duquesnoy B, Delcambre B: Dialysis-related ß2 microglobulin-amyloid arthropathy. Improvement of clinical symptoms after a switch of dialysis membranes. Clin Rheumatol, 7: 41-45, 1988.
117. Pengloan J, Blanchier D, Nivet H, Bagros Ph: Relief of hemodialysis related inflammatory shoulder pain after treatment by polysulfon membrane. Abstract Book, International Congress of Nephrology, London 1987, p 166.
118. Laurent G, Charra B, Calemard E, Uzan M, Vanel T, Terrat JC: Amélioration par la dialyse péritonéale continue ambulatoire des douleurs abarticulaires accompagnant le syndrome du canal carpien des hémodialysés. Presse Méd, 14: 2105-2106, 1985.
119. Jadoul M, Maldague B, Pirson Y, van Ypersele de Strihou C: Renal transplantation for dialysis arthropathy. Lancet, ii: 849, 1988.
120. Sethi D, Brown EA, Maini RN, Gower PE: Renal transplantation for dialysis arthropathy. Lancet, ii: 448-449, 1988.
121. Sethi E, Muller BR, Brown EA, Maini RN, Gower PE: C-reactive protein in haemodialysis patients with dialysis arthropathy. Nephrol Dial Transplant, 2: 269-271, 1988.

13

ACQUIRED CYSTIC KIDNEY DISEASE

IRENE DE LOURDES NORONHA, EBERHARD RITZ, AND RÜDIGER WALDHERR

Departments of Internal Medicine and Pathology, Ruperto Carola University - Heidelberg, Germany (FRG)

INTRODUCTION

Little recent progress has been made in understanding the pathogenesis of Acquired Cystic Kidney Disease (ACKD) in uremic patients. However, several points relating to the epidemiology and clinical consequences of this condition have been clarified and reasonable recommendations for handling of such patients can be made. This review will focus on recent reports on morphology of cysts and controversial issues of renal cell carcinoma formation in ACKD.

After the first communication of Dunnill et al (1), ACKD has been described in patients with renal insufficiency from various causes both by us (2-4) and by numerous other investigators (for review of older literature see Ref 5 and 6). Although it was originally thought that ACKD represented a new type of renal disease, our scrutiny of ancient literature showed numerous descriptions starting with an anedoctal report in 1681 (7), and culminating in a scholarly description by Frerichs in 1851 (8). The phenomenon was still known to Bell (9), but largely forgotten thereafter. The observation that cysts were common at a time when no dialysis facility was yet available clearly excludes the possibility that cysts arise as a consequence of treatment modality (10) as originally thought by many authors.

PREVALENCE

ACKD has been noted in patients on hemodialysis or CAPD and even in patients with varying stages of preterminal renal failure. Different rates of prevalence of ACKD were reported depending on the method by which the diagnosis was established, i.e. autopsy studies or studies based on imaging procedures, e.g. sonography, computed tomography or magnetic resonance imaging.

Table 1 Acquired cystic kidney disease and renal tumors reported in patients with chronic renal failure: autopsy/nephrectomy studies.

References	Number of patients examined	Patients with ACKD	Patients with ACKD and renal tumors	Patients with ACKD and renal CA	Duration of dialysis (yrs) range (mean)	Notes
	Hemodialysis					
Dunnill (1)	30	14 (47%)	6 (43%)	1 (7%)	- (3.4)	1 metastasis
Elliot (11)	18	5 (28%)	-	-	0.7-7.5 (3.5)	
Bansal (12)	52	5 (10%)	1 (20%)		3-11 (6.2)	
Hughson (13)	66	5 (8%)	1 (20%)	-	2.5-5 (3.7)	
Fayemi (14)	80	24 (30%)	9 (37%)	1 (4%)	0.8-6 (1.6)	1 metastasis
Krempien (2)	22	21 (95%)	4 (19%)	-	0.8-8.2 (2.8)	
Mirahmadi (15)	32	15 (47%)	-	-	- (3.6)	
Feiner (16)	15	5 (33%)	2 (40%)	1 (20%)	3-7 (5.3)	
Turani (17)	15	10 (67%)	3 (30%)	1 (10%)	1-10 (3.6)	
Vaziri (18)	22	11 (50%)	1 (9%)	1 (9%)	0.2-7.7 (3.7)	Tx recipients
	Peritoneal Dialysis-CAPD					
Katz (19)	15	5 (33%)	2 (40%)	-	0.3-8.4 (3.4)	1 ACKD predialysis
	Chronic Renal Failure-Predialysis					
Katz (19)	41	7 (17%)	-	-	-	
TOTAL	408	127 (31%)	29 (22.8%)	5(3.9%)	(3.7)	

Abbreviations: ACKD = Acquired Cystic Kidney Disease; CA = renal cell carcinoma; CAPD = Continuous Ambulatory Peritoneal Dialysis; Tx= renal transplantation

As shown in Table 1, in autopsy series rates of prevalence of ACKD between 8 and 95% were found in patients on dialysis. The rate is a function of duration of hemodialysis treatment, since we found that the prevalence of cysts as well as the number and the size of cysts rise with increasing duration of dialysis (4). Another factor determining prevalence of ACKD may be the type of underlying renal disease: we (4) and others noted that cysts were more common in conditions involving medullary structures (e.g. analgesic nephropathy) and rare in diabetes mellitus. Finally, Ishikawa et al (20) noted a higher prevalence of ACKD in males compared to females. The prevalence of cysts in patients on CAPD is similar to patients on hemodialysis (19), but it is markedly lower in patients who had come to death prior to renal replacement therapy (19).

Table 2. Acquired cystic kidney disease and renal tumors reported in patients with chronic renal failure-ultrasound / computed tomography studies.

References	Number of patients examined	Patients with ACKD	Patients with ACKD and renal tumors	Patients with ACKD and renal CA	Duration of dialysis (yrs) range (mean)	Notes
Hemodialysis						
Bommer (3)	14	11 (79%)	-	-	1.3-8 (5.2)	CT; cysts 3/4 Tx
Ishikawa (21)	96	41 (43%)	4 (10%)	3 (7%)	-	CT; 18 Tx
Goldsmith (22)	20	17 (85%)	-	-	6-13	US
Mickisch (4)	108	70 (65%)	1 (1%)	1 (1%)	0.5-13 (4.5)	US; cysts 8/9 Tx
Minar (23)	43	21 (49%)	-	-	-	US; cysts 4/23 Tx*
Levine (24)	30	13 (43%)	2 (15%)	-	(5.4)	CT; no cysts in 6 Tx; including pts on PD
Narasimhan (25)	83	21 (25%)	-	-	(4.0)	CT+US
Thomson (26)	79	57 (72%)	-	-	0.2-21 (5.6)	US; 8HD +CAPD
Jabour (27)	25	23 (92%)	1 (4%)	1 (4%)	>3 yrs	CT+US
	19	2 (10%)			<3 yrs	CT+US
Peritoneal Dialysis-CAPD						
Bommer (10)	65	35 (54%)	-	-	(2.8)	US
Katz (19)	7	1 (14%)	-	-	-	US
Narasimhan (25)	17	1 (6%)	-	-	(0.6)	CT+US
Thomson (26)	21	6 (29%)	-	-	0.7-5 (2.7)	US
Jabour (27)	7	7 (100%)	-	-	>3yrs	CT+US
	29	1 (3%)	-	-	<3yrs	CT+US
Smith (28)	20	5 (25%)	2 (40%)	2 (40%)	0.4-12 (5.3)	US; 4 pts HD before
Leichter (29)	15	5 (33%)	1 (20%)	-	2-6 (3.2)	US+MRI; 3 Tx;*
Chronic Renal Failure-Predialysis						
Bommer (3)	13	7 (54%)	-	-	-	CT
Mickisch (4)	120	31 (26%)	-	-	-	US
Narasimhan (25)	30	2 (7%)	-	-	-	CT+US
TOTAL	861	377 (44%)	11 (2.9%)	7 (1.8%)	(3.9)	

* in 2 patients cysts were detected prior to dialysis

Abbreviations: ACKD= acquired cystic kidney disease; CA = renal cell carcinoma; HD= hemodialysis; CAPD= continuous ambulatory peritoneal dialysis; PD= peritoneal dialysis; Tx= renal transplantation; US= ultrasound; CT = computed tomography; MRI= magnetic resonance imaging

Ultrasonography is a very sensitive procedure to detect ACKD. Using this technique between 7% (25) and 26% (4) of patients in preterminal renal failure have been reported of suffer from ACKD. On dialysis, the respective percentages increase up to 92% (27).

Till now no strict criteria for diagnosis of ACKD have been laid down. The difficulty is to distinguish between occasional solitary renal cysts and ACKD. In the study of Mickisch et al (4), parapelvic cysts and solitary renal cysts (>2.5 cm) in one of both kidneys were excluded. All other cysts were classified as ACKD. Levine et al (24) made the diagnosis of "occasional cysts" when less than 5 cysts per kidney were found; ACKD was diagnosed when multiple bilateral renal cysts were seen on computed tomography. Finally, Feiner et al (16) made the diagnosis of ACKD when 40% of the kidney was involved by cystic transformation. The crux of the matter is that more than 50% of people over 50 years of age have at least one cyst on *post mortem*. This leaves ample room for ambiguity of classification in individual cases.

Several authors reported that cysts may regress after successful renal transplantation (18, 30). This may be related to the decrease in glomerular filtration and transepithelial sodium movement. However, reversal is not uniform in all cases (31, 32).

MORPHOLOGY

ACKD is characterized by multiple bilateral cysts scattered throughout cortex and medulla. Cysts predominate in the cortex and occasionally protrude over the outer renal surface. While in general kidneys are shrunken and scarred, occasionally grotesque enlargement of kidneys secondary to cyst formation is noted and this may render difficult the distinction from adult dominant polycystic kidney disease.

The cyst wall has the characteristics of transporting epithelia. This conclusion is based (i) on ultrastructural analysis (4, 5), (ii) on analysis of cyst wall epithelial cells using segment specific monoclonal antibodies (6) and (iii) indirectly on analysis of cyst fluid composition (33).

Microdissection studies demonstrated continuity between cysts and renal tubules, suggesting that cysts begin as fusiform tubular dilatations or as saccular outpouchings, possibly arising in diverticula (16). The alternative or complementary possibility of nephronal obstruction has not been formally excluded. Because of recent speculations that cysts may arise secondary to nephronal obstruction by ß2-microglobulin derived material (34), it is of note that low ß2-microglobulin levels were found in cyst fluid of patients with ACKD (35). The role of the frequent occurrence of oxalate crystals in the lumen of cysts has not been defined: it is unknown whether deposition of oxalate represents a secondary phenomenon or whether it causes tubular obstruction. Similarly unresolved is the question whether elevated plasma oxalate levels in patient with ACKD play a pathogenetic role (36).

Most cysts are lined by flat or cuboidal epithelium but in some cysts columnar cells with clear or granular and acidophilic cytoplasm predominate. Scanning and transmission electron microscopy showed that the cells lining the cyst walls exhibit characteristic morphological features of proximal tubules, of distal segments or of collecting ducts (4); however, the majority of epithelial cells lining cysts (70-80%) stain with monoclonal antibodies (cALLa and villin; see Figure 1) which react with proximal tubular epithelial cells in normal kidney (6).

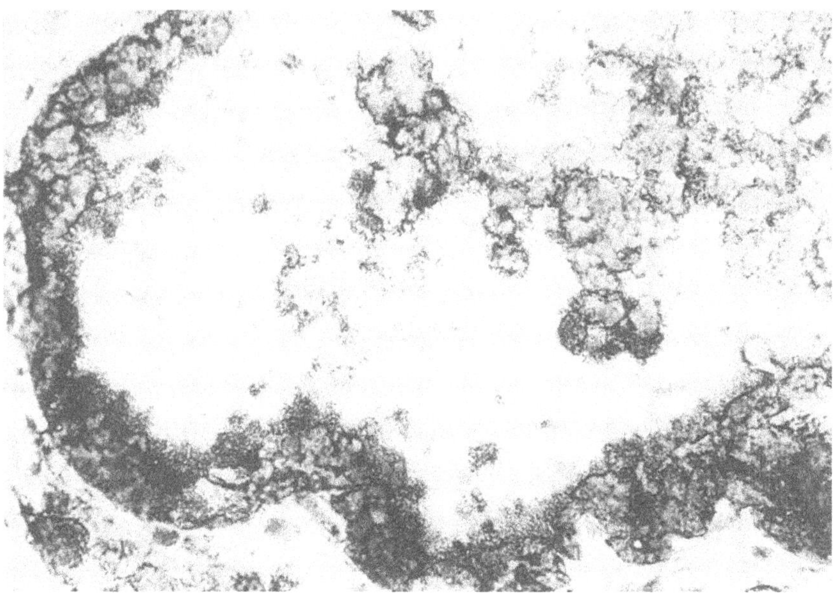

Figure 1. Cyst wall with marked staining of epithelial lining cells. Monoclonal antibody to cALLa, cryostate sections, modified PAP-method.

On careful microscopic examination (6) hyperplasia of epithelial cells covering the cyst wall is commonly observed with papillary proliferations projecting into the cystic cavities. Cytological abnormalities and microproliferates may be present even in parts of the kidney bearing no cysts (Figure 2). This observation is of potential importance for the histopathogenesis of renal tumor as discussed below.

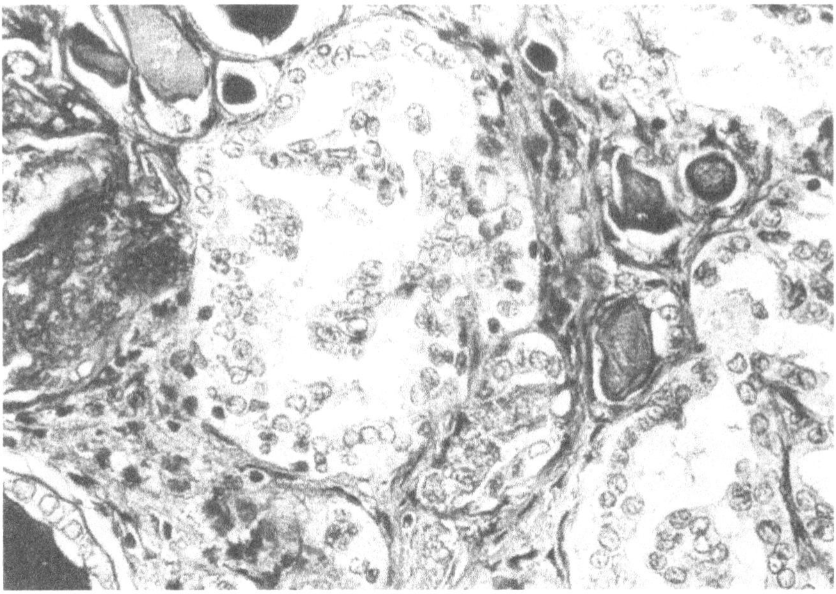

Fig 2. Papillary tubular epithelial cell hyperplasia (microadenoma) with clear cytoplasm. PAS.

CLINICAL PRESENTATION

In the majority of patients the course of ACKD is completely asymptomatic. However, in a minority of patients signs and symptoms arising from hemorrhagic complications such as *de novo* appearance of microhematuria, macrohematuric episodes, symptomatic bleeding into the cysts, perirenal hemorrhage or renal rupture are observed. To what extent this is favored by intermittent heparinization or the coagulation defect of uremia has not been established. In exceptional cases, patients may present with massive hemorrhage or shock and may require emergency nephrectomy or selective renal arterial embolization.

Infection and suppuration of cysts is not common, but has been observed by Ishikawa et al (37).

In general, no relation is found between the presence of cysts and hematocrit in dialysis patients (18, 25, 26). In some patients with advanced ACKD and in our experience particularly in patients with markedly enlarged kidneys (4) spontaneous reversal of anemia and even polyglobuly may occur.

Not infrequently, matrix stones consisting of ß2-microglobulin-derived amyloid (38) are noted in patients with ACKD. Whether this points to an obstructive origin of cysts (34) secondary to ß2-microglobulin derived microconcretions in the tubular lumen has not been clarified.

By far the most important clinical sequelae of ACKD are renal adenoma and renal cell carcinoma.

RENAL CELL CARCINOMA IN ACKD

Invasive renal cell carcinoma (RCC) was noted in the very first report by Dunnill et al (1) and later confirmed by Krempien and Ritz (2) and numerous other authors (for review see Ref 39). Common clinical presentations are macrohematuria, flank pain or renal mass. Renal mass may be either palpable or evident on imaging procedures, i.e. complex cysts on sonography or atypical masses on computed tomography or magnetic resonance tomography respectively. In some cases, metastases (40) or paraneoplastic features were presenting features at the time of diagnosis, e.g. tumor hypercalcemia (41), *de novo* hypertension (42), spontaneous reversal of anemia or even frank polyglobuly (43).

Upon morphological examination, circumscribed renal tumors are found in a high proportion of contracted cyst-bearing kidneys of patients with end stage renal failure on maintenance hemodialysis. Small tumors are conventionally designated as adenomas. In our experience, these are found in approximately 80% of dialysed patients. In an individual case the malignant potential of a given adenoma is uncertain, but the possibility of malignant growth is documented by observation of metastases.

Papillary proliferations are a common feature of renal cysts of varying etiologies including (benign) solitary cysts, polycystic kidney disease and other types of renal cysts. An increased prevalence of RCC has not been documented for any of the other conditions. In contrast, the whole spectrum of renal tumors from renal adenomas to invasive renal carcinoma is found in dialysis patients with ACKD, the two often coexisting in the same patient. Because of such coincidence, many authors concluded that renal adenoma is potentially malignant. The distinction of adenoma and RCC is usually based on size, but this distinction is clearly arbitrary. While tumors of less than 3 cm in diameter are commonly classified as adenoma, Evins et al (44) reviewed the evidence that exceptionally even tumors of less than 2 cm may metastasize.

On the basis of existing literature, it is very difficult to give a reasonable estimate of the prevalence of RCC in dialysed patients in general, i.e. with or without renal cysts. Most authors reported that clinical evidence of RCC is found in approximately 1-2% of the dialysis population. Several series in literature were undertaken to examine the overall prevalence of carcinoma in the dialysis population. In these series the prevalence of RCC was found to vary between 0.06% (45) and 4.2% (46), an average figure being approximately 0.5%. In dialysis patients the prevalence of renal tumors irrespective of size, i.e. smaller or larger than 3 cm, was given as 16.4% by Grantham et al (5), 8.9% by Waldherr et al (6), 9% by Bretan et al (47), and 19% by Gehrig et al (48). The prevalence of established RCC, i.e. > 3 cm in size, in dialysis patients with ACKD was given as 2.9% by Waldherr et al (6), 4-10% by Faber and Kupin (32) and 5.8% by Hughson et al (49). Of note is the common occurrence of bilateral tumors in patients with ACKD.

One of the largest series of RCC on record has been reported by Ishikawa (50). The author solicited information on 66,310 patients on hemodialysis by mailing a questionnaire. He identified 48 patients with RCC, 39% of whom had cysts and 21% of whom had metastases. These patients had a mean age of 50 years and a mean duration of hemodialysis of 84 months. From these figures, a prevalence of 10 cases per 100,000 patients per year was calculated which is approximately 2-4 times the expected prevalence in the general population. These figures are in good agreement with previous estimates of Ota et al (45). It is pertinent, however, to point to several biostatistical problems. Patients on maintenance hemodialysis with RCC are more likely to have macrohematuria or acute painful masses because of intermittent heparinisation. They also undergo more frequent sonographic routine examination so that the chance of detecting incidental renal carcinoma is definitely greater than in the general population.

It is also of note that incidental renal carcinoma is frequently found in patients subjected to pretransplant nephrectomy (51, 52). The remarkably low risk of late local recurrence of metastasis in these patients has been commented upon.

Renal cell carcinoma may be both of clear cell and granular cell types; more recently even spindle cell type RCC (53) has been found in dialysed patients.

The point of origin of invasive carcinoma may be the non-cystic portion of the kidney (6, 14); this finding is of note since cytological abnormalities, proliferative lesions and solid microadenoma are commonly noted even in non-cystic tubular segments of end stage kidneys (Figure 2). The observations of cytological abnormalities and papillary proliferations rasies the question whether these features (which are frequently found in end stage kidneys with cysts) must be considered as a premalignant condition. When examining epithelial cells of microadenomas in end stage kidneys, we found coexpression of the intermediate size filaments cytokeratin and vimentin (6). This is similar to the behaviour of most RCC's but unlike normal epithelial cells which commonly express only cytokeratin polypeptides. This may indicate dedifferentiation of proliferating epithelial cells in and stage kidneys. Deguchi et al (54) analysed by flow cytometry cells of RCC from dialysed patients and of patients with RCC and normal renal function. Diploid or near diploid cells were found in dialysed patients with RCC, whereas aneuploidy was common in non-uremic patients with RCC.

PATIENT MANAGEMENT

There is consensus that patients with and stage renal disease should be subjected to renal imaging procedures at regular intervals (5). Renal imaging is obligatory in the patient who has gross hematuria or *de novo* microhematuria. In agreement with previous recommendations (5), we propose to subject the patient on dialysis to annual imaging by renal sonography. Computed tomography and magnetic resonance tomography are alternative procedures. The role of fine needle aspiration analysis remains to be proven. It is of note that the results of computed tomography and sonography do not closely correlate (25, 27), so that both procedures should be used in doubtful cases. Several patients were reported in whom enlargement of lymphnodes was demonstrated by computed tomography despite no identifiable renal tumor, presumably because the latter had escaped detection in the severely deformed kidneys (40). All complex cysts or solid masses must be considered as renal tumors unless proven otherwise.

If the patient is found to have RCC, is tumor nephrectomy still worthwhile? Our own experience, reported elsewhere (42), has been encouraging: several patients survived up to 7 years post-nephrectomy and, in an individual patient, even surgical resection of a solitary pulmonary metastasis was survived for several years.

The patient who is found to have incidental RCC on pretransplant nephrectomy should not be disqualified from transplantation. Incidental RCC on pretransplant nephrectomy is found in up to 5% of patients; the remarkably low rate of local recurrence of distant metastasis has been commented upon (52). One should wait, however, two years before transplantation is performed, since most metastases occur in the first two years after tumor nephrectomy (55).

REFERENCES

1. Dunnill MS, Millard PR, Oliver D: Acquired cystic disease of the kidneys: a hazard of long term intermittent maintenance haemodialysis. J Clin Pathol, 30: 868-877, 1977.
2. Krempien B, Ritz E: Acquired cystic transformation of the kidneys of haemodialysed patients. Virchows Arch A Path Anat and Histol, 386: 189-200, 1980.
3. Bommer J, Waldherr R, Van Kaick G, Strauss I, Ritz E: Acquired renal cysts in uremic patients - *in vivo* demonstration by computed tomography. Clin Nephrol, 14: 299-303. 1980.
4. Mickisch O, Bommer J, Bachmann S, Waldherr R, Mann JFE, Ritz E: Multicystic transformation of kidneys in chronic renal failure. Nephron, 38; 93-99, 1984.
5. Grantham JJ, Levine E: Acquired Cystic Disease: Replacing one kidney disease with another. Kidney Int, 28: 99-105, 1985.
6. Waldherr R, Mickisch O, Bommer J, Ritz E: Clinical expression and impact of acquired cysts in progressive renal diseases. In: Proceedings of the Xth International Congress of Nephrology, AM Davidson (Ed), Bailliere Tindall, 1988, pp 1126-1137.
7. Wepfer JJ: Observationes medico-practicae, de affectibus capitis internis et externis. Scaphusii, Joh. Adam Ziegler, 1727.
8. Frerichs FT: Die Bright'sche Nierenkrankheit. Vieweg Verlag, Braunsschweig, 1851, pp 38.
9. Bell ET: Cystic disease of the kidneys. Am J Path, 11: 373-418, 1935.
10. Bommer J, Ritz E, Waldherr R, Mion C, Slingeneyer A: Acquired multicystic transformation of kidneys. Contr Nephrol, 48: 189-195, 1985.
11. Elliot HL, MacDougall AI, Buchanan WM: Acquired Cystic Disease of kidney. Lancet, ii: 1359, 1977.
12. Bansal WK, Ing TS, Daugirdas JT, Chejfec G, Gandhi VC, Geis WP, Hano JE: Cystic change in the kidneys of maintenance hemodialysis patients. Am Soc Artif Intern Organs J, 3: 65-68, 1980.
13. Hughson MD, Hennigar GR, McManus JFA: Atypical cysts, acquired renal cystic disease, and renal cell tumors in end stage dialysis kidneys. Lab Invest, 42: 475-480, 1980.
14. Fayemi AO, Ali M: Acquired renal cysts and tumors superimposed on chronic primary kidney diseases. An autopsy study of 24 patients. Path Res Pract, 168: 73-83, 1980.
15. Mirahmadi MK, Vaziri ND: Cystic transformation of end-stage kidneys in patients undergoing hemodialysis. Int J of Artif Organs, 3: 267-270, 1980.
16. Feiner DH, Katz LA, Gallo GR: Acquired cystic disease of kidney in chronic dialysis patients. Urology, 17: 260-264, 1981.
17. Turani H, Levi J, Zevin D, Kessler E: Acquired cystic disease and tumors in kidneys of hemodialysis patients. Isr J Med Sci, 19: 614-618, 1983.
18. Vaziri ND, Darwish R, Martin DC, Hostetler J: Acquired renal cystic disease in renal transplant recipients. Nephron, 37: 203-205, 1984.
19. Katz A, Sombolos K, Oreopoulos DG: Acquired cystic disease of the kidney in association with chronic ambulatory peritoneal dialysis. Am J Kidney Dis, 9: 426-429, 1987.
20. Ishikawa I, Onouchi Z, Saito Y, Tateishi K, Shinoda A, Suzuki S, Kitada H, Sugishita N, Fukuda Y: Sex differences in acquired cystic disease of the kidney on long-term dialysis. Nephron, 39: 336-340, 1985.
21. Ishikawa I, Saito Y, Onouchi Z, Kitada H, Suzuki S, Kurihara S, Yuri T, Shinoda A: Development of acquired cystic disease and adenocarcinoma of the kidney in glomerulonephritic chronic hemodialysis patients. Clin Nephrol, 14: 1-6, 1980.
22. Goldsmith HL, Ahmad R, Raichura N, Lal SM, McConnel CA, Gould DA, Gyde OHB, Green J: Association between rising haemoglobin concentration and renal cyst formation in patients on long term regular haemodialysis treatment. Proc EDTA, 19: 313-318, 1982.
23. Minar E, Tscholakoff D, Zazgornik J, Schmidt P, Marosi L, Czembirek H: Acquired cystic disease of the kidneys in chronic hemodialyzed and renal transplant patients. Eur Urol, 10: 245-248, 1984.
24. Levine E, Grantham JJ, Slusher SL, Greathouse JL, Krohn B: CT of acquired cystis kidney disease and renal tumors in long term dialysis patients. Am J Radiol, 142: 125-131, 1984.
25. Narasimhan N, Golper TA, Wolfson M, Rahatzad M, Bennet WM: Clinical characteristics and diagnostic considerations in acquired renal cystic disease. Kidney Int, 30: 748-752, 1986.
26. Thomson BJ, Jenkins DAS, Allan PL, Elton RA, Winney RJ: Acquired cystic disease of the kidney in patients with end-stage chronic renal failure: a study of prevalence and aetiology. Nephrol Dial Transplant, 1: 38-43, 1986.

27. Jabour BA, Ralls PW, Tang WW, Boswell WD Jr, Colletti PM, Feinstein EI, Massry SG: Acquired cystic disease of the kidneys. Computed tomography and ultrasonography appraisal in patients on peritoneal and hemodialysis. Invest Radiol, 22: 728-732, 1987.
28. Smith JW, Sallman AL, Williamson MR, Lott CG: Acquired renal cystic disease: two cases of associated adenocarcinoma and a renal ultrasound survey of a peritoneal dialysis population. Am J Kidney Dis, 10: 41-46, 1987.
29. Leichter HE, Dietrich R, Salusky IB, Foley J, Cohen AH, Kangarloo H, Fine RN: Acquired cystic kidney disease in children undergoing long-term dialysis. Pediatr Nephrol, 2: 8-11, 1988.
30. Ishikawa I, Yuri T, Kitada H, Sinoda A: Regression of acquired cystic disease of the kidney after successful renal transplantation. Am J Nephrol, 3: 310-314, 1983.
31. Arias M, de Francisco ALM, Ruiz L, Val F, Gonzalez M, Zubimendi A: Acquired renal cystic disease and renal adenocarcinoma in a long term renal transplant patient. Int J of Artif Organs, 9: 271-272, 1986.
32. Faber M, Kupin W: Renal cell carcinoma and acquired cystic kidney disease after renal transplantation. Lancet, i: 1030-1031, 1987.
33. Ishikawa I. Unusual composition of cyst fluid in acquired cystic disease of the end-stage kidney. Nephron, 41: 373-374, 1985.
34. Bommer J, Waldherr R, Ritz E: Kidney lesion in uraemic patients and ß2-microglobulin derived amyloid (Letter). Lancet, ii: 1437-1438, 1985.
35. Ishikawa I: ß2-Microglobulin level of cyst fluid in uremic acquired cystic disease of the kidney. Nephron, 44: 381, 1986.
36. Ono K, Yasukohchi A, Kikawa K: Pathogenesis of acquired renal cysts in hemodialysis patients. The role of oxalate crystal deposition in renal tubules. ASAIO Trans, 33: 245-249, 1987.
37. Ishikawa I: Uremic Acquired cystic disease of kidney. Urology, 26: 101-108, 1985.
38. Linke RP, Bommer J, Ritz E, Waldherr R, Eulitz M: Amyloid kidney stones of uremic patients consist of ß2-microglobulin fragments. Biochem Biophys Res Commun, 136: 665-671, 1987.
39. Noronha IL, Ritz E, Waldherr R, Stein G, Fassbinder W: Renal cell carcinoma in dialysis patients with acquired cystic kidney disease. Nephrol Dial Transplant, 1989 (in press).
40. Siegel SC, Sandler MA, Alpern MB, Pearlberg JL: CT of renal cell carcinoma in patients on chronic hemodialysis. Am J Radiol, 150: 583-585, 1988.
41. Thomson BJ, Allan PL, Winney R: Acquired cystic disease of kidney: metastatic renal adenocarcinoma and hypercalcaemia. Lancet, i: 502-503, 1985.
42. Fassbinder W, Hanke P, Møhring K, Klingbeil A, Ritz E: Der nierenfunktionslose Patient mit Hypernephrom: Grenzen der Tumorchirurgie aus nephrologischer Sicht. In: "Das Nierenkarzinom", v. G. Staehler (Ed), Springer Verlag, Berlin, Heidelberg, 1988, pp 35-42.
43. Ratcliffe PJ, Dunnill MS, Oliver DO: Clinical Importance of acquired cystic disease of the kidney in patients undergoing dialysis. Br Med J, 287: 1855-1858, 1983.
44. Evins SC, Varner W: Renal adenoma: a misnomer. Urology, 13: 85-86, 1979.
45. Ota K, Yamashita N, Suzuki T, Agishi TZ: Malignant Tumours in dialysis patients: a nationwide survey. Proc EDTA, 18: 724-730, 1981.
46. Miach PJ, Dawborn JK, Xipell J: Neoplasia in patients with chronic renal failure on long-term dialysis. Clin Nephrol, 5: 101-104, 1976.
47. Bretan PN, Busch MP, Hricak H, Williams RD: Chronic renal failure: a significant risk factor in the development of acquired renal cysts and renal cell carcinoma. Cancer, 57: 1871-1879, 1986.
48. Gehrig JJ, Gottheiner TI, Swenson R: Acquired cystic disease of the end-stage kidney. Am J Med, 79: 609-620, 1985.
49. Hughson MD, Buckwald D, Fox M: Renal neoplasia and acquired cystic kidney disease in patients receiving long-term dialysis. Arch Pathol Lab Med, 110: 592-601, 1986.
50. Ishikawa I: Adenocarcinoma of the kidney in chronic hemodialysis patients. Int J of Artif Organs, 11: 61-62, 1988.
51. Penn I: Transplantation in patients with primary renal malignancies. Transplantation, 24: 424-434, 1977.
52. Spees EK, Light JA, Smith EJ, Mostofi FK, Oakes DD: Transplantation in patients with a history of renal cell carcinoma: long-term results and clinical considerations. Surgery, 91: 282-287, 1982.
53. Fujimoto S, Sumiyoshi A, Yamamoto Y, Tanaka K: Renal cell carcinoma associated with acquired renal cystic disease. Int Urol Nephrol,20: 347-352, 1988.

54. Deguchi N, Tachibana M, Hata M, Tazaki H: Flow cytometry DNA analysis of neoplastic factors in the kidney of patients on hemodialysis, Xth Int Congr Nephrol. London, 26-31 July 1987, pp 498A.
55. Penn I: Renal transplantation in patients with preexisting malignancies. Transplant Proc, 15: 1079-1082, 1983.

RENAL TRANSPLANTATION

14

FINE NEEDLE ASPIRATION BIOPSY IN CLINICAL RENAL TRANSPLANTATION

GABRIEL M. DANOVITCH, CYNTHIA C. NAST AND ALAN WILKINSON

Departments of Medicine and Pathology, UCLA School of Medicine, Los Angeles, CA 90024-1689, USA

INTRODUCTION

Fine needle aspiration biopsy (FNAB) is a new technique which is being applied with increasing frequency as a clinical and investigational tool in kidney transplantation. FNAB is a means of sampling cells from the interstitium of the renal cortex in order to analyze the nature of inflammatory and toxic events occurring within the organ (1). The technique is a utilization of our increased understanding of the sequential intragraft events that occur in the rejecting allograft (2-5). FNAB owes its introduction into clinical transplantation to the work of Häyry and Von Willebrand (1, 3-6), who adapted the technique first described for renal transplants by Pasternak (7). Though it is clearly a valuable new adjunct in the diagnostic armamentarium of the transplant physician, its final place in transplant management is yet to be finally determined.

FNAB is proving to be a valuable investigational tool in transplant biology allowing sequential study and characterization of the cells infiltrating the graft by cell culture and monoclonal antibody techniques. We will discuss the technical, cytological, clinical and investigational aspects of this procedure.

TECHNIQUE

I. Clinical Procedure

The aspiration biopsy technique that is universally used is that described by Häyry and Von Willebrand (3-5). It requires no local anesthesia or prior assessment of coagulation parameters. The patient is placed supine, rotated contralateral to the allograft, with the contralateral leg bent and the ipsilateral leg straight. This position serves to make the kidney more prominent and to reduce the possibility of entering bowel. After sterile preparation the allograft is entered with a 25 gauge spinal needle with a transparent hub. The trochar is removed and the needle attached to a 10 ml plastic syringe filled with 4 ml of cold tissue culture medium (Hepes-buffered RPM1 1640 supplemented with albumin and heparin) which is fitted into an aspirator gun (Comeco, Inc., Sweden). The gun is required to provide suction to the spinal needle which is then twisted two or three times through 180° and rapidly removed. In a successful aspiration, a 10-20 μl serous specimen can often be seen in the hub of the needle, though the aspirate may be within the bore of the needle and not be visible. The specimen is then expressed through the needle into a tissue culture tube and the hub washed several times with tissue culture medium through the needle. The procedure is usually repeated and bloody specimens are discarded. The cells are then resuspended in media. A blood specimen is obtained from a finger stick and placed in approximately 2 ml of the same medium. The specimens may be processed immediately or refrigerated for up to 24 hrs.

The procedure is typically not more painful than a venipuncture. Microscopic hematuria may occur. We have observed no macroscopic hematuria or significant complications in several hundred biopsies. The patients may ambulate imme-diately after completion of the procedure.

II. Cytological Procedure

The aspirate and peripheral blood specimens are processed by the method of Häyry and Von Willebrand (6, 8, 9). The specimens are kept at 4°C until processing, which must be done within 24 hours to avoid excessive degeneration of the cells. The aspirate and peripheral blood samples are handled in the same fashion. The cells are centrifuged at 1500 rpm for ten minutes, and the supernatant is decanted and discarded. A cytocentrifuge is loaded with microscopic slides and 3 or 4 drops of the cell suspension are added to the centrifuge cups. The cells are cytocentrifuged onto the slides at 500 rpm for ten minutes. The cytospin preparations are air-dried then stained with May-Grunwald-Giemsa for interpretation. Additional cytospin slides may be made and retained for other staining procedures by storing in a dessicator.

III. Scoring

The aspirate and peripheral blood cytospin preparations are assessed quantitatively and qualitatively for their leukocytic components (6, 8). Aspirates are additionally evaluated for parenchymal cells including tubular epithelium and endothelial cells, as well as glomeruli. The aspirate is initially screened at low magnification to estimate the degree of cellularity.

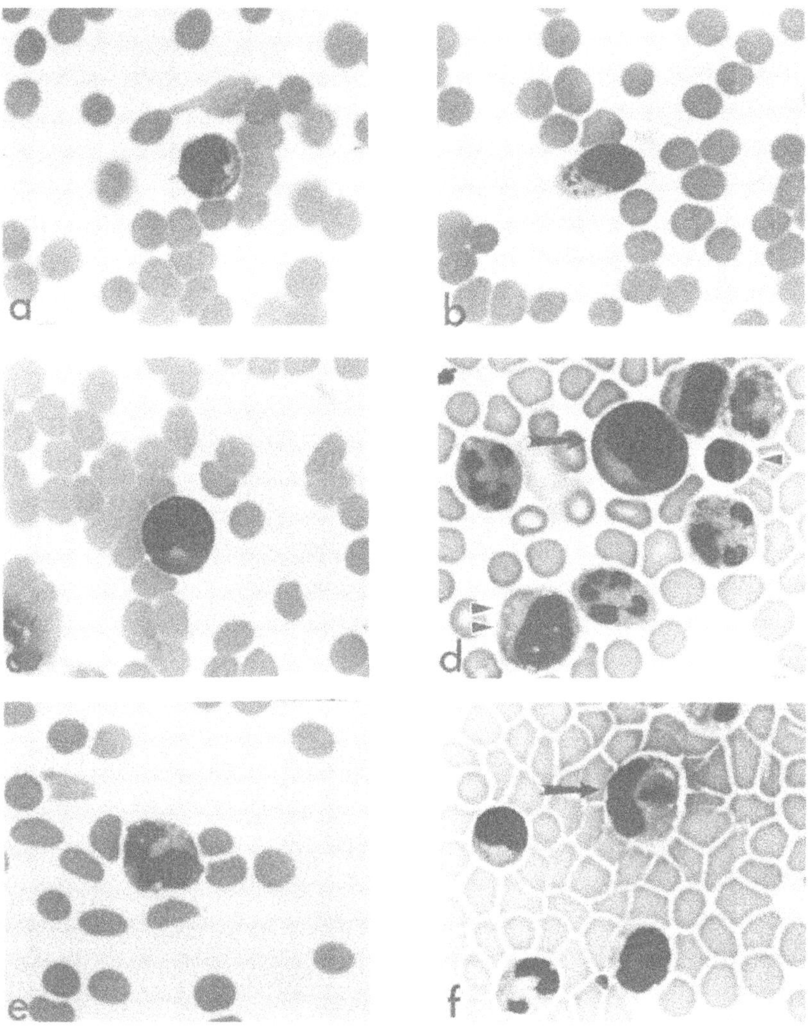

Figure 1 Leukocytes from renal allograft fine needle aspiration biopsies. (a) Lymphocyte. (b) Large granular lymphocyte containing cytoplasmic granules. (c) Activated lymphocyte. The cell is enlarged with immature nuclear chromatin. (d) Immunoblast (arrow) with abundant cytoplasm and prominent nucleoli. Note smaller adjacent normal lymphocyte (arrowhead) and activated lymphocyte (double arrowhead). (e) Monocyte. (f) Macro-phage (arrow) containing ingested material.

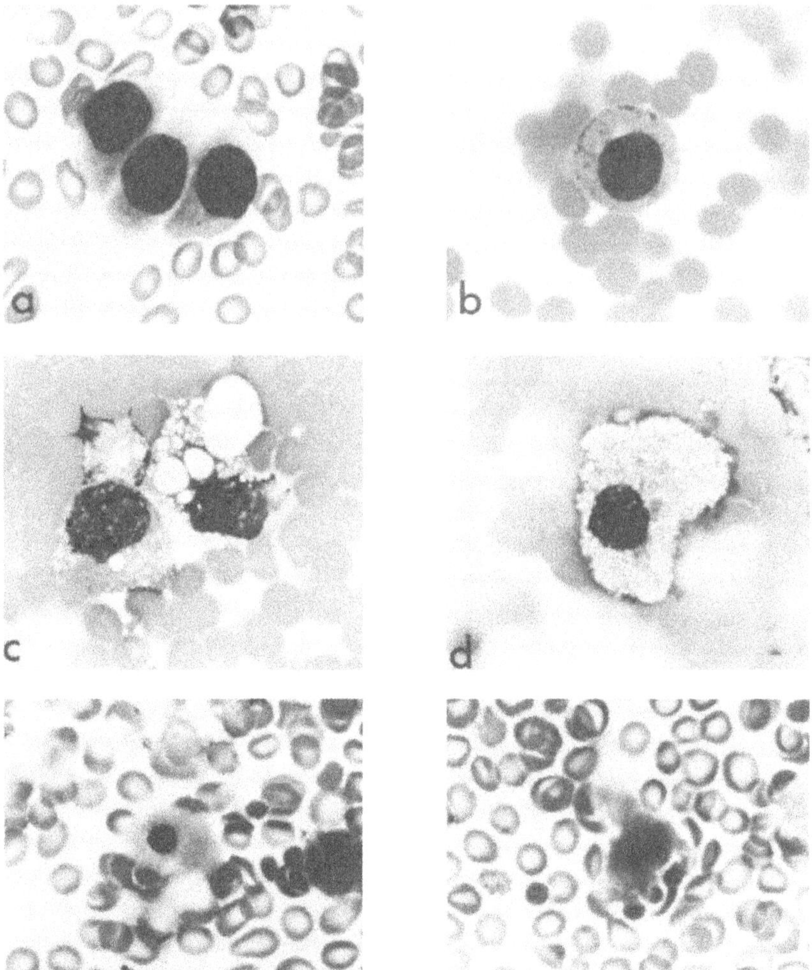

Figure 2 Parenchymal cells from renal transplant fine needle aspiration biopsies. (a) Normal tubular cells. (b) Endothelial cell containing cyto-plasmic granules. (c) Swollen tubular cells, one with irregular cyto-plasmic vacuoles. (d) Tubular cell containing cytoplasmic isometric vacuoles. (e) Degenerated tubular cell with pyknotic nucleus. (f) Necrotic tubular cell. The cytoplasmic borders are indistinct and nucleus is disintegrated.

The entire aspirate cytospin is then examined at high magnification (40x) and the total number of immunoblasts is determined, including both T and B cell immunoblasts. A 100-cell differential leukocyte count is then done separately on the aspirate and peripheral blood specimens. The peripheral blood count is subtracted from that of the aspirate, and the resulting increments multiplied by correction factors which reflect the association of that cell type with acute rejection (6, 8-10). Cell types examined and their correction factors include immunoblasts, plasma cells, and macrophages (1.0); activated lymphocytes (0.5); large granular lymphocytes and monocytes (0.2); lymphocytes, neutrophils, eosinophils and basophils (0.1) (Figure 1). Immunoblasts counted in the peripheral blood sample are added to, rather than subtracted from, those in the aspirate before correction since they are presumed to represent "spill-over" from the allograft infiltrate. The individual corrected increments are added, giving the final total corrected increment score (TCI).

Parenchymal cells are evaluated both for quantity and morphology. The number of tubular and endothelial cells are used to determine the adequacy of the aspirate; seven or more parenchymal cells per 100 leukocytes is the minimum required for an adequate sample (6, 11, 12). Clusters of three to five or more tubular cells are often counted as only two cells (11) as they likely represent epithelium from the same tubule. The presence of glomeruli ensures that a cortical aspiration was obtained. Morphologic evaluation of the parenchymal cells is done while the aspirate is screened for immunoblasts at high magnification. Tubular cell findings include normal morphology, swelling, cytoplasmic vacuolization which may be irregular or isometric, erythrophagocytosis, degeneration and necrosis, in order of increasing injury (Figure 2). Endothelial cells may be swollen or contain cytoplasmic vacuoles when damaged (Figure 2).

INTERPRETATION

Fine needle aspiration can be used to diagnose a variety of abnormalities which may be associated with renal transplant dysfunction. The FNAB findings generally fall into one of two categories; abnormal leukocytic infiltrates or alterations of parenchymal cells (6, 8) (Figure 3). Immunologic events affecting the allograft result in an alteration of the white cell infiltrates within the kidney, so called "immune activation". Immune activation is assessed using the TCI and total number of immunoblasts in the cytospin preparation (6, 9, 11). Absolute numbers vary among laboratories, but generally immune activation is defined as a total corrected increment of greater than 3.0 and/or more than three to four immunoblasts (10, 13, 14). Immune activation is most frequently due to acute rejection or viral infection. Tubular cell injury of varying degrees is the hallmark of acute tubular necrosis and cyclosporine toxicity. Bacterial infection may occasionally be recognized.

Acute transplant rejection may be diagnosed utilizing FNAB by evaluation of the degree of intragraft immune activation. The recognition of activation correlates with inflammatory infiltrates seen in renal biopsies (6, 10, 11). With severe rejection, the inflammatory infiltrate is more intense and the total corrected increment may be markedly elevated. Necrotic tubular cells and macrophages are additional findings in severe or irreversible rejection (6, 15, 16). Severe rejection may also be accompanied by immunoblasts within the peripheral blood, a "spill-over" phenomenon from the activated allograft infiltrate. The response to anti-rejection therapy can be followed by FNAB; increasing tubular cell degeneration and necrosis, macrophage infiltrates, and sustained immune activation represent persistent and worsening cellular rejection (8, 15). A decrease in the total corrected increment, absence of immunoblasts and improvement in tubular cell profile typically imply resolution of the rejection episode (6, 13).

Viral infections which may interfere with allograft function are often associated with immune activation on FNAB (6, 17, 18). An increase in both T and B cell immunoblasts and activated lymphocytes may be observed in aspirates performed during viral infections to a greater degree than during acute rejection although the graft infiltration by lymphocytes and monocytes is no different (18). The number and size of large granular lympho-cytes (natural killer cells) are elevated in both aspirate and peripheral blood specimens when there is a viral syndrome. In contrast, peripheral blood large granular lymphocytes are minimally increased in acute rejection (17). Viral infections which may produce these findings include Cytomegalovirus, Herpes simplex and Varicella zoster. *In situ* hybridization using cDNA probes against Cytomegalovirus, Herpes simplex and Epstein Barr virus have identified viral genome in renal tubular cells, even in the absence of rising serological titers and clinical symptoms (19). Viral identification in aspirate material appears to be a definitive way of diagnosing renal parenchymal infection, and a technique uniquely suited to FNAB specimens.

Acute tubular necrosis is a parenchymal cell lesion which can be diagnosed relatively easily by FNAB. Tubular cells in all phases of injury, from swelling and vacuolization to degeneration and necrosis, are evident (6, 8).

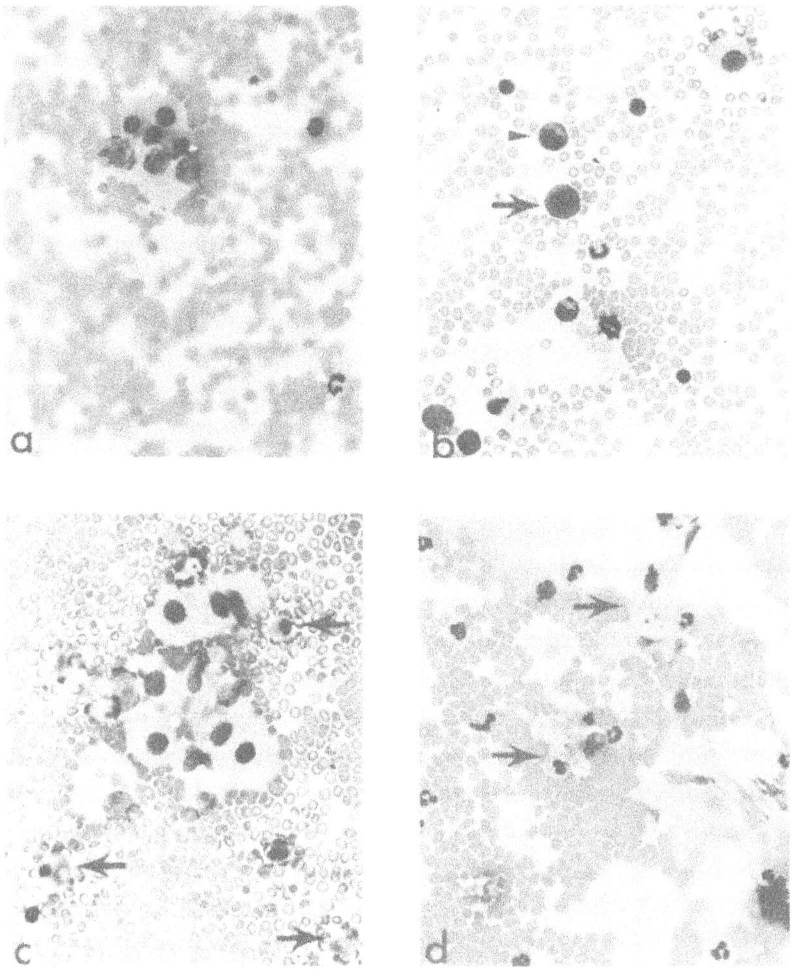

Figure 3 Renal allograft fine needle aspiration biopsies from patients with various diagnoses. (a) Quiescent graft. There are normal tubular cells with few leukocytes. (b) Acute rejection. There is increased inflammation including immunoblastic (arrow), activated lymphocytic (arrow head), and lymphocytic cells. (c) Acute tubular necrosis. There are numerous degen-erated tubular cells (arrows) without an inflammatory cell increase. (d) Acute cyclosporine nephrotoxicity. Tubular cells contain isometric vacu-oles (arrows).

Immune activation is absent, and no immunoblasts are seen in the peripheral blood. The severity of the epithelial cell injury correlates to some extent with the clinical course (20). With recovery, mitotic figures are frequently seen within the aspirate material and tubular cell findings tend to become less severe, although there is marked variability (21). At resolution, only mild swelling and rare irregular vacuolization are observed.

Acute cyclosporine toxicity is an entity frequently assessed by FNAB. Several findings have been suggested as diagnostic markers for cyclosporine toxicity. Fine isometric cytoplasmic vacuolization of tubular and occasionally endothelial cells is considered a hallmark of toxicity (16, 22, 23). This often occurs with considerable tubular cell injury exhibited as erythro-phagocytosis and degeneration (16, 20, 23). Deposits of cyclo-sporine have also been identified within tubular cells by indirect immunofluorescence in aspirates from patients with toxicity (24). After cyclosporine levels decreased the deposits could no longer be found. An isolated elevation in the graft differential lympho-cyte count in the absence of an immunoblast response has also been reported in patients receiving cyclosporine (16), and has been suggested to be a manifestation of cyclosporine toxicity (25, 26). Pitfalls in the diagnosis of acute cyclosporine toxicity exist. Early in the post-operative period, severe post-ischemic tubular cell injury may mask the morphologic evidence of cyclosporine toxicity (20). Serial FNAB may allow differentiation; isometric vacuolization with continued tubular cell damage will be observed in cyclosporine toxic patients while resolution of the cellular inju-ry will be seen in 'ATN'.

Bacterial infection can be diagnosed both by the quality of the cellular infiltrate and by identification of the infecting organism. With the exclusion of aspirates in the very early post-transplant period (16), an increase in neutrophils in the graft relative to the peripheral blood is suggestive of a bacterial infection. Definitive diagnosis can be made when there are intra- and extracellular bacteria present (27, 28). Both gram positive and gram negative bacteria have been observed in FNAB from patients with graft infections, as the Giemsa portion of the May-Grunwald-Giemsa stain will stain most bacteria. The FNAB can also be cultured for definitive bacterial identification (28) as it is obtained in a sterile fashion.

FNAB is a useful technique for interpretation of the above noted allograft abnormalities. There are, however, several entities which cannot be diagnosed by aspiration. Hemorrhage and hema-toma formation cannot be differentiated from blood contami-nation of the aspirate. Vascular rejection will not be recognized, as the cell types are no different from those in cellular rejection and their presence in vascular walls cannot be identified. Thrombosis, obstruction, and graft rupture do not result in changes identifiable by aspiration. Finally chronic alterations, whether due to chronic rejection or cyclosporine toxicity, will usually result in an inade-quate FNAB due to fibrosis without specific aspirate abnormali-ties.

Comparison of FNAB and Core Biopsy

Several studies have been performed comparing the diagnostic accuracy of FNAB to that of traditional biopsy and there has been a remarkable similarity in the degree of concordance that has been reported. The percentage of aspirations that have provided inadequate material for analyses has been reported to vary between 15 - 30% (29-32) and is determined somewhat by the experience of the individual performing the procedure. Such an occurrence is less frequent in core biopsies where it probably occurs in less than 5% of the samples. Most reports have found that acute blastogenic episodes recognized by FNAB correlate with cellular rejection diagnosed by standard histologic criteria. A high frequency of isometric vacuolization of tubular and endothelial cells correlates with similar changes in histological specimens while degenerated and necrotic tubular cells on FNAB correlate with the histologic finding of tubular necrosis. In our experience, FNAB was somewhat more effective at ruling out acute rejection than it was in ruling in rejection (31). More than 90% of episodes of graft dysfunction diagnosed histologically as 'ATN' or cyclo-sporine toxicity showed no evidence of immune activation whereas activation was present in 78% of biopsy proven rejection episodes. Koller et al (32) described 87% concordance between FNAB and core biopsy and emphasized, as have others, that repetitive FNAB allows for observation of the changing degree of immune activation, hence adding a chronologic advantage to the procedure compared to static information from a single core biopsy. Helderman et al (29) compared clinical diagnosis to aspiration diagnosis in normal and dysfunctional grafts and found that aspiration diagnosis was more than 90% sensitive and specific. Egidi et al (22) described an 85% concordance between core biopsy and FNAB. Whelchel et al (33), however, found that FNAB was only 50-60% sensitive for acute rejection and concluded that it was not diagnostically helpful or cost efficient. Much depends on the experience of the pathologist reading the specimens and the clinical circumstances in which the procedure is performed. Immunostaining for HLA-DR antigens may improve the diagnostic accuracy of FNAB (30), but this technique is not yet routinely employed for clinical transplantation. Attempts at correlating severity of rejection by core biopsy and FNAB have had variable success (34, 35) and we prefer to avoid grading rejection severity by either technique.

There are several potential reasons for discrepancy between the two procedures (Table 1). FNAB samples may be of medullary rather than of cortical origin and thus may appear inactive in the presence of cortical inflammation. The presence of tubular cell clusters may be a marker of a medullary sample and hence allow recognition of this source of error, though this finding is yet to be universally accepted (36). The serendipitous finding of an aspirated glomerulus also confirms the cortical origin of the sample. In the presence of vascular rejection, a typical blastogenic response may not be seen and the inability of FNAB to reliably diagnose humoral rejection is a recognized disadvantage of the technique which should be borne in mind when clinical and aspiration findings are divergent. Recurrence of original disease in the graft and chronic rejection are typically not recognizable by FNAB, and experience with the use of FNAB in the late transplant course is limited (37). Evidence of immune activation by FNAB in the absence of histological evidence of acute rejection is a less frequent finding that may be induced by CMV infection (22, 38), hence producing a potentially confusing clinical picture.

Table 1. Potential causes of discrepancy between FNAB and clinical and core biopsy diagnosis.

Aspiration of medullary sample
Focal pattern of immune infiltrate
Vascular rejection
Misreading of borderline samples
Recurrence of original disease
Cyclosporine induced lymphocytosis
Viral-induced lymphocytosis
Aspiration at site of previous core biopsy
Erroneous clinical or biopsy diagnosis
'Spontaneous' resolution of rejection

Clinical Use of FNAB

In clinical transplantation FNAB helps fill a diagnostic void in the differential diagnosis of acute rejection, cyclosporine toxicity and tubular necrosis. In the cyclosporine era the clinical differentiation of these syndromes may be difficult. Clinicians may use non-invasive yet poorly specific techniques such as ultrasound, magnetic resonance imaging and isotope scanning, or core biopsy which is accurate yet invasive and not suitable for frequent repetition.

The absence of complete parallelism between FNAB and core biopsy together with qualitative differences in the information obtained prevents FNAB from replacing core biopsy in clinical transplantation. Rather than being regarded as competing procedures they should be used in a complementary fashion in clinical management. FNAB is most useful in the early transplant course when lesions such as chronic rejection and recurrent nephropathy are typically not relevant. Repeated FNABs during the post transplant period may confirm clinically diagnosed ATN with or without cyclosporine toxicity or suggest development of clinically covert rejection. FNAB during early episodes of graft dysfunction may be valuable in the differentiation of cyclosporine toxicity from acute rejection, without need to resort to renal biopsy. Occasional cases of pyelonephritis have been diagnosed by finding polymorphs and bacteria in the aspirate (27, 28). Immunohistochemical staining for early and late CMV antigens may be a valuable and rapid way to recognize CMV disease. We perform FNAB in all cases where CMV is suspected and the confirmation of the diagnosis may have a critical impact on the management of immunosuppression.

The morphologic picture observed by FNAB may be markedly influenced by the immunosuppressive regimen that is employed (38). The cyclosporine associated changes in graft parenchymal cells noted above may be partially overcome by high dose steroids (39). Patients not receiving cyclosporine may have higher levels of T- cell immunoblasts during rejection episodes, reflecting the more specific nature of cyclosporine immunosuppression. Sequential FNABs have shown that the first episode of immune activation occurs significantly earlier in patients who are immunosuppressed with cyclosporine alone. Comparative analysis of aspirates should thus take into account the immunosuppressive regimen that is being used. Analysis of aspirates provides justification for the combined immunosuppressive drug regimens that are now typically employed in clinical transplantation.

FNAB as a Research Tool

Fine needle aspiration is a useful method for the investigation of cell types and markers in immunologic responses to transplantation. The subsets of cells infiltrating renal allografts in various clinical settings can be ascertained utilizing monoclonal antibodies against specific cell markers (6, 30, 39, 40). Flow cytometry can be utilized in assessing aspirates for more complete evaluation of the relative numbers of cells involved in rejection episodes, such as CD4, CD8 and subsets of these cell types (41). Comparison of aspirate and peripheral blood infiltrates may also help establish cellular reactions in rejection and other immunologic events. Aspirate material may be used for the evaluation of gene expression on cells in rejection and other conditions. The degree of expression of class II HLA antigens, production of interleukins and presence of interleukin and other receptors can be assessed and compared to concomitant clinical events (41, 42). Cells obtained in fine needle aspiration may also be cultured, with phenotypic and functional assays utilized to evaluate cellular response in rejection or cyclosporine toxicity (43, 44). Aspirated cells clearly provide a unique opportunity to view immunologic responses in allografts.

REFERENCES

1. Häyry P, Von Willebrand E, Ahonen T, Lautenschlager I and Neskinen R: Aspiration cytology in organ transplantation. Transpl Rev, 1: 133-157, 1977.
2. Strom TB, Tilney NL, Carpenter CB and Busch GJ: Identity and cytotoxic capacity of cells infiltrating renal allografts. New Engl J Med, 292: 1257-1263, 1975.
3. Von Willebrand E, Soots A and Häyry P: *In situ* effector mechanisms in rat kidney allograft rejection: I. Characterization of host cellular infiltrate in rejecting allograft parenchyma. Cell Immunol, 46: 309-326, 1979.
4. Häyry P, Von Willebrand E and Soots A: *In situ* effector mechanisms in rat kidney allograft rejection: III. Kinetics of the inflammation response and generation of donor-directed killer cells. Scand J Immunol, 10: 95-108, 1979.
5. Von Willebrand E and Häyry P: Composition and *in vitro* cytotoxicity of cellular infiltrates in rejecting human allografts. Cell Immunol, 41: 358-372, 1978.
6. Häyry P and Von Willebrand E: Transplant aspiration cytology. Transplantation, 38: 7-12, 1984.
7. Paternack A: Fine needle aspiration biopsy of human renal homografts. Lancet, ii: 82-84, 1968.
8. Von Willebrand E: Fine needle aspiration cytology of human renal transplants. Clin Immunol Immunopathol, 17: 309-322, 1980.
9. Häyry P and Von Willebrand E: Practical guidelines for fine needle aspiration biopsy of human renal allografts.Ann Clin Res, 13: 288-306, 1981.
10. Häyry P and Von Willebrand E: Monitoring of human renal allograft rejection with fine needle aspiration cytology. Scand J Immunol 13:87-97, 1981.
11. Belitsky P, Campbell J and Giopta R: Serial biopsy controlled evaluation of fine-needle aspiration in renal allograft rejection. Lab Invest, 53: 580-585, 1985.
12. Von Willebrand E, Zola H and Häyry P: Thombocyte aggregation in renal allografts. Transplantation, 39: 258-262, 1985.
13. Cooksey G, Reeve RS, Nicolopoulos N, Burden RP, Cotton RE and Blamey RW: Monitoring the response to treatment of renal allograft rejection with fine needle aspiration cytology. Trans Proc, 17: 2085-2086, 1985.
14. Tufveson G, Backman V, Claesson K, Frodin L, Stenquist B and Wahlberg J: Renal transplant cytology: impact of different immunosuppressive protocols and biopsy techniques. Trans Proc, 17: 2087-2088, 1985.
15. Häyry P and Von Willebrand E: Diagnostic evaluation of the in situ inflammatory response of renal allograft rejection. Proc EDTA, 17: 418-423, 1980.
16. Häyry P: Monitoring of renal allografts by transplant aspiration cytology. Triangle, 21: 111-120, 1982.
17. Nguyen L, Hammer C, Dendorfer U, Castro L, Schleibner C and Land W: Changes in large granular lymphocyte size and number in kidney transplant patients during rejection and viral infection. Trans Proc, 17: 2110-2111, 1985.
18. Ouziala M, Santelli G, Charpentier B and Fries D: Diagnostic value of fine needle aspiration biopsy during viral infections in renal transplant recipients. Trans Proc, 17: 2098-2099, 1985.
19. Arndt R, Heinzer P, Huland H, Lohning T and Kramer-Hansen H: Identification of virus DNA in kidney transplants by fine-needle aspiration biopsy. Trans Proc, 20: 581-583, 1988.
20. Stadler J, Heidecke C-D, Plorack G and Holscher M: Postischemic injury and acute tubular necrosis: diagnostic and prognostic value of fine-needle aspirates. Trans Proc, 20: 687-689, 1988.

21. Baumgartner D, Burger HR, Binswanger U and Largiader F: Routine fine needle aspiration biospy adds clinically relevant information for evaluation and treatment of renal transplant recipients with primary oliguria. Trans Proc, 17: 2080-2081, 1985.
22. Egidi F, Banfi G, Bogetic J, Passerini P and Ponticelli C: Correlation between fine needle aspiration biopsy and renal biopsy in renal transplantation. Trans Proc, 20: 592-594, 1988.
23. Yussim A, Shapira Z, Shmueli D, Heibronn YD, Kaufman L and Servaclio C: The impact of transplant aspiration cytology in management of cyclosporin-A treated renal transplant recipients. Trans Proc 19:1658, 1987.
24. Von Willebrand E and Häyry P: Cyclosporin-A deposits in renal allografts. Lancet, ii: 189-192, 1983.
25. Egidi F, Torantino A, DeVecchi A, Zubani R and Ponticelli C: Patterns of inflammation in fine needle aspiration biopsies in renal transplant patients treated with different immunosuppressive regimens. Trans Proc, 17: 2091-2092, 1985.
26. O'Brien JP, Horsburgh T, Veitch PS and Bell PRF: Experience with fine needle aspiration biopsies from renal transplant patients on different immunosuppressive regimens. Trans Proc, 17: 2089-2090, 1985.
27. Surackno S, Van Oers MHJ and Wilmink JM: Early diagnosis of bacterial infection of renal allografts by fine needle aspiration biopsy. Lancet, i: 686-687, 1986.
28. Hernandez JA, Glennie J, Toto R, Sagalowsky A, Davidsen I and Helderman JH: A novel use of fine-needle aspiration biopsy: documentation of acute pyelonephritis of the transplanted kidney. Trans Proc, 20: 632-634, 1988.
29. Helderman JH, Hernandez J, Sagalowsky A, Davidson I, Glennie J, Womble D and Toto RD: Confirmation of the utility of fine needle aspiration biopsy of the renal allograft. Kidney Int, 34: 376-381, 1988.
30. Bishop GA, Hall BM, Waugh J, Phillips T, Horuath JS, Duggin GG, Johnson JR, Ross-Sheil AG and Tiller DJ: Diagnosis of renal allograft rejection by analysis of fine needle aspiration biospy specimens with immunostains and simply cytology. Lancet, ii: 645-649, 1986.
31. Danovitch GM, Nast C, Rosenthal and Wilkinson A: Fine needle aspiration biopsy in the diagnosis renal transplant dysfunction. Am Soc Transpl Phys, 134: 65, 1988 (Abstract).
32. Koller C, Hammer C, Govew M, Land W, Hillerbrand D, Castro LA, Badier J and Weber B: Correlation between core biopsy and aspiration cytology. Trans Proc, 16: 1298-1300, 1984.
33. Whelchel JD, Delaney VB, O'Brien D, Ling B, Fekete P and Campbell WG: Efficacy and cost of the various tests used in the diagnosis of rejection in cadaveric renal transplant recipients. Kidney Int, 35: 526, 1989.
34. Boshkos C, Steinmuller DR, Nouick AC, Streem S, Cunningham PJ, Fishleder A and Dlugosa B: Correlation between fine needle aspiration biopsies with core biopsies after renal transplantation. Trans Proc, 20: 592-594, 1988.
35. Manalich R, LaGarde M, Wellar C and Jiminez P: Intrarenal inflammation during rejection crises in renal allografts: comparison between fine needle aspiration cytology and renal biopsy. Trans Proc, 20: 601-602, 1988.
36. Hammerer P, Arndt R, Krämer-Hansen H, Huland H and Khosterhalfen H: Consecutive selective aspiration cytology of renal cortex and renal medulla in kidney transplants. Trans Proc, 20: 577-578, 1988.
37. Yussim A, Kaufman L, Shmuely D and Shapira Z: Aspiration cytology in late cellular rejection. Trans Proc, 20: 621-622, 1988.
38. Häyry P, Von Willebrand E, Ahonen J, Eklund B, Calmela K, Hîckerstedt K, Peterson E and Koskinies S: Effects of cyclosporine, azathioprine, and steroids on the renal transplant, on the cytologic patterns of intragraft inflammation, and on the concomitant rejection associated changes in recipient blood. Trans Proc, 20: 153-162, 1988.
39. Taube D, Welsh K, Hobby P, Williams DG: Human renal allograft and peripheral blood T-lymphocyte subpopulations during the onset and treatment of rejection. Clin Nephrol, 22: 127-132, 1984.
40. Bolton EM, Thompson JF, Wood RFM, Morris PJ: Immunoperoxidase staining of fine-needle aspiration biopsies and needle core biopsies from renal allografts. Transplantation, 36: 728-730, 1983.
41. Fuggle SV, McWinnie DL and Morris PJ: Precise specificity of induced tubular HLA-class II antigens in renal allografts. Transplantation, 44: 214-220, 1987.
42. Helderman JH, Hernandez J, Glennie J and Womble D: The interleukin-2 receptor detected by fine needle aspiration specimens. Trans Proc, 20: 675-676, 1988.

43. McKenna RM, Heiman D, Rush DN and Jeffery JR: Limiting dilution analysis of the frequency of functional T cells in human renal allograft fine needle aspirates. Trans Proc, 20: 207-208, 1988.

44. Goldman M, Vandervorst P, Abramowicz D, Vereerstraeten P, Kinnaert P, Schandene L, Dupont E, Wybran J, Toussaint C: Interleukin-2 release assay in limiting dilution microcultures: possible application to fine needle aspiration of kidney transplants. Trans Proc, 17: 2117-2118, 1985.

DIAGNOSTIC METHODS IN NEPHROLOGY

15

CAN INTRAVENOUS UROGRAPHY BE REPLACED BY SONOGRAPHY?

ERNESTO TOMEI AND HEDVIG HRICAK

University of Rome, "La Sapienza", Italy and University of California School of Medicine, Department of Radiology, Box 0628, San Francisco, California 94143-0628, USA

INTRODUCTION

For the last four decades, intravenous urography (IVU) has been considered indispensable in evaluation of the urinary tract. Since the introduction of cross-sectional imaging modalities (diagnostic ultrasound [US] computed tomography [CT] and magnetic resonance imaging [MRI]), however, the role of IVU has changed (1), and the number of studies performed around the country is decreasing. Technical advances in radiology have improved diagnostic evaluation, facilitated interventional approaches for diagnosis and treatment, and refined the assessment of therapeutic results. In order to avoid duplication and efficiently achieve the best outcome with this vast array of imaging options, it is necessary to understand the advantages and limitations of each (2). This review provides a comparison of the use of IVU and US in nephrology, and discusses the optimal diagnostic choice in various clinical situations.

TECHNICAL NOTES AND ANATOMY

Intravenous Urogram

Intravenous urography (IVU) is an established technique which has undergone few changes in the last twenty years (3). It provides primarily morphologic information, although some functional information — limited to excretion — may also be realized. Cross-sectional anatomy is not displayed with IVU, and exposure to ionizing radiation and injection of iodine-containing contrast media are necessary.

Use of contrast media may produce minor reactions (nausea, vomiting, urticaria, itching and sneezing); moderate reactions (nephrotoxicity, congestive heart failure, pulmonary edema); and severe reactions (bronchospasm, anaphylaxis and even death). The reported mortality during excretory urography ranges from 1 in 17,000 to 1 in 14,000. The Mayo Clinic reported four deaths in a series of 300,000 consecutive urographies, or 1 in 75,000 (4). All four patients who died were 50 years or older, had a history of hypersensitivity, and a respiratory component to the reaction. Although the incidence of minor and moderate reactions to contrast media has been significantly reduced by the introduction of nonionic contrast media, reduction in the number of severe reactions has not been definitely established because at present the numbers are too low to draw conclusions (5).

The timing of the film sequence during IVU is governed by the rate of contrast injection (infusion versus bolus). With the bolus method, there is a higher plasma contrast media concentration providing an excellent nephrogram. Since a small volume of contrast media is injected, however, abdominal compression is needed for calyceal, pelvic and ureteral visualization. Although the infusion method results in a lower peak contrast media concentration, the average level is maintained over a longer period of time. Because a larger volume of contrast media is injected, there is calyceal distention and ureteral visualization is routinely present.

IVU is used to evaluate kidney size, shape, and orientation; the appearance and homogeneity of the nephrogram phase; symmetrical excretion; and the appearance of the calyces, pelvis and ureters. Although assessment of the urinary bladder by IVU is crude, it can be informative.

Diagnostic Ultrasound

Diagnostic ultrasound (US) is noninvasive, does not use ionizing radiation, and does not require the use of potentially nephrotoxic iodine contrast agents. Moreover, it provides multiplanar tissue display, is relatively inexpensive, and can be portable. US allows only morphologic assessment, however, and no functional information is obtained. Ultrasound is also an operator-dependent technique.

A number of established US scanning approaches to evaluate the kidneys have been described. The kidneys are routinely imaged in two planes (customarily the longitudinal and transverse) which are perpendicular to one another. The right kidney is best viewed in the parasagittal plane, using the liver as an acoustic window. Images of the left kidney require a more posteriorly-placed transducer (between the mid and posterior axillary line) in order to avoid the bowel gas of the left colon interposed between the kidney and abdominal surface. This approach results in a more coronal view of the left kidney, and the left renal cortex may appear thicker than the right. This discrepancy in cortical thickness should not be misinterpreted as cortical thinning or atrophy of the right kidney. The posterior oblique longitudinal scan is useful in studying the renal parenchyma and hilus in their vertical axes and is well suited to the evaluation of hydronephrosis.

Sonograms are routinely used to assess kidney size, cortical thickness, echogenicity, and corticomedullary differentiation. Renal echogenicity is a subjective visual assessment and should be evaluated in comparison with the echogenicity of the liver on the right and the spleen on the left. Although nonspecific, an increase in renal echogenicity is a uniformly abnormal finding (6). In the adult, the normal renal cortex appears less echogenic than the adjacent liver. It is important to note that assessment of renal echogenicity is not reliable when the internal standard — the liver — is altered by primary hepatic disease. Fatty infiltration especially is associated with increased hepatic echogenicity. The echogenicity of the left kidney is compared to the spleen. Because the spleen is normally more echogenic than the liver, it is more difficult to detect mild abnormalities in the echogenicity of the left kidney. Since renal medical disease is bilateral, however, this is rarely a significant drawback.

The normal medullary pyramids appear hypoechoic relative to the renal cortex and in the majority of normal individuals, the cortex and medulla can be differentiated on a sonogram. The hypoechoic pyramids should not be mistaken for the sonolucent, dilated, fluid-filled calyces seen in hydronephrosis. Using real-time imaging, the pyramids can be recognized by their regularly spaced anatomic distribution, by their continuity with the peripheral cortical parenchyma, and by demonstration of a bright reflection from the arcuate artery at the corticomedullary junction. In addition, the normal renal sinus can be identified since it demonstrates echogenic and compact echo patterns due to sinus adipose tissue, pelvic blood vessels, and collapsed collecting structures. The renal arteries and veins can be visualized, extending from the renal hilum to the aorta and inferior vena cava respectively. The ureters cannot be seen unless distended. When examining the kidney for congenital anomalies or acute renal failure, examination of the pelvis is essential. The fluid-filled urinary bladder is easily identified and, when distended, the ureter at the ureterovesical junction can be demonstrated.

ACUTE RENAL FAILURE (ARF)

To expedite the evaluation of ARF, the causes of renal failure are usually categorized as pre-renal (renal hypoperfusion), intrinsic (renal medical disease), or post-renal (urinary obstruction). Pre-renal factors are the major causes of acute kidney failure in the in-patient setting. The pre-renal causes of ARF are best evaluated and treated without the use of radiology. In intrinsic causes of renal failure, the clinical as well as the radiologic characterization of renal medical disease is nonspecific (Figure 1). Diagnosis requires renal biopsy after which treatment can be initiated. Because renal biopsy is invasive, the evaluation of renal medical disease is usually deferred until pre- and post-renal causes of renal failure have been excluded.

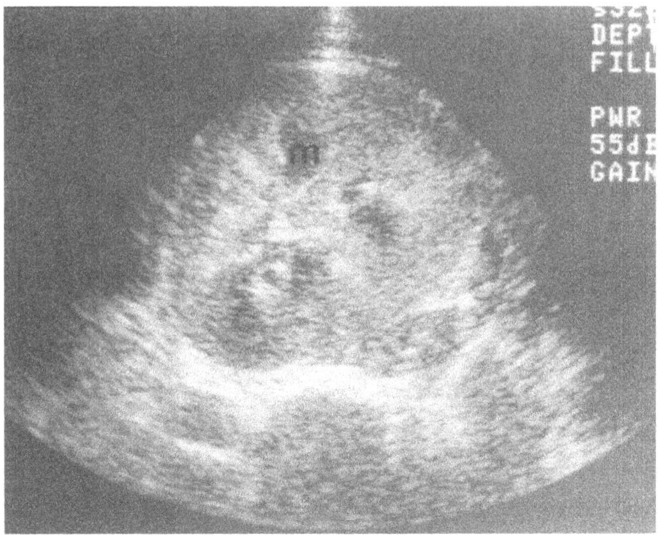

Figure 1 Lupus glomerulonephritis: Enlarged kidney with increased echogenicity. The medullary pyramids (m) appear sonolucent. While the sonographic features of this kidney are very abnormal, the finding is nonspecific (e.g. see Figure 17).

Although renal obstruction, the cause of post-renal ARF, is the least common of the three (1-10%), it is potentially curable and can be surgically corrected if diagnosed early. It is difficult to identify urinary obstruction clinically, and radiologic evaluation is necessary. Although high-dose contrast urography has for years been the initial method of examination, decreased renal function - causing poor renal opacification and excretion during IVU - has often resulted in nondiagnostic studies. Consequently, ultrasonography has now replaced excretory urography as the initial radiologic method for evaluation (7). With ultrasonography, there is no need for contrast media, and the display of renal morphology is independent of renal function.

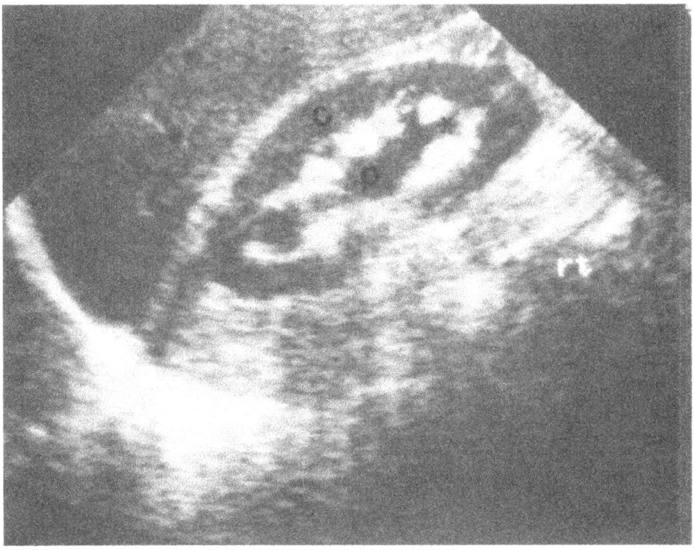

Figure 2 Mild hydronephrosis: Echogenic sinus fat is preserved. Cortex (C), Calyce (*), Pelvis (P)

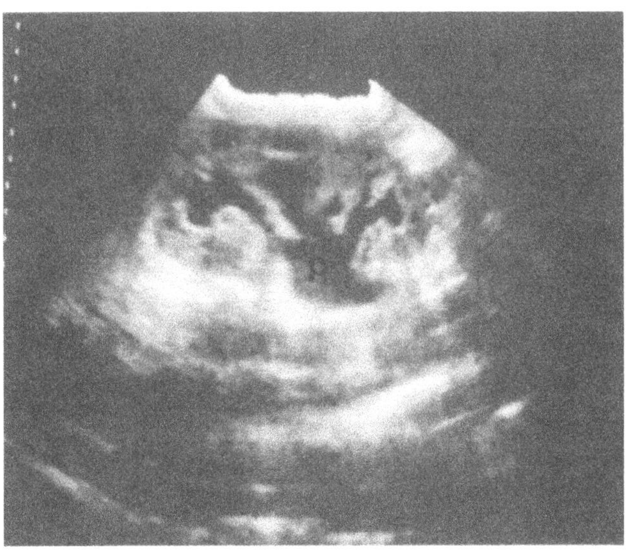

Figure 3 Moderate hydronephrosis: Distention and rounding of intrarenal collecting system. Calyce (*), Pelvis (P)

Ultrasound is highly accurate in the detection of hydronephrosis, with a sensitivity estimated at between 90% and 100% (8). Hydronephrosis is diagnosed when the compact sinus complex echo is separated by branching unechoic (fluid-filled) calyces, infundibula, and pelves. The blunted configuration of the dilated calyx may also be discerned. The degree of dilatation is judged subjectively. Mild hydronephrosis is characterized by fluid-filled intra-renal collecting structures which are not significantly distorted but are slightly separate from the sinus fat (Figure 2). In moderate hydronephrosis, there is obvious distention and rounding of the intrarenal collecting structures with well preserved cortical thickness (Figure 3). The diagnosis of severe hydronephrosis is usually reserved for those cases in which the sinus fat is virtually replaced by rounded and dilated infundibula and calyces in a kidney in which there is significant cortical thinning (Figure 4).

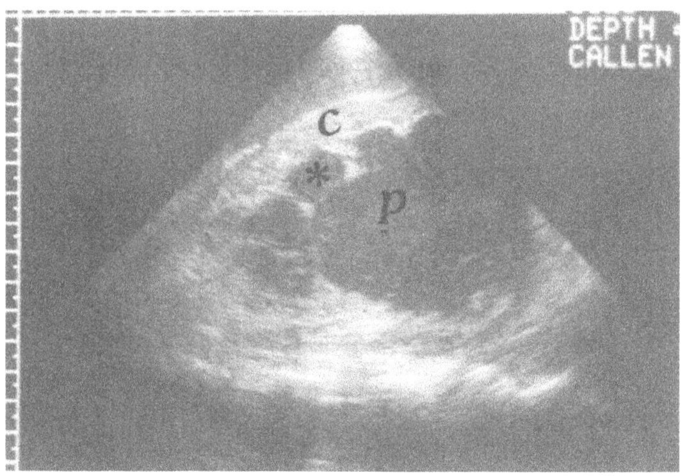

Figure 4 Severe hydronephrosis: Renal sinus fat is replaced by distended, rounded infundibula and calyces (*) in a kidney with significant cortical thinning. The echogenicity of the cortex (C) is increased. Pelvis (P)

Although the morphologic display by ultrasound is excellent, it is important to emphasize that the detection of hydronephrosis is not exclusive to urinary tract obstruction (9) and that the severity of hydronephrosis does not correlate with the degree of renal failure. Hydronephrosis is a descriptive term indicating dilatation of the collecting system. It may be caused by obstruction; high output urinary flow; or nonobstructive entities such as vesicoureteral reflux, dilatation secondary to reflux from an interposed ileal loop, post-obstructive renal atrophy, or congenital megacalyces. When hydronephrosis is demonstrated on sonography, correlation with the clinical findings and previous radiographs, if available, should be performed. If there is suspicion that the hydronephrosis is due to urinary obstruction, the diagnosis needs to be confirmed by contrast studies such as IVU or antegrade (Figure 5) or retrograde pyelogram.

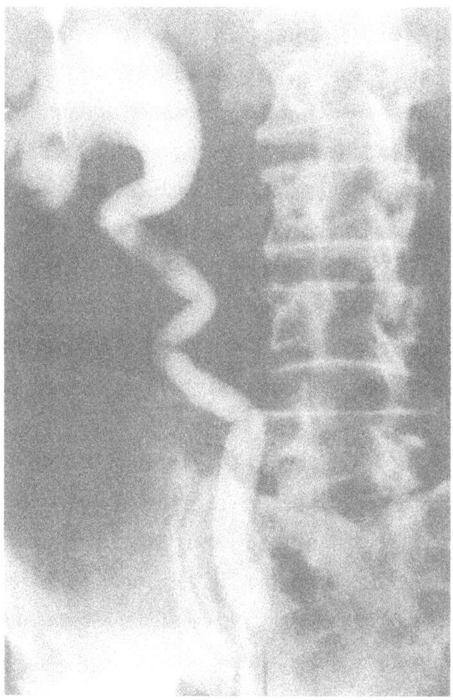

Figure 5 To confirm the diagnosis of urinary obstruction, contrast injection in this patient and antegrade pyelogram is necessary.

When two functioning kidneys are present, obstruction must be bilateral to cause renal failure. Therefore, the obstruction is usually at the level of the bladder and/or pelvic inlet. The most common causes of bilateral obstruction are malignancies involving the pelvis, prostate, uterus, ovaries, cervix, or rectum. Mechanical obstruction at the bladder neck (prostatic hypertrophy or neoplasm) or functional bladder neck obstruction (neurogenic bladder) are also relatively common causes. Bilateral extrinsic compression of the ureters secondary to retroperitoneal fibrosis or pelvic lipomatosis are also important, but less common causes of obstructive uropathy. The varying nature of pelvic diseases in these cases underscores the importance of careful scanning of the pelvis and bladder once hydronephrosis is detected. Frequently, dilated hydroureters can be followed into the pelvis to the level of an obstructing mass. Scanning of the pelvis and examination of the architecture of the distal ureters and bladder are optimally performed through the acoustic window of a filled bladder.

CHRONIC RENAL FAILURE (CRF)

CRF is the end point of many renal diseases. Glomerular nephritis is a heterogeneous group of glomerular disorders accounting for 41.6% of CRF; cardiovascular diseases and hypertension account for 13.5%, urinary tract disease for 10.5%, congenital abnormalities for 7.6%, diabetes for 7.2%, and infections for 6.1% (10). In chronic glomerulonephritis, the kidneys are small, suggesting underlying irreversible disease, and can be seen either on plain films or with sonography. Since IVU is compromised by poor renal function and subsequent insufficient excretion, it has no role in the evaluation of chronic failure. Diagnostic ultrasound allows assessment of kidney size and cortical thickness, as well as evaluation of cortical echogenicity (Figure 4).

Cortical echogenicity can be graded as normal 0 when the echo amplitude of the renal cortex is less than that of adjacent liver. It is judged grade I when the amplitude of the cortical echoes equals that of the liver, grade II when cortical amplitude is greater than that of liver but less than that of the renal sinus, and grade III when the echogenicity of the renal parenchyma is markedly increased, approaching that of the renal sinus fat. A significant correlation has been found between cortical echogenicity and the prevalence of global sclerosis, focal tubular atrophy, and the number of hyaline casts per glomerulus. However, although cortical echogenicity corresponds to the severity of histopathologic changes, it does not allow specific diagnosis (11). There are no distinct sonographic features that enable diagnosis of specific renal medical disease, and renal biopsy remains essential. Ultrasound does, however, have a role in guiding the biopsy needle and, if needed, in the evaluation of possible complications secondary to biopsy. Furthermore, after the initial histopathologic diagnosis has been obtained, sonography can be used to monitor the progression of disease by assessment of renal size and echogenicity on sequential films.

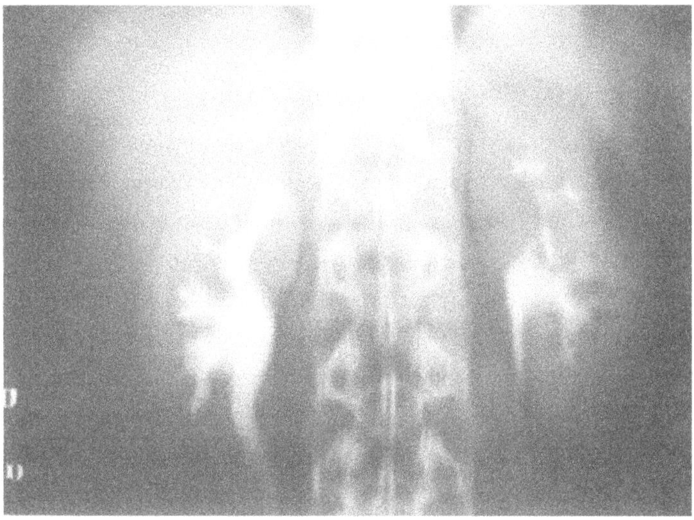

Figure 6A Mild blunting of calyces with adjacent thinning of the cortex is well seen with intravenous urogram.

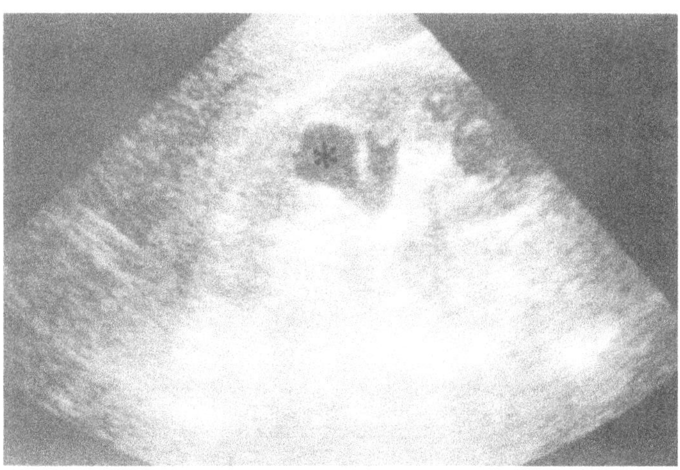

Figure 6B Blunted calyces (*) can be studied with ultrasound but it requires expertise.

In chronic glomerulonephritis where poor or no excretion has been described, IVU findings include symmetrically small kidneys and normal shape of the collecting system. The findings do not offer specificity.

HYPERTENSION

For many years, hypertensive IVU has been considered to be the screening modality for renovascular hypertension. The hypertensive urogram consists of a bolus or injection of contrast medium, followed by a rapid sequence of films — one each minute for the first three minutes, followed by films at 5, 10, 15, and 30 minutes. Findings indicative of renovascular hypertension include a difference in kidney length of 1.5 cm or greater, a delay in the appearance of the collecting system, and hyperconcentration of the contrast medium in the collecting system on the delayed films. In a study of 416 patients (12) with proven renovascular hypertension and a renal artery stenosis greater than 50%, IVU studies were true-positive in 59% of cases and false-negative in 41%. Similar results were reported by Thornbury et al (13). They found that IVU examinations failed to confirm the diagnosis in 41.6% of patients with a high degree of arterial stenosis. They also stressed that only 0.8% of all patients with hypertension had a positive urogram, and that of these, only 24% were candidates for surgery. Results from a study at the Mayo Clinic (14) indicated that only 0.18% of patients with renal hypertension detected by IVU had surgically correctable disease. It must be concluded, therefore, that hypertensive urography is a test whose time has past.

Although sonographic findings in patients with renal hypertension have been reported, ultrasound has not replaced IVU as the diagnostic procedure of choice in suspected renovascular hypertension. The modality now preferred is digital arteriography with assays of venous renin activity. Sonography, however, can demonstrate the physical causes of hypertension such as perirenal hematoma (Page Kidney) or acute renal vein thrombosis.

INFECTIONS

Renal infection may be localized or it may involve the entire kidney and perirenal fossa. Sonography and CT have now replaced IVU as the preferred diagnostic approach in the evaluation of renal infection. IVU is not helpful in the evaluation of renal infection. In 75% of patients with proven renal infections, the IVU was completely normal (15). IVU findings in renal infection may include enlargement of the kidney, striated nephrogram, delayed excretion of contrast material, and either a spidery appearance of the collecting system (secondary to interstitial edema) or a dilated collecting system (when a concomitant urinary obstruction is present) (Figures 6A and B). Calyceal distortion due to stricture has been reported in 68% of cases of renal tuberculosis.

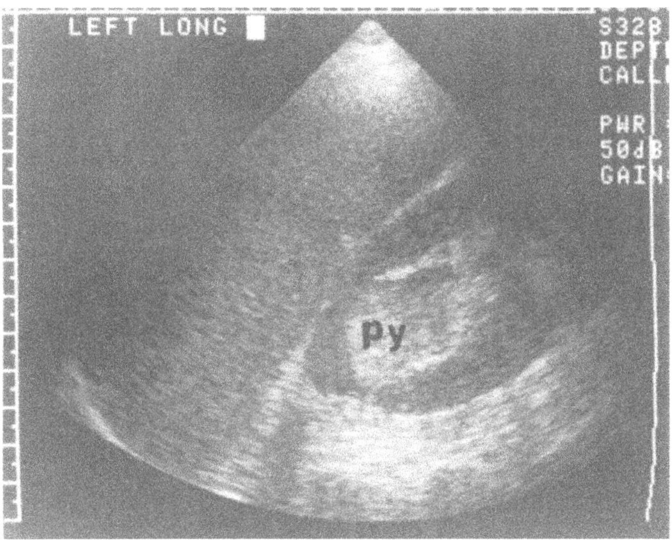

Figure 7 Pyonephrosis (pus in the collecting system), dilated upper pole collecting system demonstrates internal echoes indicative of pyonephrosis (Py).

Sonographic findings may vary, depending on the type of infection (Figure 7). With sonography, the internal architecture of the kidney can be assessed, allowing differentiation between a localized and a diffuse renal process and demonstrating extension of the infection to the perirenal space. Renal enlargement with hypoechoic parenchyma has been reported in acute pyelonephritis. In focal bacterial nephritis, the sonogram may demonstrate localized areas of decreased echogenicity indistinguishable from tumor (Figure 8). A perinephric abscess may be seen as an anechoic or hypoechoic region with or without internal echoes. The distinction between sterile and pyogenic perinephric fluid collections cannot be made with sonography.

The sonographic appearance of renal inflammatory disease is not specific, and a normal sonogram does not exclude the presence of disease. The presence and extent of parenchymal or perinephric infection are detected more accurately with contrast-enhanced CT. However, once the diagnosis has been established, resolution of disease can be monitored with sonography when sequential renal studies are performed. While CT is superior to US in the demonstration of parenchymal inflammatory disease, US is quite useful in the detection of pyonephrosis.

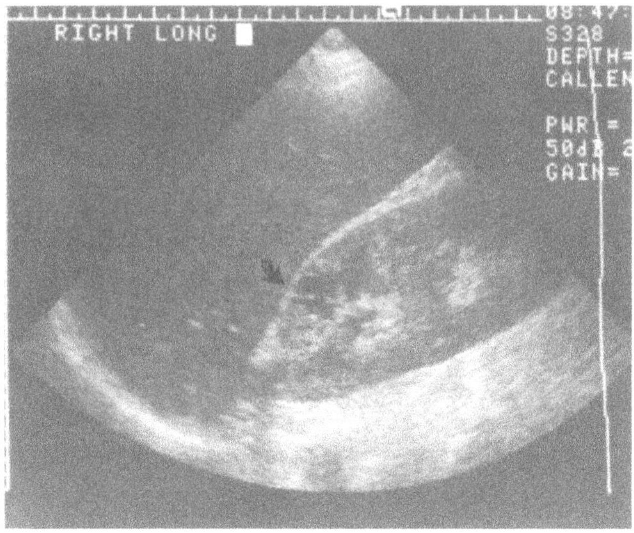

Figure 8 Focal bacterial nephritis: Small area of heterogeneous echogenicity in the cortex (curved arrow) cannot be distinguished from tumor.

Evaluation of recurrent urinary tract infections (UTI) in women is a distinct clinical problem. Ten to 20% of women experience a UTI during their lifetimes. Women with recurrent infections do not develop morphologic changes and IVU is not particularly accurate in identifying these infections (16). In a study of 164 women (16), no significant urographic findings were discovered to justify the use of this examination, and the examination results had no impact on treatment. When IVU, cystography and cystoscopy were evaluated in a prospective study of women with a history or clinical evidence of persistent UTI, it was found that the probability of finding abnormalities with these modalities was very low. Urography can be used in patients with a history of risk factors such as urinary infection in childhood, fever, stones, neurological bladder, and a history of genitourinary surgery.

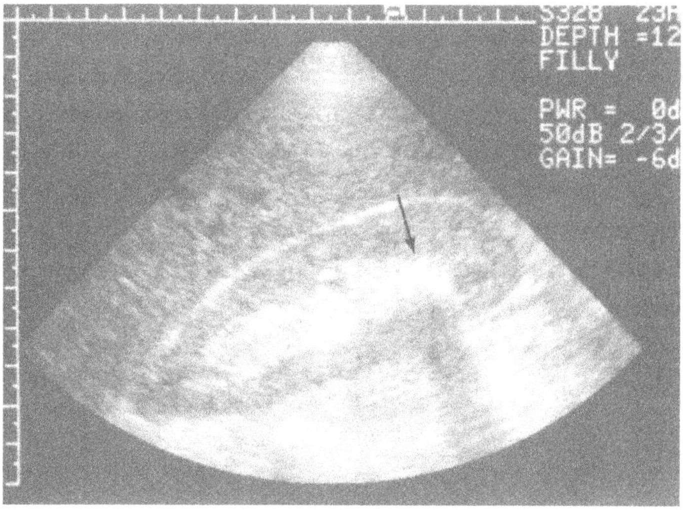

Figure 9 Typical appearance of a renal stone (arrow) in otherwise normal kidney.

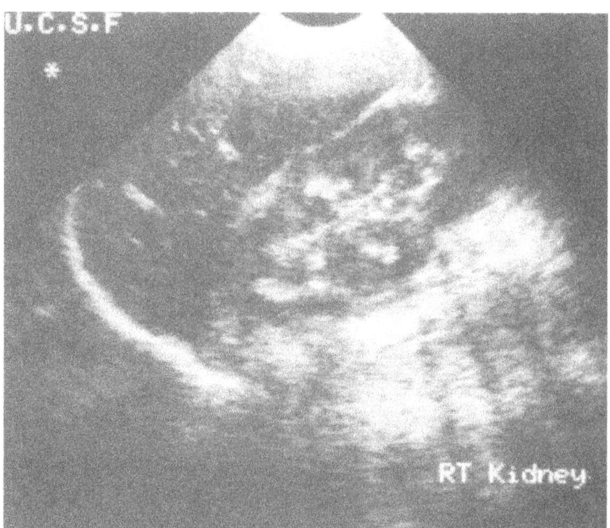

Figure 10 Multiple echogenic foci causing acoustic shadowing in the medullary pyramids of the kidney indicative of nephrocalcinosis.

CALCULI

In the routine workup of a patient with renal colic, a plain film of the abdomen was, and still is, the initial examination of choice. About 85% of urinary calculi contain calcium and are therefore visualized on plain film of the abdomen. Depending on the plain film findings and the clinical symptoms, the next step in the diagnostic workup was traditionally the excretory urogram. Ultrasonography, however, is now being advocated as a viable alternative to IVU (18) (Figures 9 and 10). In obstructive uropathy, ultrasound demonstrates hydronephrosis and may display the calculus itself. However, obstructive calculi are most commonly located at the ureteropelvic or ureterovesical junctions, and assessment of these two locations by ultrasound requires experience and expertise (Figure 11). Early indications that IVU is superior to ultrasound in the detection of calculi should change as experience with ultrasound in this application increases (19).

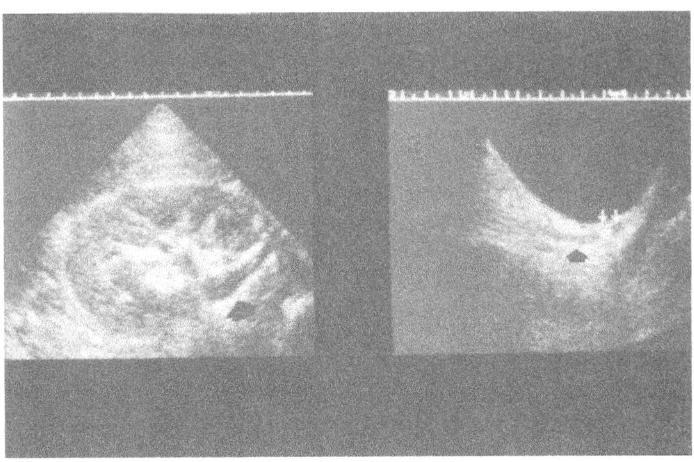

Figure 11 Mild dilation of ureter (arrowhead) due to a stone at the ureteropelvic junction.

When using ultrasound in the diagnosis of renal calculi, it is important to remember that ultrasound may be misleading when the obstruction is either partial or there has been forniceal rupture due to severe obstruction which results in urinary decompression and absence of hydronephrosis. Hydronephrosis may also be absent in cases of pelvic calculi, when the symptoms may precede calyceal dilatation. Therefore, negative findings by ultrasound in the presence of clinical symptoms suggesting calculus obstruction should not preclude further evaluation by IVU.

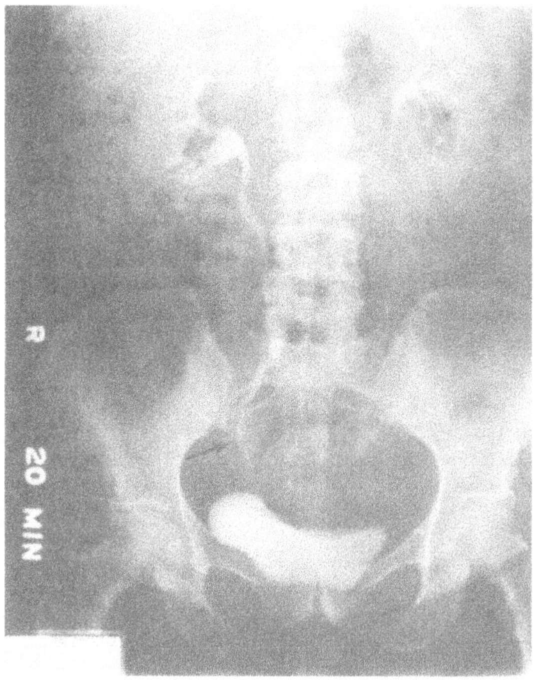

Figure 12 Mild obstruction due to a calculus in the distal right ureter (arrow) with very mild hydronephrosis.

IVU still remains the most accurate modality for the diagnosis of urinary calculus obstruction (Figure 12). In obstruction, IVU findings consist of a prolonged nephrogram, delayed excretion of contrast media and pelvocaliceal and ureteral dilation. Since the concentrating ability of the kidneys is diminished, the excreted contrast media is less radio-opaque, and becomes even more faint as it is further diluted by the urine in the dilated collecting system. A combination of plain film of the abdomen and US is used in the followup of the patient after lithotripsy. Residual stone disease, presence of hydronephrosis or perirenal fluid collections are accurately assessed by US (Figure 13).

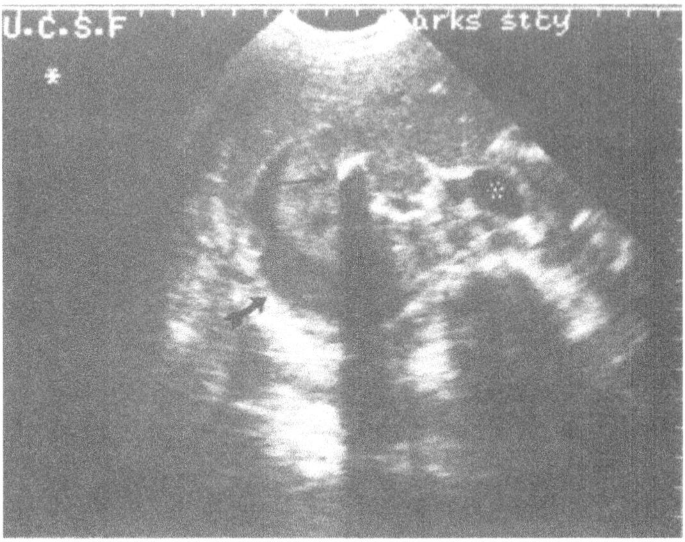

Figure 13 Residual stone (thin arrow), hydronephrosis (*) and perirenal fluid collection (big arrow) after lithotripsy.

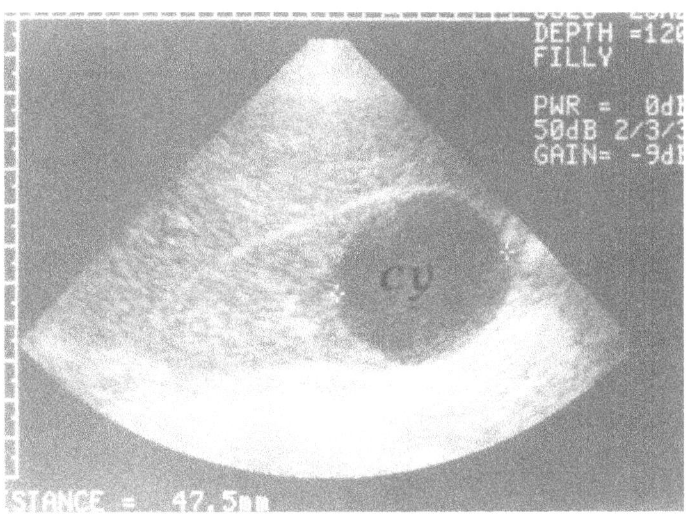

Figure 14 Typical benign cystic (Cy) lesion of the kidney.

RENAL MASSES

IVU is still considered to be the best initial study in the search for renal masses. However, a normal IVU does not exclude the presence of a renal mass, and even when a mass is detected, it is not possible to differentiate between cystic and solid lesions with IVU. Even when a mass appears on sequential IVUs, it is risky to assume that it represents a simple cyst because renal cell carcinomas, particularly of the cystic type, may be very slow growing. Further studies such as US, CT or MRI are necessary to determine the character of the mass. If IVU findings suggest a cystic mass, ultrasound is the next imaging examination of choice. If a solid lesion is suspected, however, the examination to follow should be CT.

Sonographic criteria for the diagnosis of a simple cyst include the absence of internal echoes, a smooth and well defined wall, and acoustic enhancement behind the posterior wall (Figure 14). With ultrasonography, cystic renal masses can be differentiated from solid renal masses (Figures 15 and 16) with an accuracy of 97% (20). Renal cysts may show a complex pattern of echogenicity due to previous hemorrhage, or they may have a calcified wall, making an accurate diagnosis difficult. Atypical renal cysts, such as those with a thickened wall and internal echoes, require further evaluation with CT or biopsy.

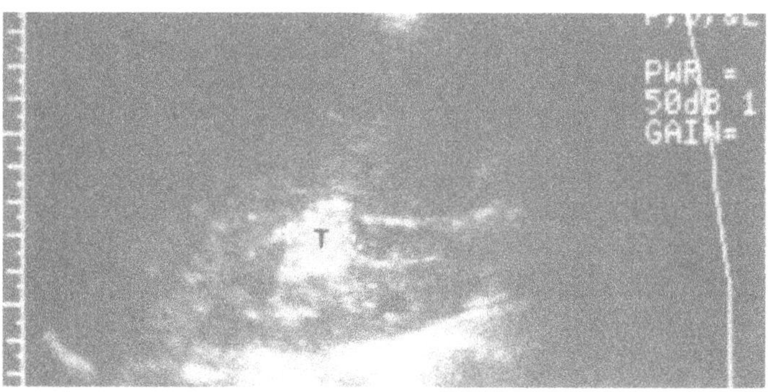

Figure 15 Hyperechoic mass which at surgery was proven to be renal cell carcinoma (T). This sonographic appearance is not specific. Renal cell carcinoma may be hypo- or isoechoic.

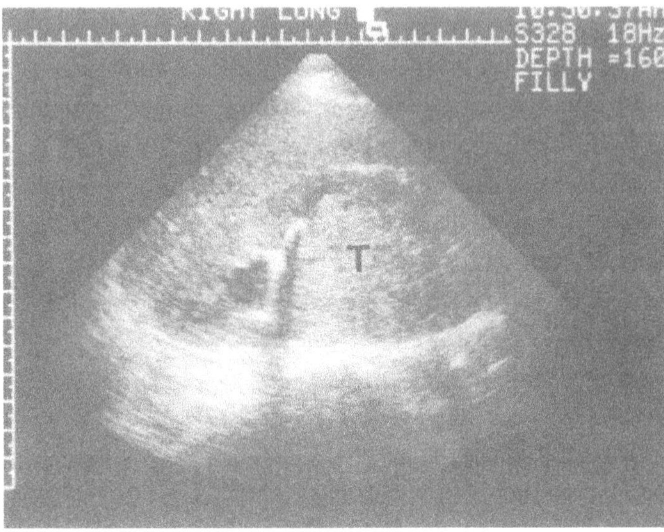

Figure 16 Tumor (T) (renal cell carcinoma) in the lower pole of the right kidney demonstrated ill-defined margin and echo pattern.

Sonographic evaluation of solid renal masses has an accuracy superior to 90%. With solid lesions smaller than 2 cm (21), however, sonography is not useful and CT must be used to clarify the diagnosis of renal space occupying lesions.

RENAL TRANSPLANTATION

IVU has a very minor role in the evaluation of renal transplants. Because of the possible nephrotoxic effects of contrast media (22), use of IVU is limited to the evaluation of persistent hematuria and urinary tract obstruction, after dilatation of the collecting system has been demonstrated by ultrasound or nuclear medicine.

Because of the superficial location of the transplanted kidney, sonographic images are of high quality and ultrasound is highly accurate in distinguishing urologic from parenchymal causes of decreased renal function (23). Perinephric fluid collections are accurately displayed, but differentiation between lymphocele and urinoma requires clinical correlation. If a urinoma is suspected, further studies, preferably nuclear medicine or IVU, are suggested. Sonographic diagnosis of hematoma, especially acute hematoma, may be difficult because the echogenicity of fresh blood is similar to that of the surrounding tissue, and the diagnosis is often made only by the kidney displacement. In these clinical situations, CT is the imaging modality of choice. Subacute and chronic hematoma are more easily identified by ultrasound, but differentiating between a hematoma and an abscess may be difficult. Again, clinical correlation is crucial. Ultrasound is also sensitive in diagnosing hydronephrosis (Figure 17) of the transplanted kidney (24), but similar to the native kidney, hydronephrosis may be of obstructive or nonobstructive etiology. If obstruction is suspected, further studies such as antegrade pyelogram or IVP are indicated. At present, ultrasound is not helpful in the diagnosis of renal arterial occlusion, but as experience is gained with the Doppler ultrasound, this application may be expanded.

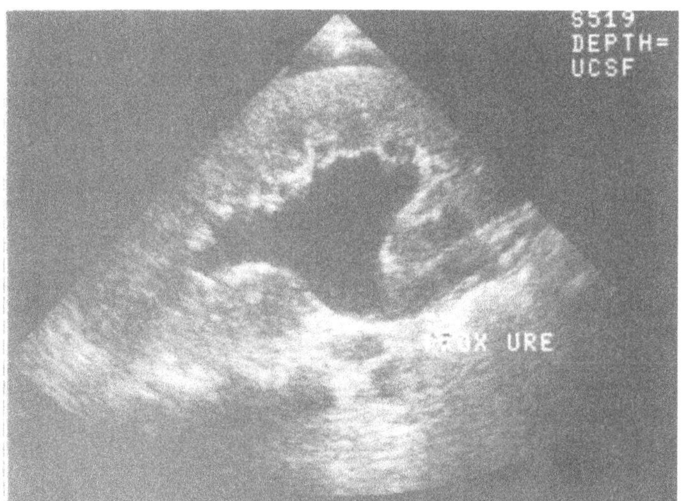

Figure 17 Hydronephrosis in a transplanted kidney.

Ultrasound can also be used in the evaluation of post-transplant renal failure due to renal medical problems. Although renal morphology and anatomy remain normal in acute tubular necrosis, a variety of sonographic features associated with acute rejection have been reported. These include enlargement and decreased echogenicity (increased prominence) of medullary pyramids (Figures 18 and 19), decreased amplitude of renal sinus echos (decreased fat), thickening of renal pelvic and infundibula walls, and generalized transplant enlargement (edema). If all of the morphologic features of rejection are present, acute rejection can be predicted with 100% accuracy. Sensitivity of the test is low, however, since all features were present in only 21% of patients with acute rejection. It has also been noted that when the donor was less than five years of age, sonographic abnormalities in transplant morphology were not helpful in the diagnosis of rejection .

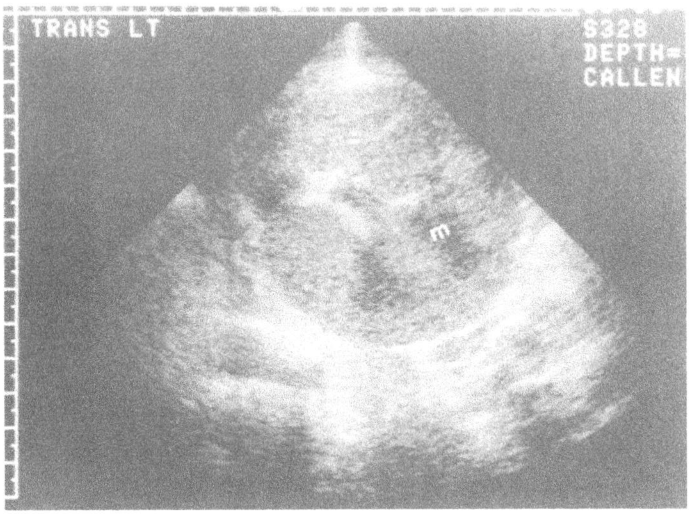

Figure 18 Renal enlargement and prominence of pyramids (m) are nonspecific signs of transplant rejection (see also Figure 1).

Doppler ultrasound waveform analysis can be used to evaluate vascular resistance peripheral to the sampling side, and its use has been publicized in the diagnosis of rejection (19). Several ways of quantifying Doppler changes have been reported, but the most practical is the resistive index. Using the resistive index, the sensitivity of Doppler ultrasound has been reported to be 60% for interstitial rejection and 82% for vascular rejection. The specificity of the test is reported to be 95-96%. The Doppler resistive index is an excellent predictor of acute rejection and, when combined with morphologic changes, it can be useful in the diagnosis of acute rejection. However, because sonographic findings in patients with acute rejection, normal transplants, or other parenchymal abnormalities (such as cyclosporin nephrotoxicity) overlap, a definite diagnosis of acute rejection can be made by sonograms in only a relatively small number of patients (25). At this point, accurate diagnosis of parenchymal disease in many cases still requires transplant biopsy.

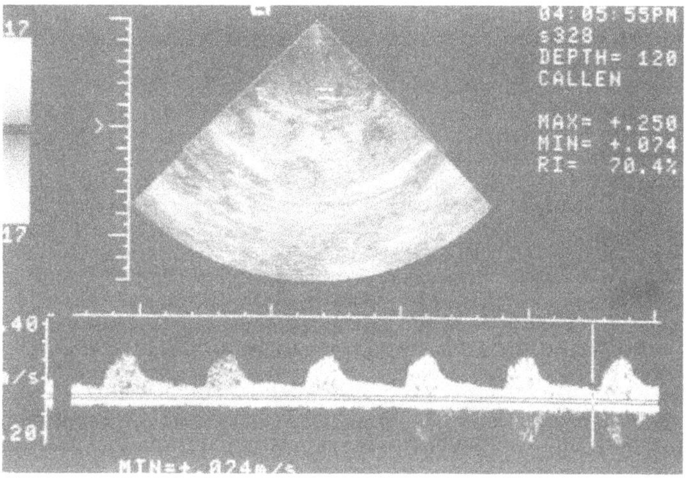

Figure 19 Transplanted kidney: morphologic features of kidney enlargement, increased prominence of medullary pyramids and decreased amplitude of renal sinus echos supplemented by Doppler findings of abnormal resistive index are highly suggestive of acute rejection.

REFERENCES

1. Jacobson HG, Edeiken J: The changing indications for excretory urography. JAMA, 254(3): 403-405, 1985.
2. Aslaksen A, Gothlin JH: Ultrasonography versus excretory urography: Value in urological disease. Europ J Radiol, 8: 179-180, 1988.
3. Hattery R, Williamson B Jr, Hartman GW, LeRoy AJ, Witten DM: Intravenous urographic technique. Radiology, 167: 593-599, 1988.
4. Hartman GW, Hattery RR, Witten DM, Williamson B Jr: Mortality during excretory urography: Mayo Clinic experience. Am J Radiol, 139: 919-922, 1982.
5. Jacobsson BF, Jorulf H, Kalantar MS, Narasimham DL: Nonionic versus ionic contrast media in intravenous urography: Clinical trial in 1,000 consecutive patients. Radiology, 167: 601-605, 1988.
6. Hricak H: Renal ultrasound, in Sarti DA (ed): Diagnostic Ultrasound. Text and Cases 2nd ed. Chicago, Year Book Medical Publishers, 350-364, 1987.
7. Rosenfield AT, Siegel NJ: Renal parenchymal disease: Histopathologic-sonographic correlation. Am J Radiol, 137: 793-798, 1981.
8. Lee JKT, Baron RL, Melson GL, et al: Can real-time ultrasonography replace static B-scanning in the diagnosis of renal obstruction? Radiology, 139: 161-165, 1981.
9. Cochlin D LL, Wake A, Salaman JR, Griffin PJA: Ultrasound changes in the transplant kidney. Clin Radiol, 39:373-376, 1988.
10. Wineman R: End stage renal disease: Dialysis & Transplant, 7:1034-1037, 1978.

11. Hricak H, Cruz C, Romanski R, Uniewski MH, Levin NW, Madrazo BL, Sandler MA, Eyler WR: Renal parenchymal disease: Sonographic-histologic correlation. Radiology, 144: 141-147, 1982.
12. Kaufman JJ: Renovascular hypertension: The UCLA experience. J Urol, 121: 139-144, 1979.
13. Thornbury JR, Stanley JC, Fryback DG: Hypertensive urogram: A non-discriminatory test for renovascular hypertension. Am J Radiol, 138: 43-49, 1982.
14. Tucker RM, Labarthe DR: Frequency of surgical treatment for hypertension in adults at the Mayo Clinic for 1973 through 1975. May Clin Proc, 52: 549-555, 1977.
15. Wicks JD, Thornbury JR: Acute renal infections in adults. Rad Clin North Am, 17: 245, 1979.
16. Fowler JE Jr, Pulaski ET: Excretory urography, cystography, and cystoscopy in the evaluation of women with urinary tract infection: A prospective study. N Eng J Med, 304: 462-465, 1981.
17. Fair WR, McClennan BL, Jost RG: Are excretory urograms necessary in evaluating women with urinary tract infections? J Urol, 121: 313-315, 1979.
18. Jagjivan B, Moore DJ, Naik DR: Intravenous urography in the investigation of the urinary tract. Br J Surg, 75(3): 246-248, 1988.
19. Middleton WD, Dodds WJ, Lawson TL, Foley WD: Renal calculi: Sensitivity for detection with US. Radiology, 167: 239-244, 1988.
20. Pollack HM, Bamier MP, Arges PH, James P, Mulhern CB, Gleman BG: The accuracy of grey-scale renal ultrasonography in differentiating cystic neoplasm from benign cysts. Radiology, 143(3): 741-745, 1982.
21. Warshauer DM, McCarthy SM, Street L, Bookbinder MJ, Glickman MG, Richter J, Hammers L, Taylor C, Rosenfield AT: Detection of renal masses: Sensitivities and specificities of excretory urography/linear tomography, US, and CT. Radiology, 169: 363-365, 1988.
22. Miller DL, Chang R, Wells WT, Dowjat BA, Malinosky RM, Doppman JL: Intravascular contrast media: Effect of dose on renal function. Radiology, 167: 607-611, 1988.
23. Hricak H, Cruz C, Eyler WR, et al: Acute post-transplantation renal failure: Differential diagnosis by ultrasound. Radiology, 139: 441-449, 1981.
24. Hricak H, Cruz C, Eyler WR, Madrazo BL, Sandler MA: Post-transplant renal failure: Differential diagnosis by ultrasound-experimental and clinical obstructions. Med Ultrasound, 6: 1, 1982.
25. Genkins SM, Sanfilippo FP, Carrol BA: Duplex Doppler sonography of renal transplant. Am J Radio, 152: 535-539, 1989.

INDEX

[Page numbers following (T) refer to Tables; page numbers following (F) refer to Figures]

GPSR Compliance
The European Union's (EU) General Product Safety Regulation (GPSR) is a set of rules that requires consumer products to be safe and our obligations to ensure this.

If you have any concerns about our products, you can contact us on

ProductSafety@springernature.com

In case Publisher is established outside the EU, the EU authorized representative is:

Springer Nature Customer Service Center GmbH
Europaplatz 3
69115 Heidelberg, Germany

www.ingramcontent.com/pod-product-compliance
Ingram Content Group UK Ltd.
Pitfield, Milton Keynes, MK11 3LW, UK
UKHW020238160926
475610UK00001B/37
9781461288022